Surgical Management of Pheochromocytoma and Retroperitoneal Paraganglioma

Jin Wen
Editor

Surgical Management of Pheochromocytoma and Retroperitoneal Paraganglioma

中国协和医科大学出版社
Peking Union Medical College Press
Springer

Editor
Jin Wen
Department of Urology
Peking Union Medical College Hospital
Beijing, China

ISBN 978-981-99-8423-7   ISBN 978-981-99-8421-3 (eBook)
https://doi.org/10.1007/978-981-99-8421-3

Peking Union Medical College Excellent Textbook Project
National High Level Hospital Clinical Research Funding (2022-PUMCH-C-044)

Jointly published with Peking Union Medical College Press
The print edition is not for sale in China (Mainland). Customers from China (Mainland) please order the print book from: Peking Union Medical College Press.

This Springer imprint is published by the registered company Springer Nature Singapore Pte Ltd.
The registered company address is: 152 Beach Road, #21-01/04 Gateway East, Singapore 189721, Singapore

Foreword

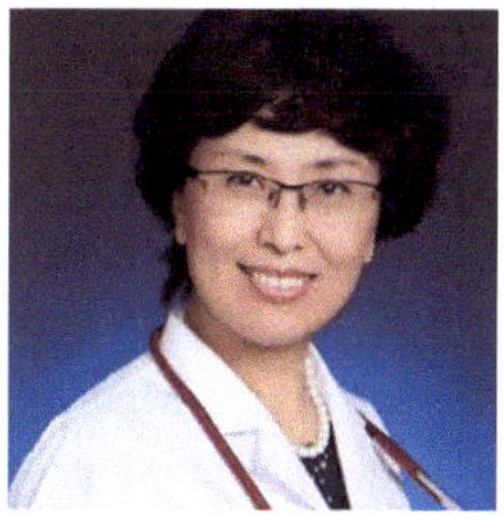

Rare diseases generally refer to diseases with a very low incidence. According to the definition of the World Health Organization, rare diseases are diseases with 0.65‰ to 1‰ of the total population. At present, there are more than 7000 rare diseases known in the world, of which about 80% are hereditary diseases caused by gene defects, and there is no effective drug treatment for the vast majority of rare diseases. It is estimated that there are more than 20 million rare disease patients in my country, and more than 200,000 children with rare diseases are born every year. Compared with common diseases, the level of related medical research on rare diseases is obviously lagging. Due to the limited understanding of the pathogenesis of many rare diseases and insufficient diagnostic methods, 40% of rare disease patients have been misdiagnosed at least once, and many patients have been misdiagnosed for a long time. I searched for a doctor but couldn't get a clear diagnosis. In addition, there are still some patients who suffer from the lack of effective treatment, or the unaffordable cost of treatment despite being diagnosed. Rare disease patients often become socially disadvantaged groups due to their illness. In addition to scientific significance, the research on rare diseases also has great significance in sociology and ethics.

In recent years, the state has vigorously supported basic and clinical research on rare diseases, including rare diseases in the "13th Five-Year Plan" development plan, and related fields have gradually developed and expanded, fully reflecting the state's care for vulnerable groups and the principle of social equity. In 2018, five ministries and commissions jointly released the first batch of rare disease catalogs in my country, filling the gap in the identification standards of rare diseases in my country for many years. Peking Union Medical College Hospital has compiled and published my country's first batch of rare disease catalog definitions and rare disease diagnosis and treatment guidelines, and elaborated the clinical manifestations, differential diagnosis, treatment methods, etc. Which clearly illustrates the diagnosis and treatment path for rare diseases with a clear flowchart.

Pheochromocytoma/retroperitoneal paraganglioma is a rare disease with variable tumor size and location and dangerous clinical symptoms. Peking Union Medical College Hospital has treated patients from all over the country, concentrated a wide variety of cases with complex manifestations, and accumulated a lot of experience in clinical diagnosis and treatment. In the multidisciplinary team consultation including urology, endocrinology, anesthesiology, ICU, respiratory medicine, neurology, dermatology, ophthalmology, stomatology, pathology, imaging, and other departments, we found that in the form of cases, according to the patient's medical history, clinical manifestations, imaging manifestations, MDT discussion, and the order of treatment methods can provide a relatively comprehensive understanding of the disease; and on this basis, the "Pheochromocytoma/Retroperitoneal Paraganglioma Surgery" was compiled. The book of "Surgical management of pheochromocytoma and retroperitoneal paraganglioma" was compiled on this basis. The cases in this book are all selected from the difficult cases in the Department of Urology of Peking Union Medical College Hospital. It is rich in content and has accurate data. It systematically shows the main points of analysis, diagnosis, and treatment of difficult diseases. Which can be used as a reference for doctors engaged in clinical work, as well as for medical students to consult and learn. It is my sincere hope that this book can enhance the medical staff's understanding of the disease and make a certain contribution to the progress of the diagnosis and treatment of rare diseases in my country.

Shu Yang Zhang

Peking Union Medical College Hospital
Chinese Academy of Medical Sciences
Beijing, China

China Rare Disease Alliance
Beijing, China
Nov 2022

Editorial Board

Preface

Pheochromocytoma/Retroperitoneal Paraganglioma Surgical Diagnosis and Treatment Strategy adopts a format that is different from textbooks. We select representative cases, show their diagnosis and treatment process, and describe the clinical thinking process in the diagnosis and treatment. In this way, we present the book to the readers. This unique form of arrangement can not only consolidate the theoretical knowledge of clinical medical students, urological graduate students, advanced physicians, and urologists who have a certain level of theory and clinical practice, but also reproduce the collection, testing, and analysis of case data for each disease. The process of analyzing imaging results and making diagnosis and treatment is very important for cultivating their clinical active thinking ability and creative ability.

The theoretical part of this book mainly refers to the papers and reviews written by the editors in recent years. The selected cases are also real cases of urological surgery in Peking Union Medical College Hospital after team discussion. This form can not only show the problems that junior doctors may encounter in disease diagnosis and treatment and may remind readers to avoid the same mistakes in future clinical work, but also reflect the scientific and careful clinical diagnosis and treatment thinking of senior doctors in disease diagnosis and treatment.

Due to the limitations of the author's diagnosis and treatment experiences or professional level, some cases may not be perfect, and the content of the book may have some deficiencies and omissions. I urge readers to criticize and correct them so that it can be revised and improved in the next edition.

Beijing, China
Nov 2022

Jin Wen

Acknowledgments

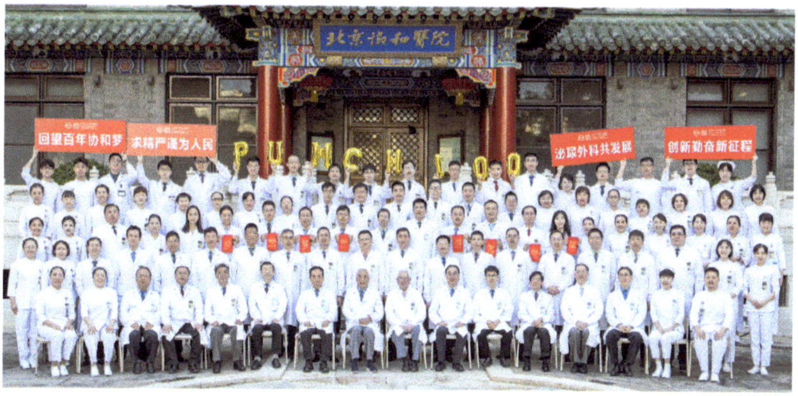

I am indebted to all the authors who have contributed new chapters describing the novel topics covered in this book, *Surgical Strategies for Pheochromocytoma/Paraganglioma*. These researchers have lighted the candles of knowledge so that the entire community can tap into their light and break through knowledge barriers, especially through the participation of a group of eminent/prominent urologists, clinicians, and academicians. I express my special gratitude to the reviewers for offering help and valuable comments to improve chapter contents and enhance their scientific importance. This work would not have been possible without the acceptance of the publisher, Springer, and the entire technical team, which has taken diligent care during the different stages of writing, evaluation, and correction, in addition to the stages of preparation and publication. For this, I would like to express my sincere thanks to both the publishing house and the technical team. I would also like to extend my special thanks to the translators team, which spared no effort to ensure the success of this work, and to all the members of the editorial committee who mobilized all their technical and scientific efforts for the realization of this work.

Jin Wen

I am indebted to all the authors who have contributed new chapters describing [illegible]

[illegible] scientific efforts for the realization of this work.

[illegible]

Contents

1 **Principles of Diagnosis and Treatment of Pheochromocytoma and Retroperitoneal Paraganglioma** 1
Han Zhong Li, Jian Hua Deng, Jin Wen, He Xiao, Yong Qiang Li, Xing Cheng Wu, Xue Bin Zhang, Peng Hu Lian, and Yin Sheng Zhang

2 **Overview of Pheochromocytoma and Retroperitoneal Paraganglioma**........................... 7
Zhi Gang Ji, Wen Da Wang, Jin Wen, Zhen Yu Zhang, Hong Bo Zhang, Xin Rong Fan, Yi Zhou, and Jing Min Zhou

3 **Surgical Treatment of Pheochromocytoma and Retroperitoneal Paraganglioma**...................... 23
Yu Shi Zhang, Zi Xing Ye, Jin Wen, Yuzhi Zuo, Jie Dong, Juan Sun, Yi Qiao, Chang Liu, Ying Jie Li, and Yong Huang

4 **Multidisciplinary Treatment of Adrenal Pheochromocytoma**.................................... 29
Wei Gang Yan, Dong Wang, Jin Wen, Zhong Ming Huang, Hou Feng Huang, Yi Xie, and De Xin Dong

5 **Multidisciplinary Treatment of Paragangliomas in the Vascular Area of the Epigastric Region** 73
Guang Hua Liu, Yi Zhao, Jin Wen, Zhi En Zhou, GuoYang Zheng, Yang Zhao, Ting Kai Yang, Xin Zhao, Wei Feng Xu, and Qing Zhen Wen

6 **Multidisciplinary Treatment of Paragangliomas in the Vascular Area of the Epigastric Region** 95
Quan Zong Mao, Shi Jun Wang, Jin Wen, Hua Fan, and Xiao Qiang Xue

7 **Multidisciplinary Treatment of Paragangliomas in the Lower Abdominal Vascular Area** 127
Bing Bing Shi, Zhi Jun Zhang, Jin Wen, Rui Qiang Zhang, Xue Min Gao, Meng Chao Wei, and Nan Lei

8 **Multidisciplinary Treatment of Pelvic Paraganglioma and Metastatic Pheochromocytoma** 155
Shi Rong, Lin Ma, Jin Wen, Hong Jun Li, Su Yan, Zhan Wang, Hai Wang, Xu Wang, and Guo Rong Li

Editor and Contributors

About the Editor

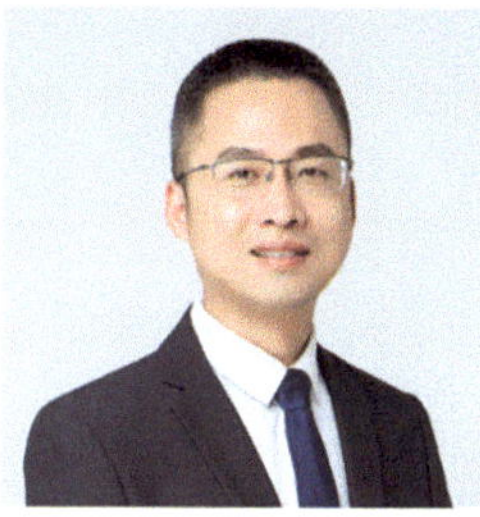

Jin Wen is an Assistant to the Chief of Urology Department of Peking Union Medical College Hospital, Chief Physician, Master Tutor, Senior Visiting Scholar of Memorial Sloan-Kettering Cancer Center (MSKCC) in New York, USA. In 2004, he obtained a PhD in Urology. He has been engaged in clinical work related to urological diseases. He keeps improving his surgical techniques, especially in the minimally invasive treatment of adrenal diseases. He has accumulated rich experience and achieved good results.

He is currently the national youth committee member of the Urology Branch of the Chinese Medical Doctor Association, the deputy head of the Laser Collaboration Group, a member of the International Exchange Committee of the Urology Branch of the Chinese Medical Association, a youth member of the Beijing Medical Association Organ Transplantation Branch, a member of the Beijing Medical Award Foundation Urology Branch and Member of the second committee of Beijing Medical Association, Medical Science Branch.

With good scientific research ability and organization and coordination ability, he has successively received funding from Peking Union Medical College Hospital Youth Fund, Young Teacher Training Fund, and Chinese Academy of Medical Sciences Clinical Transformation Fund. In 2017, he was selected as the "Sino-French Outstanding Young Scientists Exchange Program" of the Ministry of Science and Technology and visited the Saint-Etienne University Hospital in France. He has published more than 30 research papers in domestic core journals and foreign SCI journals, obtained 3 invention patents, and edited the medical monograph *Surgical Treatment Strategies for Pheochromocytoma/Paraganglioma*.

core journals and foreign SCI journals, obtained 3 invention patents, and edited the medical monograph *Surgical Treatment Strategies for Pheochromocytoma/Paraganglioma*.

About the Honor Consultants

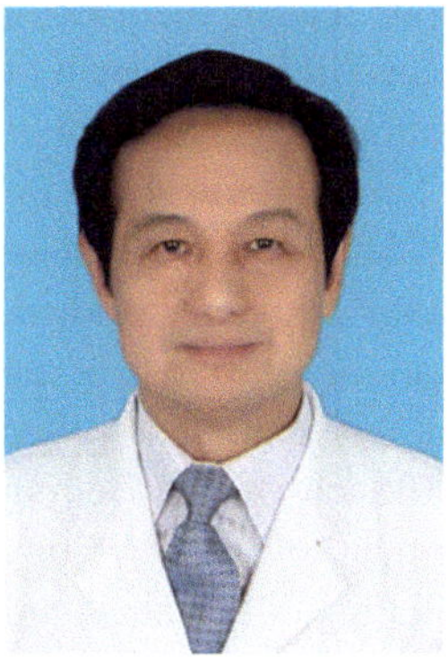

Han Z. Li is a Chief Physician, Professor, PhD tutor, and Doctoral Supervisor of Urology Department of Peking Union Medical College Hospital, Director of Department of Surgery, Peking Union Medical College Medical School, Academic Leader of Urology Department, recipient of Government Allowance of the State Council; Honorary Professor of the University of Hong Kong; Chairman of the Urology Branch of the Beijing Medical Association, Chairman of the Urology Branch of the Beijing Medical Association, Chairman of the Expert Committee, Deputy Head of the Minimally Invasive Group and Deputy Head of the Oncology Group of the Urology Branch of the Chinese Medical Association, Urology of the Chinese Medical Association Member of the Standing Committee of the Surgeon's Association, Deputy Editor-in-Chief of *Chinese Journal of Urology*, Deputy Editor-in-Chief of *Union Medical Journal*, editorial board member of *Chinese Journal of Surgery*, and Deputy Editor-in-Chief of *Beijing Medicine*.

He has won the China Medical Science and Technology Award, the Huaxia Medical Science and Technology Award, "Top Ten Health Guards in the Capital," "National Health System Advanced Worker," "Golden Cystoscopy Award," "Golden Lancet Award," "Chinese Physician Award," "Beijing University," , "Teaching Famous Teacher Award," "Peking Union Medical College Teacher Morality Pioneer." He has published more than 300 professional papers at home and abroad, including dozens of SCI papers and more than 10 monographs.

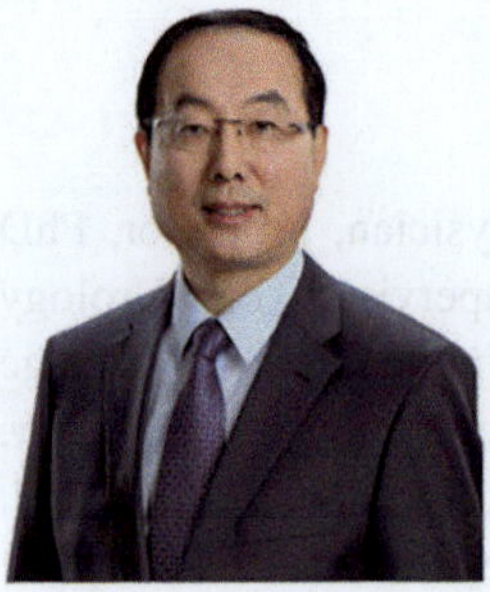

Zhi Gang Ji is a chief physician, professor, PhD tutor, director of the Department of Urology, Peking Union Medical College Hospital, Chinese Academy of Medical Sciences; academic leader; member of the Standing Committee of the Urology Branch of the Chinese Medical Association, Vice President of the Urology Branch of the Chinese Medical Doctor Association, and Vice President of the Chinese Medical Association Andrology Branch President, President-designate of the Andrology Branch of the World Chinese Physician Association, Vice Chairman of the Urology Branch of the Beijing Medical Association, Chairman of the Urology Expert Committee of the Beijing Medical Award Foundation, and Deputy Head of the Oncology Group of the Urology Branch of the Chinese Medical Association, Deputy Head of Robotics Group of Urology Branch of Beijing Medical Association, Review Expert of Drug Evaluation Center of State Food and Drug Administration, Health Care Consultation Expert of Central Health Bureau; Editorial Board Member of *Chinese Journal of Urology*, *Chinese Journal of Medicine*, *Journal of Clinical Urology*, *Modern Journal of Urogenital Oncology*, *Chinese Journal of Surgery* correspondent editor, *International Journal of Surgery* correspondent editor.

He has won the China Medical Science and Technology Award. He has presided over and completed a number of clinical scientific research work. He has published more than 200 professional articles and written 6 monographs.

Principles of Diagnosis and Treatment of Pheochromocytoma and Retroperitoneal Paraganglioma

1

Han Zhong Li, Jian Hua Deng, Jin Wen, He Xiao, Yong Qiang Li, Xing Cheng Wu, Xue Bin Zhang, Peng Hu Lian, and Yin Sheng Zhang

Pheochromocytoma and retroperitoneal paraganglioma (PPGL) are neuroendocrine tumors derived from the neural crest cells of sympathetic and parasympathetic chain, including PPGL located in the adrenal medulla (85–90%) and PPGL located outside the adrenal gland (10–15%), the most common parts of which are located along with the abdominal aorta, bladder, chest, head, neck, and so on (Fig. 1.1). PPGL accounts for about 0.2–0.6% of hypertensive patients, with an annual incidence of about 0.8/100,000.

Han Zhong Li and Jian Hua Deng contributed equally to this work.

H. Z. Li · J. H. Deng · J. Wen (✉) · H. Xiao · Y. Q. Li
X. C. Wu · X. B. Zhang · P. H. Lian · Y. S. Zhang
Department of Urology, Peking Union Medical College Hospital, Beijing, China

J. Wen (ed.), *Surgical Management of Pheochromocytoma and Retroperitoneal Paraganglioma*,
https://doi.org/10.1007/978-981-99-8421-3_1

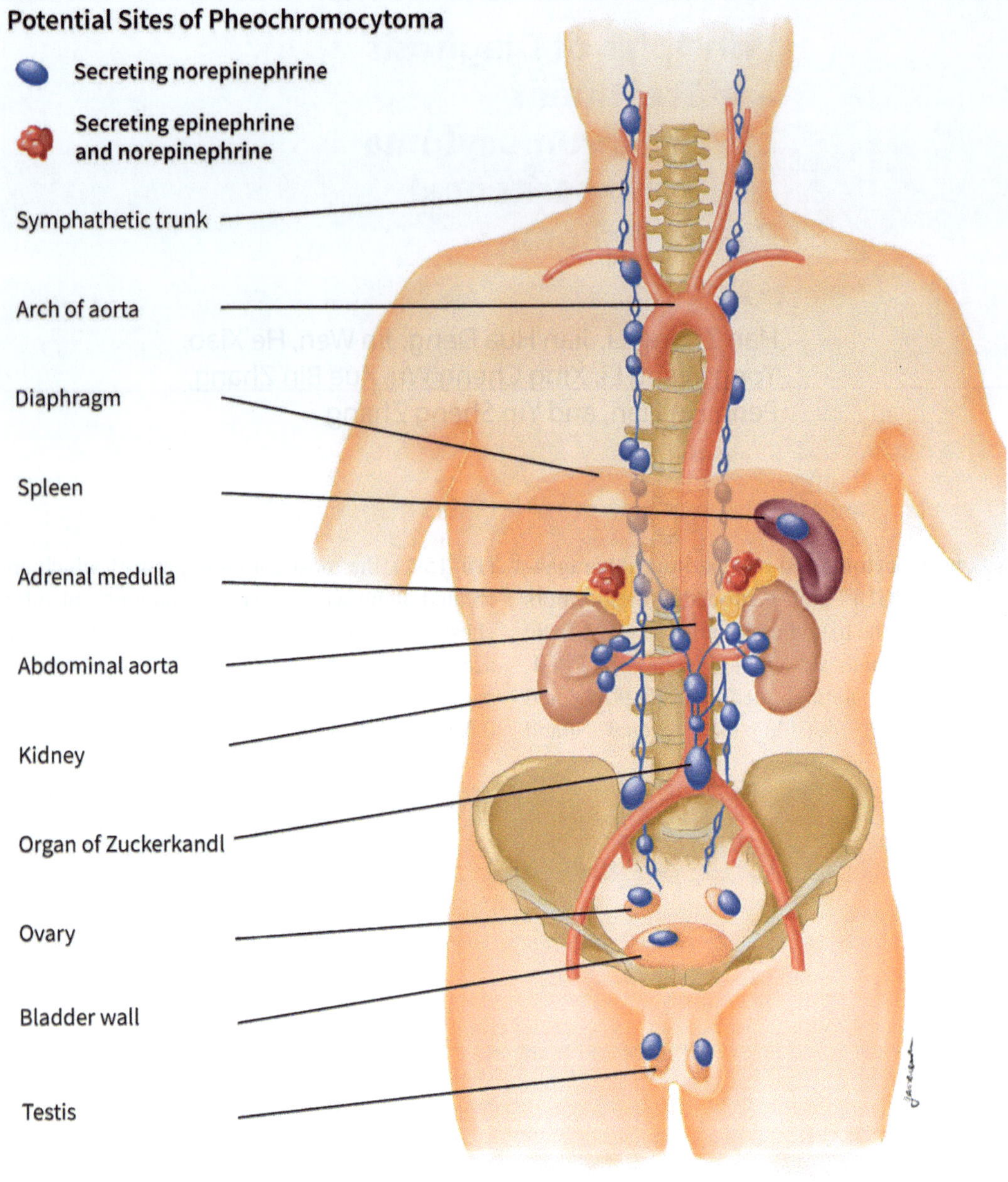

Fig. 1.1 Occurrence sites of pheochromocytoma/paraganglioma

1.1 Clinical Manifestations

Pheochromocytoma and retroperitoneal paraganglioma (PPGL) secrete catecholamines. The main clinical manifestations are persistent or intermittent hypertension, palpitations, headache, and other symptoms (nausea, fatigue, sweating, abdominal pain, chest pain, arrhythmia, etc.) Life-threatening symptoms such as heart failure and myocardial infarction may occur. The currently recommended laboratory test method is the determination of plasma/urine catecholamine or intermediate metabolites methoxyephrine or methoxyphenylephrine. The latest evidence shows that the sensitivity and specificity of plasma testing are better than urine testing and the detection of epinephrine in plasma has a lower false-positive probability than epinephrine in urine. Free epinephrine, norepinephrine and 3-Determination of methoxytyramine are the preferred plasma test. Increased concentrations of two or more catecholamine metabolites are highly suggestive of PPGL.

CT (computed tomography) and MRI (magnetic resonance imaging) are commonly used imaging localization methods for clinical diagnosis of PPGL. On contrast-enhanced CT, tumor enhancement is obvious, and cystic degeneration, calcification, and hemorrhage may be found in the tumor. If the above imaging tests have no positive findings, 131I-m-iodobenzylguanidine (etaiodobenzylguanidine, 131I-MIBG) and somatostatin receptor imaging can be performed. The sensitivity and specificity of 131I-MIBG imaging in the diagnosis of pheochromocytoma were 82.41% and 100%, respectively. According to literature reports, the reason for the false negative may be related to, in some cases, insufficient uptake of the tracer by the tumor or by the patient taking reserpine, cocaine, amphetamine, and other drugs that affect the body's uptake of MIBG. Extensive necrosis and bleeding in tumors with a diameter of less than 2.0 cm or large tumors can easily lead to false negatives.

Fluorodeoxyglucose (18F-FDG) PET-MRI or 18F-FDG PET-CT can accurately visualize tumor histology, further assess the extent of disease, and is more sensitive than MIBG and CT/MRI in detecting metastatic disease. The latest data show that 68Ga-DOTATATE PET/CT is significantly better than the abovementioned examinations in the detection of metastatic PPGL lesions and has gradually become the preferred method of examination for metastatic PPGL.

PPGL is a highly hereditary tumor that is inherited in approximately 40% of patients. So far, more than 20 pathogenic genes have been identified, mainly including SDHB, SDHD, VHL, RET, TMEM127, and so on. The patient's genotype is related to clinical phenotype, such as tumor location, type of catecholamine secretion, tumor metastasis, and prognosis. Compared with sporadic tumors, patients with hereditary catecholamine-secreting tumors are generally younger, and their incidence is higher in patients with family history, bulky tumors, and multiple tumors. SDHB gene mutation carriers during diagnosis or follow-up indicate a high risk of malignant PPGL. Because the genetic data of patients are closely related to the clinic, genetic screening and enhanced follow-up should be carried out for families carrying PPGL-related gene mutations to facilitate early diagnosis of the disease and timely intervention.

At present, there are still many basic research issues that need to be discussed. It is necessary to establish a clinical data database of PPGL, as well as a database of patients' blood and tissue specimens, to lay a good foundation for further clinical and basic research of PPGL. To use the research results on VEGF, HIF, mTOR, and other signaling pathways to apply targeted drug therapy to clinical practice, extensive and in-depth basic research on the pathogenesis of PPGL is also required. In addition to the establishment of primary cultures of human PPGL, systematic studies should also be carried out in terms of genetics, epigenetics, signaling pathways, and targeted drugs.

1.2 Treatment

1.2.1 Preoperative Management

The impact of hypercatecholamineremia produced by PPGL on patients includes the following aspects: firstly, the greatest impact on blood pressure, serious cardiovascular, and cerebrovascular accidents is not uncommon; secondly, there is damage to cardiac function and structure caused by catecholamine cardiomyopathy; thirdly, it is the mass effect of the huge tumor that squeezes the surrounding organs and the possibility of invasion and metastasis of some PPGLs.

The incidence of paroxysmal hypertension in patients is 25–40%. The incidence of persistent hypertension is about 50%, of which 50% have paroxysmal exacerbation. About 70% of patients have orthostatic hypotension. For a small number of patients, blood pressure is normal. Surgery to remove the tumor is one of the most effective treatments, but it is risky. Perioperative mortality can be as high as 45% in patients with complex PPGL without systemic preoperative adjustment and treatment of concurrent disease. Some tumors appear to be in a "quiescent state" without secreting hormones, but under stress conditions such as anesthesia and other organ surgery, they can induce hypertensive crisis or shock state. Enough attention should be paid to these tumors.

Alpha-blockers are usually prescribed for 2–4 weeks, depending on symptom severity, cardiac function status, and catecholamine levels. The criteria for adequate drug preparation are:

1. Blood pressure is controlled at about 130/80 mmHg; blood pressure is stable, and the original orthostatic hypotension is reduced.
2. Heart rate is less than 80 beats/min, with no palpitations, sweating, etc.
3. Hypermetabolic symptoms are improved or disappear.
4. Recovery of blood volume and improvement of peripheral circulation.

Alpha-blockers can reduce blood pressure, dilate the vascular bed, and gradually increase blood volume. The commonly used drug is phenoxybenzamine, which is usually taken for 2–4 weeks. After the patient has normal blood pressure control, blood volume recovery, weight gain, warm extremity skin, improved microcirculation, and improvement of hypermetabolic syndrome and abnormal glucose metabolism, surgery can be considered.

Catecholamine cardiomyopathy caused by high concentrations of catecholamines on myocardial damage can usually be relieved after the use of alpha-blockers and cardioprotective therapy. Arrhythmias, heart failure with pulmonary edema, myocardial infarction, and generalized or focal ventricular wall motion abnormalities may be improved. Such patients should be prepared for 3–6 months before surgery and then undergo surgery after the myocardial damage has recovered to a better state. Life-threatening cases of PPGL with a high level of catecholamine secretion are common during the onset of catecholamine cardiomyopathy, during interventional therapy, during induction of surgical anesthesia, and in the case of circulatory instability due to insufficient volume after surgery. These patients should be treated with caution.

In addition, a multidisciplinary discussion of mechanism needs to be established before surgery. A multidisciplinary collaborative team including urology, endocrinology, basic surgery, anesthesiology, ICU, radiology, pathology, etc., through careful preoperative discussion, repeatedly deduces intraoperative and postoperative possibility of complex PPGL. Various situations that may occur during and after PPGL surgery can be successfully handled for treating difficult and high-risk patients with PPGL tumors. Preoperative fingernail fold microcirculation detection, adequate preoperative drug preparation, and proper perioperative management are the keys to reducing surgical risks and making the surgery successful.

1.2.2 Surgical Management

Surgical resection is a radical cure for PPGL, but surgery and anesthesia are of high risk. Adequate preoperative preparation can effectively reduce the occurrence of various perioperative complications. Since the 1990s, the Department of Urology of Peking Union Medical College Hospital has taken the lead in carrying out laparoscopic adrenal tumor resection in China. Since 2003, Peking Union Medical College Hospital has focused on the clinical practice of laparoscopic surgery to remove adrenal PPGL with a sum of successful experience of 211 cases of laparoscopic surgery to remove PPGL. We focus on the safety and feasibility of this technology to lay a foundation for further work. Since December 2012, Peking Union Medical College Hospital has successively introduced 3D laparoscopic and da Vinci robotic surgery systems, which have advantages in the identification and dissection of blood vessels and organs around PPGL and have achieved satisfactory results.

PPGL is rich in blood supply, and larger tumors are more prone to hemodynamic instability. Therefore, the operation is difficult, and the perioperative mortality is high. The application of some new technologies, such as image reconstruction technology and robotic laparoscopy, reduces tumor extrusion, avoids secondary damage to large blood vessels and important organs, greatly improves the success rate of surgery, and is worthy of promotion. Laparoscopic surgery can reduce the amount of intraoperative blood loss and has obvious advantages for bilateral, multifocal, and deep tumors. Repeated squeezing of the tumor should be avoided as much as possible during the operation.

3D laparoscopic or robotic surgery has advantages for vessel identification and suturing, which can maintain the blood supply of the residual normal adrenal gland as much as possible and can also shorten the operation time. Some huge tumors are embedded with the inferior vena cava, abdominal aorta, pancreas, duodenum, etc. Open surgery is required, or laparoscopic surgery is converted to open surgery. Therefore, the operator should also have a solid foundation in open surgery. Complex and difficult cases involve the identification of catecholamine cardiomyopathy, improvement of cardiac function, blood pressure management, blood sugar regulation, electrolyte imbalance adjustment, anesthesia coordination, use of vasoactive drugs, and many other aspects.

For suspected locally advanced tumors or advanced tumors with metastases that can be resected by surgery, perioperatively combined organ resection should be considered, which will reduce the effect of catecholamines on the cardiovascular system and reduce mortality.

1.2.3 Postoperative Management

Due to the high risk of PPGL surgery, patients should be monitored at least for blood pressure, heart rate, and blood glucose fluctuations in an intensive care unit after surgery. After complete resection of the primary tumor, patients with PPGL are at risk of tumor recurrence and metastasis. Genetic testing of PPGL patients and their families is recommended, and plasma or urine catecholamines are tested annually to screen for local or metastatic recurrence, as well as new tumors. Patients with PPGL surgery should be followed up for at least 10 years, and high-risk patients (young patients, patients with genetic diseases, patients with larger tumor volumes, etc.) should be followed up every 6 months and followed up annually for life. For patients after bilateral PPGL surgery, in addition to monitoring blood pressure, it is also necessary to pay attention to the detection of adrenal corticosteroids. If necessary, the physiological requirements of glucocorticoids should be actively supplemented for patients with irregular morphology, large volume, positive SDHx gene mutations, and immunohistochemical staining suggestive proliferative activity. ^{131}I-MIBG imaging should be regularly performed to exclude recurrence and malignant metastasis.

Metastatic PPGL can be treated with nuclide ^{131}I-MIBG, which can be selectively absorbed by PPGL tissue to emit β Radiation, acting on tumor cells to achieve a therapeutic effect. Palliative chemotherapy mostly uses cyclophosphamide, vincristine, and dacarbazine (CVD) regimens. In addition, sunitinib has been reported in the treatment of liver metastases from PPGL. For metastatic PPGL, low chemotherapy response rates, due to abundant blood transport and radiotherapy insensitivity, still need to be further explored such as metastatic law, abnormal protein expression, and gene mutation characteristics, to make a breakthrough in treatment.

In summary, surgery is the first treatment of PPGL. Adequate preoperative preparation, meticulous intraoperative procedures, and close postoperative monitoring are essential for successful surgery of pheochromocytoma/paraganglioma. Accumulated experience continues in the treatment of metastatic PPGL lesions with 131I-MIBG, and the trend of tumor volume changes in metastatic lesions is regularly monitored by using 68Ga PET-CT imaging. With the further deepening of molecular biology research, future genetic diagnosis will affect the formulation of treatment plans and will guide the application of targeted therapeutic drugs.

Further Reading

Alobuia WM, Ammar S, Tyagi M. Probability of positive genetic testing in patients diagnosed with pheochromocytoma and paraganglioma: criteria beyond a family history. Surgery. 2021;169(2):298–301.

Armaiz-Pena G, Flores SK, Cheng ZM. Genotype-phenotype features of germline variants of the TMEM127 pheochromocytoma susceptibility gene: a 10-year update. J Clin Endocrinol Metab. 2021;106(1):e350–64.

Deng J, Li H. Pheochromocytoma/Paraganglioma mutation-associated genetic syndrome. Med J Peking Union Med Coll Hosp. 2015a;6(03):161–5.

Deng J, Li H. Advances in genetic research of pheochromocytoma/paraganglioma. CMJ. 2015b;95(15):1193–5.

Fan H, Li H, Ji Z, et al. Perioperative management of pheochromocytoma/paraganglioma with catecholamine cardiomyopathy. Chinese J Urol. 2018;39(05):333–7.

Gild ML, Naik N, Hoang J. Role of PET/CT in preoperative assessment of phaeochromocytoma and paragangliomas. Clin Endocrinol(Oxf). 2018;89(2):139–47.

Grodski S, Jung C, Kertes P, et al. Phaeochromocytoma in pregnancy. Intern Med J. 2006;36(9):604–6.

Han-zhong L, Wei-gang Y, Wei W, et al. Adrenal incidentalomas: report og 126 cases. Chin J Surg. 2004;02:33–5.

Jin W, Zhigang-Ji, Xiao H, et al. Laparoscopic surgery for adrenal Pheochromocytoma and Paraganglioma: report of 211 cases. Med J Peking Union Med Coll Hosp. 2010;1(01):72–6.

Jin C, Shao Y, Zeng Z, et al. Analysis of clinical efficacy of 131I-meta-iodobenzylguanidine in the treatment of malignant pheochromocytoma/paraganglioma. Chinese J Urol. 2015;36(01):24–8.

Kotecka-Blicharz A, Hasse-Lazar K, Handkiewicz-Junak D, et al. 131-I MIBG therapy of malignant pheochromocytoma and paraganglioma tumours—a single-Centre study. Endokrynol Pol. 2018;69(3):246–51.

Ma X, Zhang X, et al. Synonymous mutations in the Von-Hippel Lindau gene cause familial pheochromocytoma. Basic Med Clin Practice. 2020;40(11):1489–93.

Mannelli M, Bemporad D. Diagnosis and management of pheochromocytoma during pregnancy. J Endocrinol Investig. 2002;25(6):567–71.

Phoon JW, Kanalingam D, Chua HL. Adrenal tumours in pregnancy: diagnostic challenge and management dilemma. Singapore Med J. 2013;54(7):e141–5.

Wen J, Li H, Ji Z, et al. Clinical study of 3D laparoscopic surgery for adrenal pheochromocytoma/paraganglioma. Chinese J Urol. 2015;36(07):511–3.

Wen J, Li H, Ji Z, et al. Analysis of 35 cases of adrenal pheochromocytoma/paraganglioma with 3D laparoscopic surgery. Basic Med Clin Practice. 2016;36(07):1014–6.

Yalniz C, Morani AC, Waguespack SG. Imaging of adrenal-related endocrine disorders. Radiol Clin North Am. 2020;58(6):1099–113.

2 Overview of Pheochromocytoma and Retroperitoneal Paraganglioma

Zhi Gang Ji, Wen Da Wang, Jin Wen,
Zhen Yu Zhang, Hong Bo Zhang, Xin Rong Fan,
Yi Zhou, and Jing Min Zhou

2.1 Section 1: Cystic Pheochromocytoma/Retroperitoneal Paraganglioma

Cystic PPGL is rare, and clinical manifestations are often atypical. Clinicians have conducted more frequently diagnostic screenings for adrenal cystic mass due to the potential risks and possible serious consequences of preoperative missed PPGL. The number of patients diagnosed with cystic PPGL is gradually increasing.

2.1.1 Clinical Manifestations

Cystic changes in PPGL are the result of tumor mucoid degeneration or necrosis after local bleeding, a process that begins with intrafocal bleeding and then local necrosis, the trigger mechanism of which may be that the tumor volume is too large, resulting in insufficient blood supply to the tumor. Most patients with cystic PPGL have no obvious clinical symptoms, mainly because the number of catecholamine-secreting cells decreases significantly with the increase of the cystic region of extensive necrosis in the center of the mass.

This results in tumors consisting mainly of non-biologically active interstitial cells, and catecholamines and their metabolites in cysts are not released into the blood circulation before the tumor is isolated. These factors also lead to the laboratory test negative in most cystic PPGL patients. Some patients with cystic PPGL have been found to complain of abdominal pain, which may be due to factors that cause cystic changes. Some degree of pain may occur at any stage of the cysticization process, so chronic abdominal or lumbar pain may be a more common symptom of cystic PPGL. Clinically, cystic PPGL is easily misdiagnosed as kidney tumors, liver abscesses, liver cysts, and distal pancreatic masses.

2.1.2 Treatment

In view of the clinical manifestations of occult cystic PPGL, which leads to preoperative omission and misdiagnosis, adequate preoperative preparation before surgical treatment is extremely important. Currently, preoperative drug preparation for PPGL is the α-blocker of choice, with the main drugs being the non-selective α-receptor blocker phenol benzylamine and the selective α-1 receptor blockers such as doxazo-

Zhi Gang Ji and Wen Da Wang contributed equally to this work.

Z. G. Ji · W. Da Wang · J. Wen (✉) · Z. Y. Zhang · H. B. Zhang · X. R. Fan · Y. Zhou · J. M. Zhou
Department of Urology, Peking Union Medical College Hospital, Beijing, China

J. Wen (ed.), *Surgical Management of Pheochromocytoma and Retroperitoneal Paraganglioma*,
https://doi.org/10.1007/978-981-99-8421-3_2

sin, piperazosin, and trazosin. α-receptor blockers can prevent complications caused by intraoperative catecholamine secretion. If the α-receptor blockers do not control blood pressure ideally or patients cannot tolerate the adverse reactions of α-receptor blockers, calcium ion antagonists can be added or used alone. Commonly used drugs such as nifedipine, amlodipine, and nicardipine, calcium antagonists, can block the entry of calcium ions into the chromeochromocytes, thereby inhibiting the release of catecholamines. When patients develop tachycardia, β-blockers should be added to combat reflex tachycardia caused by α-blockers. The mostly used drug is propranolol, and β-blockers alone cannot be used without α-blockers to control blood pressure. Otherwise, it will lead to hypertensive crises and even cardiac arrest.

Because most of the catecholamines secreted by cystic PPGL are metabolized in the tumor, only a small amount is released into the bloodstream, resulting in patients' often negative preoperative laboratory tests. It is difficult to be accurately diagnosed before surgery. It is often accurately diagnosed when hemodynamic abnormalities occur during surgery. The key to successful surgery lies in the correct exposure of the mass and the prevention of rupture of the tumor envelope. It is also not advisable to attempt to aspirate the cyst fluid during surgery, as the cyst contains a large amount of catecholamines that may cause severe acute hypotension after being pumped. During surgical removal of the tumor, when unexpected hypertension is found, the surgical team must immediately consider the diagnosis of PPGL.

Ligation of the adrenal central vein prevents most catecholamines from entering the bloodstream, reducing the risk of intraoperative hypertensive crisis. Laparoscopic adrenalectomy is safe and effective for tumors with a maximum tumor diameter of less than 12 cm. The advantages of laparoscopic surgery are less postoperative pain, a lower incidence of postoperative intestinal obstruction, better cosmetic results, and faster recovery, but it is more likely to lead to cyst rupture. At present, there are four cases of translaparoscopic resection of PPGL with a diameter of >10 cm, of which two cases were operated by transperitoneal approach and one case by retroperitoneal approach. Another case was not known what kind of approach to use, but bilateral adrenalectomy was performed. These patients had preoperatively elevated urine or plasma epinephrine, clearly diagnosed as PPGL. Therefore, all patients received adequate preoperative α- and/or β-blocker therapy, the surgical process was smooth, no serious perioperative complications occurred, and postoperative recovery was good. A study comparing transabdominal-approach laparoscopic surgery with transperitoneal approach laparoscopic surgery showed that retroperitoneal approach surgery took less time and had less postoperative pain and that postoperative patients recovered faster their diet and had a lower incidence of complications. Another study of PPGL patients undergoing laparoscopic surgery grouped according to tumor diameter showed that patients with larger tumor diameter (≥6 cm) had higher preoperative doses of oral benzylamine and higher levels of urinary norepinephrine and epinephrine at 24 h and patients with tumors ≥8 cm in diameter required more intraoperative transfusions and longer periods of monitoring in intensive care units.

If locally advanced malignancy is suspected preoperatively or if metastatic lesions can be surgically removed, combined organ resection should be chosen, which reduces the effect of catecholamines on the cardiovascular system and reduces mortality. Palliative care should be done when advanced malignancy has local infiltrates or distant metastases that cannot be surgically removed. Surgery for complex cystic lesions such as diaphragm, thick-walled, calcified, strengthened cystic walls, or solid masses inside the lesions is usually recommended in patients diagnosed with adrenal cystic mass. Surgery should also be performed in patients with obvious clinical symptoms, such as chronic abdominal pain without other clear causes or symptoms caused by tumor compression of other organs.

PPGL is a catecholamine-secreting neuroendocrine tumor. Its incidence is not high, and cystic PPGL is even rarer. Patients usually have no obvious clinical symptoms. Preoperative laboratory tests are often no positive findings. It is difficult to confirm the diagnosis before surgical treatment. CT, MRI, and other imaging tests can find that there is cystic mass in the adrenal region suggestive of PPGL. Surgery is the preferred treatment for cystic PPGL. Adequate preoperative preparation, intraoperative meticulous manipulation, and postoperative close monitoring are extremely important for the successful treatment of cystic PPGL. Clinicians should pay more and more attention to such diseases. With more recent research results, more accurate diagnosis and treatment methods on cystic PPGL will appear in the future, thereby significantly improving the efficacy and reducing the incidence of postoperative complications.

2.2 Section 2: Functionally Quiescent Pheochromocytoma/Paraganglioma

Functionally quiescent PPGL is defined as clinically asymptomatic or without typical symptoms of hypercatecholamineremia such as episodic palpitations, headache, profuse sweating, and persistent or fluctuating hypertension. If these patients are not accurately diagnosed before surgery, blood pressure may fluctuate violently during surgery. In severe cases, hypertensive crisis may occur and even endanger the life of patients. In recent years, with the popularization of physical examination and the continuous progress of imaging technology, the accidental discovery of adrenal accidental tumor is increasing year by year. It has been reported in the literature that about 8.5% of adrenal accidental tumors are functionally quiescent PPGL. This type lacks typical paroxysmal hypertension and symptoms such as headache, palpitations, and excessive sweating and is prone to misdiagnosis or delayed diagnosis. However, functionally quiescent PPGLs can still be lethal. Therefore, asymptomatic tumor does not mean no function, and some patients can induce hypertension and even pheocytoma crisis under special circumstances (such as surgical stimulation, etc.).

2.2.1 Clinical Manifestations

Functional static PPGL can be divided into two forms: (1) concealed functional PPGL, which refers to PPGL that does not usually show signs of high blood pressure but can rapidly rise in blood pressure under stress conditions such as severe trauma, infection, and surgery, and (2) no functional PPGL. No functional pheochromocytoma refers to the type without perioperative blood pressure fluctuations. Since it is difficult to predict whether PPGL patients without a history of hypertension will experience a sudden increase in blood pressure under stress conditions such as surgery before surgery, the two are collectively referred to as functionally quiescent PPGL.

The lack of typical clinical manifestations of functionally quiescent PPGL may be due to the following reasons: although the tumor contains a large amount of catecholamine hormones, most of them are metabolized inside the tumor. A relatively small number of vasoactive substances and a large amount of inactive metabolites are secreted into the circulatory system. For relatively large tumors, they are more prone to hemorrhage and necrosis. Their function is affected. For some patients, stress conditions, especially when the cardiovascular system is not sensitive to catecholamines. However, under certain tumor is squeezed during surgery, the release of catecholamines can be 1000 times larger than usual, resulting in large fluctuations in blood pressure, which brings great difficulty to the surgery.

The detection of functionally quiescent PPGL patients largely relies on imaging examinations. Older hemorrhage, necrosis, or cystic degeneration often occurs in patients with large tumor diameters. B-ultrasound usually shows mixed echoes. Enhanced CT often shows heterogeneous enhancement inside the tumor. However, it is difficult to make a qualitative diagnosis based on imaging examinations alone. Endocrine testing is necessary for quiescent PPGL, but its diagnostic value is limited.

Because the endocrine examination of functionally quiescent PPGL often suggests normal or mildly elevated blood and urine catecholamines, further diagnosis relies on 131I-MIBG and somatostatin receptor imaging. 131I-MIBG is an adrenergic neuron blocking agent that is taken up by chromaffin cells via a sodium ion and energy-dependent amine uptake mechanism (type I) to visualize tumors. For functionally quiescent PPGL, 131I-MIBG imaging is the only effective diagnostic method. Therefore, for functionally quiescent PPGL, if preoperative imaging is highly suspected to be PPGL, even if there is no positive indication on endocrine examination and somatostatin receptor imaging, further 131I-MIBG imaging should be performed.

2.2.2 Treatment

Surgery to remove the tumor is the treatment of choice. Laparoscopic surgical resection of functionally quiescent PPGL is an ideal surgical approach. For patients with functionally quiescent PPGL, strict drug preparation to reduce the risk of surgery should be performed before surgery, and alpha-blockers such as doxazosin mesylate and phenoxybenzamine are usually used for 2–4 weeks to perform preoperative volume expansion to correct the potential hypoglycemia of patients, to reduce the fluctuation range of intraoperative blood pressure, and to reduce the probability of blood transfusion. For all patients with static PPGL, intraoperative anesthesia must be prepared strictly according to the routine of PPGL. The anesthesia method is intravenous-inhalation compound anesthesia. Intrajugular or subclavian vein puncture is used to measure central venous pressure, or floating catheter is used to measure pulmonary artery wedge pressure and record urine volume. Arterial pressure measurement is used to observe the instantaneous change of blood pressure during operation. Continuous ECG monitoring and opening of multiple venous accesses can be used to correct blood pressure abnormalities by giving different concentrations of antihypertensive or vasopressor drugs during and after surgery. During the specific operation, if the tumor is tightly adhered to the surrounding tissue and/or large blood vessels during the operation, which makes the separation difficult, laparoscopic surgery should be converted to open surgery in a timely manner.

To sum up, a part of quiescent PPGL may appear "pheochromocytoma crisis" under stress state, such as unexplained sudden increase in blood pressure and cold sweat under trauma, infection, surgery, etc. and other stress states, such as coma, convulsions, pulmonary edema, heart failure, and other crises. Even if there is no history of hypertension, the possibility of "static PPGL" should still be considered, and corresponding rescue should be made, and then the corresponding examinations should be carried out according to the diagnostic steps of PPGL for a clear diagnosis. The disease has different degrees of blood pressure fluctuations during the operation. If the symptoms and minor endocrine changes that are often ignored by patients and clinicians are observed before the operation, the clinicians can fully understand the disease before the operation and can deal with the corresponding situation calmly during the operation.

2.3 Section 3: Pheochromocytomas/Paragangliomas with Catecholamine Cardiomyopathy

PPGL can secrete catecholamines, mostly norepinephrine (NE). Hypercatecholamineemia can cause clinical symptoms such as hypertension, palpitations, and sweating. Catecholamine cardiomyopathy is a serious complication of PPGL and can even lead to death, but it is often clinically overlooked or misdiagnosed. Therefore, it is necessary to identify and accurately diagnose catecholamine cardiomyopathy.

2.3.1 Clinical Manifestations

Common structural and functional abnormalities of the heart in catecholamine cardiomyopathy are symmetrical left ventricular hypertrophy and decreased left ventricular systolic function, which in severe cases cause acute left heart failure. They can also be manifested as dilated, hypertrophic obstruction, ventricular hypertrophy, or diffuse or segmental ventricular wall movement disorder that is inconsistent with the distribution of coronary arteries.

Catecholamines can produce direct myocardial damage by calcium overload, oxidative stress, induction of apoptosis, pro-fibrosis, and activation of the renin-angiotensin-aldosterone system. They can also cause microcirculation dysfunction by increasing myocardial oxygen consumption, inducing coronary artery spasm and endothelial injury, which result in myocardial ischemia and aggravating myocardial damage. The actual incidence of catecholamine cardiomyopathy may be higher than generally recognized. According to autopsy studies, 50–60% of patients who die of PPGL have myocarditis manifestations, typically manifested by focal degeneration, cardiomyocyte contraction band necrosis, inflammatory cell infiltration, and later fibrosis is more prominent.

Meune et al. also found that some patients with PPGL, despite normal echocardiographic findings, were pervasive in subclinical left ventricular systolic dysfunction and were associated with the risk of intraoperative circulatory failure. Paul et al. believed that after high catecholamine activation of myocardial β-2-adrenergic receptors, Gs in the intracellular signaling pathway were converted to Gi, resulting in negative inotropic effects on the myocardium at this site, and postoperative cardiac function was restored. The reason may be mainly that β-2AR-Gi has a protective and anti-apoptotic effect on the myocardium.

2.3.2 Treatment

In terms of treatment, regular α-blockers (phenoxybenzamine 5–10 mg, once every 8 h), β-blockers (metoprolol tartrate 12.5–25 mg, one to two times a day), and calcium antagonists (nifedipine 10–30 mg, once a day) are given for 3 months. Suspected pulmonary infection is treated with sensitive antibiotics, cardiotonic, diuretics, and other drugs. After the blood pressure and heart rate are stable, the peripheral circulation is increased, the body weight is increased, and the cardiac function is significantly improved by echocardiography.

Patients with quiescent PPGL do not have typical endocrine dysfunction, and imaging tests do not indicate rich blood circulation of the tumor. Most of them are not prepared for preoperative drugs, but they are prone to hypertensive crisis during the anesthesia induction stage or when the tumor is touched. Opioid sedatives, dopamine receptor antagonists, and sympathetic tone-increasing muscle relaxants and sympathomimetic amine vasoactive substances used in the induction of anesthesia can induce large releases of catecholamines. Any patient with suspected PPGL requires improved endocrine and nuclear medicine tests. Then surgery is performed after aggressive drug preparation to avoid severe catecholamine cardiomyopathy as much as possible.

The severity of catecholamine cardiomyopathy is not associated with endocrine examination. Previous studies have reported 15 patients with PHEO, 6 of whom present with left ventricular hypertrophy. But their plasma NE or epinephrine levels are not correlated with measurements of left ventricular structure. Predisposition factors suggestive of catecholamine cardiomyopathy still need to be further studied.

In summary, catecholamine cardiomyopathy is a serious comorbidity of PPGL. Patients with PPGL with catecholamine cardiomyopathy need to be fully prepared with adequate medication if the diagnosis is clear. Aggressive symptomatic treatment is required when cardiac dysfunction occurs, and cardiac dysfunction can be effectively improved after tumor resection. Patients with functional quiescent PPGL are at high risk during the perioperative period, and patients with functionally quiescent PPGL require aggressive drug preparation before surgery.

2.4 Section 4: Pheochromocytoma/Retroperitoneal Paraganglioma in Pregnancy

PPGL is specific during pregnancy, with an incidence of about 0.007%. The secretion of catecholamines causes hypertension, which is extremely harmful to pregnant women and fetuses during pregnancy. Improper disposal may cause serious consequences of maternal or fetal death. Its diagnosis and treatment should be paid attention to. Pregnancy PPGL can cause placental ischemia, placental abruption, fetal intrauterine growth retardation, fetal hypoxia, and even fetal death in the fetus. It can cause uncontrollable hypertension, hypertensive crisis, heart failure, pulmonary edema, cerebrovascular accident, and so on. Moretti et al. pointed out that in cases of pregnant PPGL that were not diagnosed and treated in time, the maternal mortality rate was 17–24%, and the fetal mortality rate was 50–62%. In cases of timely diagnosis and treatment, maternal mortality rate decreased to 1–5%, and fetal mortality rate decreased to 14–15%.

2.4.1 Clinical Manifestations

The clinical manifestations of pregnancy with pheochromocytoma are no different from those of pheochromocytoma in general. They are mostly hypertensive, episodic, or persistent and may be accompanied by a triad of episodic headache, palpitations, and sweating. Other symptoms are a head dizziness, nausea, fatigue, anxiety, etc. These symptoms are easily confused with gestational hypertension syndrome and preeclampsia, making diagnosis difficult or leading to misdiagnosis.

The distinction between pregnancy with pheochromocytoma and preeclampsia should be noted:

1. The former can appear at any stage of pregnancy by careful request of medical history and may manifest before pregnancy. The latter occurs after 20 weeks of pregnancy.
2. The former can be presented as onset hypertension with triple signs. The latter is persistent.
3. The former rarely has proteinuria. The latter is often accompanied by proteinuria.
4. The former persists hypertension after childbirth, and the latter hypertension can return to normal.

Therefore, for those who have hypertension in the early stage of pregnancy and whose hypertension is difficult to control; those with typical episodic headache, palpitations, and sweating symptoms; and those whose postpartum symptoms have not disappeared, pheochromocytoma may be considered.

Diagnosis of pregnancy with pheochromocytoma includes both qualitative diagnosis and diagnosis for localization. Qualitative diagnosis includes the determination of blood and urinary catecholamines and their metabolites. Normal pregnancy or preeclampsia does not affect catecholamine concentrations. Twenty-four-hour urinary catecholamines are more frequently used due to their high sensitivity and high diagnostic value. B ultrasound examination is easy to perform and harmless to the fetus. It is an important means of examination. Most of the lesions are first found by B ultrasound examination. The disadvantage is poor sensitivity, especially for extra-adrenal pheochromocytoma. CT is an important means of localization diagnosis of pheochromocytoma with high sensitivity. It can find tumors >1 cm in diameter and accurately localize them. However, due to the disadvantage of exposing the fetus to radiation, it is limited in the application of pregnancy cases. MRI avoids the possible effects of radiation on the fetus and is highly sensitive and accurately positioned, making it a good diagnostic tool. In addition, MRI testing for pheochromocytoma T2 is often (?) an abnormally high signal, which is also helpful for the qualitative diagnosis of tumors. Nuclear medicine tests such as 131I-MIBG imaging and somatostatin receptor imaging are good qualitative and diagnostic methods for localization. They are only used to determine cases of termination of pregnancy or postpartum.

2.4.2 Treatment

Surgery is the treatment of choice. Adequate medication preparation is required prior to surgery. Alpha-blockers should be used to control blood pressure. In cases of pregnancy, drugs such as phenolic benzylamine and piperazine are safe. Beta-blockers are used to treat cases of rapid heart rate but should be used after a receptor blocker to avoid inducing episodes of hypertension.

There is controversy about the timing and method of surgery in pregnancy cases. At present, the second trimester of pregnancy is considered to be an ideal time for surgery. Because pregnancies are relatively stable during this period, the incidence of spontaneous miscarriage is low, the early organ development of the fetus is basically complete, and the size of the uterus has little impact on the operation currently.

The timing of surgery should be determined according to the physiological characteristics of early, middle, and third trimester pregnancy and the functional status of pheochromocytoma. In cases of first trimester pregnancy, blood pressure can be controlled using drugs such as alpha-blocker until post-second trimester surgery. If the patient chooses to miscarry, pheochromocytoma surgery may be performed electively after drug preparation. In cases of the second trimester, pheochromocytoma surgery can be performed after drug preparation. In cases of third-trimester pregnancy, blood pressure should be controlled with medication as much as possible and maintained until full-term pregnancy before surgery. Pheochromocytoma may be surgically removed at the same time as delivery. Natural labor and delivery of child should be avoided as caesarean sections have a lower risk of maternal mortality than vaginal deliveries.

Laparoscopic surgery has been shown to be a safe and effective treatment for pheochromocytoma with the following advantages:

1. Reduced surgical trauma.
2. Reduced intraoperative bleeding.
3. Avoidance of excessive squeezing of the tumor and reduced intraoperative hemodynamic fluctuations.
4. Reduced use of postoperative analgesic medications.
5. Retroperitoneal laparoscopy avoids interference with the uterus by the transperitoneal route.

However, there are little experiences in pregnant cases. The following controversies exist:

1. The effect of pneumo-abdominal pressure on uterine blood circulation
2. Preterm labor induced by increased abdominal pressure
3. Fetal acidosis caused by hypercapnia
4. Increased abdominal pressure inducing hypertension attacks
5. Fetal hypoxia due to decreased cardiac output caused by pneumoperitoneal pressure

In short, for pregnant women who have hypertension in the first trimester of pregnancy or typical episodic hypertension or who are accompanied by a triad of headache, palpitations, and sweating and hypertension after childbirth, the possibility of pheochromocytoma should be considered, and related tests should be carried out. Timely diagnosis can greatly reduce the maternal and fetal mortality rate. Management should be based on the period of pregnancy and on the functional status of the pheochromocytoma. The second trimester is an ideal time for surgery. Laparoscopic surgery is a safe and effective option for the treatment of pregnant pheochromocytoma.

2.5 Section 5: Paraganglioma of the Urinary Bladder

Paraganglioma of urinary bladder is rare in clinical practice. It is first reported by Zimmerman in 1953, accounting for about 1% of paragangliomas and 0.06% of bladder tumors, with an age of onset of 20–40 years old. The sex ratio of male/female is 1:3.

2.5.1 Clinical Manifestations

2.5.1.1 Cause

Bladder PPGL originates from paraganglion cells in the bladder wall and can occur at all levels and at any part of the bladder wall, with more common in the anterior, posterior, and apical walls. The cause of bladder PPGL is unknown and may be genetically related. Family history exists in 10–20%. The main reason for the occurrence of most familial paragangliomas is VHL (von Hippel-Lindau gene), succinate dehydrogenase subunit complex B (SDHB), succinate dehydrogenase subunit complex C (SDHC), and succinate dehydrogenase subunit complex D (SDHD) gene site mutations, which are also marker gene fragments of sporadic PPGL and which may be related to the site of tumorigenesis. Patients with mutations at the SDHB locus have usually larger tumor in size and are more likely to be malignant than sporadic and more likely to invade surrounding tissue organs. Detecting the expression of the SDHB protein by immunohistochemistry is very useful for determining the genetic background of tumors and predicting which tumors have a higher risk of malignancy.

2.5.1.2 Pathology and Pathophysiology

Bladder PPGLs are located under the mucosa or intramuscular layer of the bladder wall. More than 90% involve the muscular layer, and 37% can penetrate the entire bladder layer or invade the pelvic wall. Generally, the surface of the tumor is covered with intact mucous membranes, or ulceration is formed. Most tumors are less than 4 cm in diameter and up to 15 cm in size. It is leafy, with clear boundaries and surrounding tissues, homogeneous sections, and a red or yellowish-brown appearance. As seen under the microscope, most of the tumor cells are more uniform, oval or polygonal, arranged in a nest shape, and partially arranged in a cord or acinar-like, with obvious blood sinus separation between the cells. The nucleus is located in the center of the cell. The nucleus varies in size. Sometimes, nuclear atypia is visible, and nuclear division is rare. Tumor cells are rich in clear cytoplasm, containing basophilic or eosinophilic fine particles. Some melanin particles are visible. Immunohistochemical examination shows a positive expression of neuroendocrine marker SEs, support cell S-100 protein, chromochromin A, serotonin, and somatostatin, while some epithelial markers such as CK, EMA, and CEA are negative. Most bladder PPGLs are histologically benign, and a few (about 1a) are malignant. Electron microscopy shows neuroendocrine granules with dense cores visible in the cytoplasm. There are cell connections between cells. Immunohistochemical S-100 protein staining and electron microscopy show the presence of support cells, which suggest benign tumors.

The bladder PPGL is classified as functional and non-functional according to the secretion of catecholamines (CA). About 75% of bladder PPGL secrete CA, such as norepinephrine (NE) and epinephrine (E), and rarely dopamine (DA). The methylaniline-based ethanol-converting enzyme that converts NE to E is lacking in extra-adrenal pheochromophilus cells. Therefore, the CA secreted by bladder paragangliomas is dominated by NE. During or after urination, the tumor is squeezed, which leads to releasing large amounts of catecholamines, resulting in paroxysmal increases in blood pressure or persistent increases in blood pressure and paroxysmal exacerbations or even syncope. Rupture of the tumor surface can cause hematuria. When the tumor is located in the neck of the bladder, it causes obstruction to the bladder outlet. Difficulty in urinating may appear. Some tumors compress the ureteral bladder entrance, which causes obstruction of the upper urinary tract and causes hydrohydration of the ureter and kidneys.

2.5.1.3 Symptoms

According to the secretion of CA, bladder PPGL is divided into functional tumors and non-functional tumors. Clinical manifestations of nonfunctional bladder PPGL are occult. Possible clinical manifestations include (1) intermittent painless whole-course gross hematuria, with an incidence of about 60%; (2) urinary frequency and urgency; (3) poor urination; and (4) dilated hydrops in the kidneys and ureters, accompanied by lumbar swelling and discomfort. Functional bladder PPGL may not only have the above manifestations but also a series of symptoms due to excessive secretion of CA. Paroxysmal increase in blood pressure during or after urination is accompanied by headache, palpitations, and sweating. Some may appear with dizziness, blurred vision, and syncope, as well as hypertensive crisis, acute heart failure, shock, pulmonary edema, and acute renal failure. Other conditions that cause outbreaks include overfilling of the bladder, sexual intercourse, defecation, ejaculation, cystography, and cystoscopy. Other manifestations include orthostatic hypotension and elevated blood sugar.

2.5.1.4 Adjunctive Testing

Urinary CA measurement includes:

1. Retention of 24-h urine is used for the measurement of CA, manifested as NE elevation. When NE is more than four times higher than the control, it can be diagnosed.
2. Urinary E/NE is decreased.
3. The comparison of CA is carried out 3 h before urination and 3 h after urination.

Ultrasonography shows a mound or nodule-like mass, raised in the bladder cavity, with a wide basal base, smooth and continuous mucous membranes, and low echogenic spotting and uniform distribution inside the tumor. There are star-like blood flow signals inside the mass. The tumor blood supply is characterized by a low resistance index (RI). Advanced bladder paragangliomas can destroy the bladder mucosa, and ultrasound shows roughness and disruption of the mucosa.

For CT examination, flat scan shows low-density shadow of the bladder wall, fringing smoothness, and moderate uniform intensification after reinforcement.

For MRI examination, T1WI mass shows a slightly higher signal. No clear vascular flow signal is seen internally. The enhanced scan mass is significantly strengthened, which is characteristic.

Valk et al. reported in 1981 that PPGL was diagnosed by the 131I-MIBG method. 131I-MIBG has a strong affinity with chromophilus tissue and can be diagnosed qualitatively and locally at the same time. Its diagnosis of the localization of multiple and metastatic PPGLs is more advantageous than CT. It has been reported that 131I-MIBG is more sensitive to the diagnosis of PPGL, has less effect on germ cells, and is more suitable for the diagnosis of young patients.

Somatostatin receptor imaging (OTC) is suitable for localization staging of neuroendocrine tumors. In the diagnosis of PPGL, it has more advantages than 131I-MIBG. These two methods can complement each other during the diagnosis process.

For 18F-FDG PET-CT, Pacak et al. reported that PET for the diagnosis of pheochromocytoma was made and correctly localized. The diagnosis for bladder PPGL has a high sensitivity. The fusion of PET and CT is more advantageous, which can accurately locate the metastatic foci of malignant PPG and which is conducive to the clinical correct treatment and follow-up observation of the treatment effect.

Cystoscopy is the main method of diagnosing PPGL of the bladder. It presents with a mass in the bladder wall with a broad basal base and a rich blood supply. In the early stage, the smaller tumors have a mucosal bulge-like lesion. The mucosa is intact and smooth, and the surface mucosa of the larger tumors can be wrinkled and ulcerative. In cases of clinical suspicion of paragangliomas of the bladder, it is better to undergo cystoscopy after drug preparation, or no preoperative cystoscopy is performed. During cystoscopy, the bladder should not be overfilled, nor should a biopsy of the mass be advocated in order not to induce seizures and accidents.

2.5.2 Treatments

Bladder PPGL is not sensitive to chemoradiotherapy. Treatment is mainly surgery. The overall effect in surgical treatment of PPGL depends on factors such as preoperative readiness, intraoperative anesthesia management, and postoperative support for respiratory and circulatory function.

2.5.2.1 Preparation of the Drug

Regardless of whether the preoperative diagnosis of functional bladder PPGL is made, as long as the possibility of bladder PPGL is clinically considered, it is recommended to perform preoperative drug preparation, generally more than 2 weeks, often for 2–4 weeks. Adequate drug preparation can significantly reduce the mortality rate of surgery. The commonly used drug is a long-acting non-selective α-blocker—phenol benzylamine. The initial dose is 5–10 mg, two times per day, adjusted once every 2–3 days, each time increasing by 10–20 mg, according to blood pressure and symptoms to specific adjustment. The general dose is 30–60 mg/day or 1 mg/kg body weight. In most cases, the drug does not exceed 120 mg/day. If necessary, it should be prepared in combination with other drugs, such as calcium channel antagonists, β-blockers, etc.

2.5.2.2 Anesthesia Management and Coordination During Surgery

Functional bladder PPGL may occur during surgical anesthesia such as sharp rise and fall in blood pressure, severe arrhythmias, and other drastic hemodynamic changes. Because the risk is large, it is necessary for the anesthesiology department and the operating department to cooperate closely and deal with it properly in order to successfully complete the operation. More than half of the cases have nonspecific CA cardiotoxic manifestations. The degree of damage to important organs such as cardiovascular disease needs to be carefully assessed during preoperative visits, and long-acting antihypertensive drugs and β-receptor blockers need to be discontinued before surgery in cases of catecholamine cardiomyopathy to prevent prolonged hypotension due to the vasodilatory effect and myocardial inhibition of the drug after tumor removal.

2.5.2.3 Choice of Surgical Modalities

Depending on the size, location, and locality of the tumor, transurethral electroresection or laser resection, partial bladder resection, or total cystectomy may be selected. Most scholars advocate complete removal of the tumor by partial removal of the bladder, with the option of open surgery or laparoscopic surgery. Since most of the bladder PPGL is in the muscular layer, transurethral resection is at risk of incomplete resection. If the tumor is preoperatively judged to be nonfunctional and the tumor is small, transurethral surgery may be attempted. The resection should be treated as a malignant tumor of the bladder with a 2 cm from the edge of the tumor and deep into the muscle layer. Our experience is that using a 2 μm laser treatment is safer and more effective. The entire piece of the tumor and surrounding bladder tissue can be removed, which can achieve the effect of partial removal of the bladder.

Total bladder surgery is mainly used in cases where the lesion is widespread, bladder retention is impossible, and lymph node metastasis is present. Bilateral pelvic lymph node dissection is performed. For patients with extensive lesions or metastases, chemoradiation and chemotherapy can be performed. The commonly used chemotherapy regimen is CVD (cyclophosphamide, vincristine, dacarbazine), with an effective rate of 57.1%. Targeted drug therapy can be tried. Radiotherapy also has certain value of clinical application. 131I-MIBG is mainly used for bladder PPGL with extensive metastases, which significantly prolong the survival of patients with a median survival of 4.7 years. After treatment, a regular and long-term follow-up is required. Follow-up includes monitoring blood pressure, 24-h urinary CA, regular ultrasound, cystoscopy, etc.

2.6 Section 6: Metastatic Pheochromocytoma/Retroperitoneal Paraganglioma

In 2017, the World Health Organization (WHO) classification of neuroendocrine tumors abolished the "benign PPGL" and "malignant PPGL" in the 2004 WHO classification and named it PPGL uniformly. Genetic screening can identify about 40% of PPGL and paragangliomas. Metastatic PPGL is defined as the appearance of metastatic foci in areas without chromophilus tissue, such as bone, liver, lungs, lymph nodes, brain, or other soft tissues. After complete resection of the primary tumor, patients with PPGL are at risk for tumor recurrence and metastasis. Postoperative testing of plasma or urine catecholamines is recommended annually to screen for local or metastatic recurrence and emerging tumors. Patients at high risk (young, hereditary disease, large-volume PPGL) should be followed up every 6 months. All patients undergoing surgery should be followed up for at least 10 years.

2.6.1 Clinical Manifestations

18F-FDG PET-CT can be used to screen for metastatic PPGL. For patients with SDHDx mutations, the effect of 18F-FDG PET-CT is more pronounced, with detection rates of 100% and 92% in primary and metastatic lesions, respectively. The plasma concentration of chromogranin A (CgA) can be used as a detection marker of functional activity in patients with PPGL. Therefore, screening and follow-up programs should include four markers, epinephrine (E), norepinephrine (NE), 3MT (3-methoxytyramine), and CgA. Quantitative determination of epinephrine, norepinephrine, and 3MT in serum and urine is the gold standard for diagnosis and the primary indicator for screening and follow-up of patients with PPGL. Measurements of epinephrine and norepinephrine above three to four times the upper limit of the normal reference range are typical features of PPGL.

At present, the genetic changes of metastatic PPGL have been well understood. In addition to 131I-MIBG radionuclide therapy and chemotherapy, gene diagnosis and targeted drug therapy have become possible. Metastatic PPGL accounts for 10–17%. Its pathogenesis is related to mutations in the gene encoding succinate dehydrogenase gene subunit B (SDHB) in 43–71% of adults and in 70–82% of children. SDHB gene mutation is present in patients with metastatic PPGL. Para-aortic metastases are often confused with primary lesions. It is difficult to identify. Attention should be paid to the diagnosis.

According to the intracellular signaling pathways involved in gene mutations, there are two categories. The first involves pseudo-hypoxia pathways, which promote hypoxia-related growth factors by activating hypoxia-inducing factors, such as vascular endothelial growth factor (VEGF), platelet-derived factors, etc. The expression of tumor growth stimulates tumor growth, including VHL, SDHx (SDHA, SDHB, SDHC, SDHD, SDHAF2), and genes such as *HIF2A*, *FH*, *PHD1*, *PHD2*, *MDH2*, and *KIF1Bβ*. The second type is kinase pathways, which promote tumor growth by activating mitogen-activated protein kinase (MAPK) and/or AKT-mTOR signaling pathways, including genes such as *NF1*, *RET*, *HRAS*, *MAX*, and *TMEM127*. The frequency of germline mutations is 10.3% in SDHB, 8.9% in SDHD, 7.3% in VHL, 6.3% in RET, and 3.3% in NF1. Mutation frequencies of other genes such as *SDHC*, *SDHA*, *MAX*, and *TMEM127* are less than 2%. Among them, SDHB mutations are clearly associated with tumor metastasis. About 40% of patients with SDHB mutations have metastasis. In addition, some tumors have epigenetic changes such as hypermethylation and miRNA changes.

Patients with PPGL are at risk for tumor recurrence and new tumors after primary tumor resection, especially those with tumor seeding at the time of surgery. Non-PPGL tumors can occur in patients with certain syndromes such as von Hippel-Lindau syndrome, multiple endocrine neoplasia (MEN2), neurofibromatosis 1 (NF1), or PPGL with hereditary PPGL. These include kidney cancer, medullary thyroid cancer, or other cancers, which are more common in younger patients and patients with hereditary influence, bulky tumors, multiplex, or PPGL. Mitochondrial dysfunction caused by mutations in SDH is associated with hypoxia and angiogenic pathways, apoptosis tolerance, and developmental upregulation of neural precursor cells, leading to PPGL formation. *SDHB* gene mutation carriers are at high risk for metastatic PPGL during diagnosis or follow-up.

Histologically, the pheochromocytoma of the adrenal gland scaled score (PASS) is used to score 12 pathological features including tumor cell morphology and invasiveness. Tumor diameter is currently one of the most reliable indicators for predicting metastasis tendency of PPGL in clinical practice. Tumor diameter >5 cm is considered to be significantly correlated with malignant invasion and metastasis. The PPGL with a PASS score of 4 or more is more aggressive, with a sensitivity of 100% and a specificity of 75%. Kimaru et al. proposed a new grading system GAPP (Grading System for Adrenal pheochromocytomas and PGL). GAPP is a clinical-biochemical-pathological grading system that classifies PPGL into well differentiated (WD), moderately differentiated (MD), and poorly differentiated (PD). In the GAPP system, the metastasis probability of each stage is different, which are 4%, 60%, and 82%, respectively for WD, MD, and PD. The 5-year survival rate of each stage is also different, which is, respectively, 100%, 67%, and 22% (PD) for WD, MD, and PD. In addition, the Ki-67 index can be used to evaluate the clinical diagnosis and prognosis of metastatic PPGL. Because the Ki-67 index is often low, it cannot be used alone to determine the prognosis. The expression of EM66, S-100, NSE, etc. is decreased in malignant. However, the observation results are all based from small sample studies, and the follow-up time is short. Its clinical application value still needs to be further explored.

The sensitivity and specificity of 131I-MIBG imaging for localizing PPGL can reach 77–88% and 96–100%, respectively. But the sensitivity of MIBG in diagnosing malignant metastatic PPGL is only 56%. Using radionuclide-labeled somatostatin receptor (SSTR) analogs such as somatostatin receptor imaging to specifically bind to SSTR on the tumor surface to make tumor imaging can be used as a supplement to negative MIBG imaging. For extra-adrenal metastatic lesions and head and neck PPGL, the sensitivity can reach 90%. 68Ga-DOTATATE PET/CT imaging is expected to become a routine functional imaging method for diagnosing PPGL in the future. Its clinical application value needs further study.

2.6.2 Treatment

Surgical resection of primary and metastatic lesions is still the mainstay of treatment. Although surgical debulking does not prolong survival, it can help control blood pressure and other related symptoms and may be beneficial for postoperative chemoradiotherapy or nuclide therapy. Nuclide therapy is used in inoperable or in multiple metastases, MIBG imaging, or SSTR imaging positive. The most commonly used drug is 131I-MIBG, which can be selectively absorbed by PPGL tissue, emits β rays, and acts on tumor cells to achieve therapeutic effects. High-dose 131I-MIBG treatment can prolong survival and relieve symptoms. In the short term, the effect is good, 75% effective for symptoms, 45% for hormone, 30% for the tumor volume partial response rate and 5% for the complete response rate. However, the long-term efficacy is not good. There are almost all recurrences or metastasis within 2 years. The main side effects are the suppression of thyroid function and bone marrow. External beam radiation therapy is used for tumors that cannot be surgically removed and to relieve pain from bone metastases. However, it may worsen hypertension.

Chemotherapy recommends a CVD regimen (cyclophosphamide + vincristine + dacarbazine) with an effective rate of about 50%. However, most relapse within 2 years. The combination with MIBG may improve efficacy. Anti-angiogenic targeted drug therapy may be effective. There are no data to confirm the survival benefit or relapse-free survival benefit of adjuvant therapy with 131I-MIBG after resection of metastatic focus. In patients with multiple liver metastases who cannot undergo surgical resection or non-surgical ablation, case studies have shown that trans-arterial chemoembolization (TACE) is beneficial, reducing tumor volume and improving symptoms. As with other topical treatments, TACE may induce a large number of catecholamine secretions and hypertensive crises. Preoperative preparation of drugs is required. In an early study, five of the seven PPGL patients receiving sunitinib monotherapy were stable, but no objective remission was observed. In addition to hypertension, the most common side effects of sunitinib treatment are diarrhea, hand-foot syndrome, aphthous sores, and fatigue.

All patients receiving PPGL treatment should be followed up for at least 10 years to monitor local or metastatic recurrence or new tumors. Patients at high risk (young, with genetic disease, large-volume tumors, and/or paragangliomas) should be followed up for life. Kaplan-Meier analysis is still needed to estimate the probability of recurrence of sporadic and hereditary PPGLs, as well as the assessment of the distribution of events between these metastatic recurrences and new tumors. Cohorts are established to document clinical, biochemical, imaging, or tumor features associated with recurrence and to identify how to tailor follow-up of individual patients.

Although the incidence of recurrent metastases of PPGL is as low as about 1%, more than 40% are metastatic relapses. If the primary tumor is >5 cm in diameter or young patients (<20 years), the risk of new or recurrent tumors at 5 years is 27%. For patients with PPGL, the risk of new or recurrent tumors in 5 years is about 20–25%. The risk of recurrence in elderly patients with PPGL in 5 years is about 10%. Prognosis depends on tumor burden, site of metastasis, and rate of progression. Patients with metastases to the brain, liver, and lungs tend to have a worse prognosis than those with isolated bone lesions. Personalized estimates on PPGL patients of surgical treatment are based on age, genetic testing, tumor site, and size of the risk of new events. More in-depth studies of the specific molecular pathway may explain the changes that lead to metastatic PPGL. A variety of molecularly targeted therapy drugs may be offered in the future to successfully treat metastatic lesions.

Further Reading

Akkuş G, Evran M, Sert M. Multidisciplinary approach for patients with functional and non-functional adrenal masses and review of the literature. Health Sci Rep. 2017;20(1):e22. https://doi.org/10.1002/hsr2.22.

Al-Zahrani AA. Recurrent urinary bladder paraganglioma. Adv Urol. 2010;2010:912125.

Amar L, Bertherat J, Baudin E, et al. Genetic testing in pheochromocytoma or functional paraganglioma. J Clin Oncol. 2005;23:8812–8.

Andreoni C, Krebs RK, Bruna PC, et al. Cystic phaeochromocytoma is a distinctive subgroup with special clinical, imaging and histological features that might mislead the diagnosis. BJU Int. 2008;101:345–50.

Antedomenico E, Wascher R. A case of mistaken identity: giant cystic pheochromocytoma. Curr Surg. 2005;62:193–8.

Asai S, Katabami T, Tsuiki M, et al. Controlling tumor progression with cyclophosphamide, vincristine, and Dacarbazine treatment improves survival in patients with metastatic and Unresectable malignant Pheochromocytomas/Paragangliomas. Horm Cancer. 2017;8:108–18.

Babińska A, Siekierska-Hellmann M, Blaut K, et al. Hormonal activity in clinically silent adrenal incidentalomas. Arch Med Sci. 2012;8(1):97–103.

Bishnoi K, Bora GS, Mavuduru RS. Bladder paraganglioma: safe and feasible management with robot assisted surgery. J Robot Surg. 2016;10(3):275–8.

Bouassida M, Samet A, Mseddi MA, et al. Laparoscopic treatment of a cystic pheochromocytoma of 6cms: a challenging case. Urol Case Rep. 2019;26:100978.

Bruynzeel H, Feelders RA, Groenland TH, et al. Risk factors for hemodynamic instability during surgery for pheochromocytoma. J Clin Endocrinol Metab. 2010;95:678–85.

Burnichon N, Rohmer V, Amar L, et al. The succinate dehydrogenase genetic testing in a large prospective series of patients with paragangliomas. J Clin Endocrinol Metab. 2009;94:2817–27.

Cascón A, Comino-Méndez I, Currás-Freixes M, et al. Whole-exome sequencing identifies MDH2 as a new familial paraganglioma gene. J Natl Cancer Inst. 2015;107:djv053.

Clements HA, Wilson MS, Smith DM. Incidental giant cystic pheochromocytoma: a case report and review of the literature. Scott Med J. 2020;65:64–70.

Costa Almeidal C, Silva M, Carvalho L, et al. Adrenal giant cystic pheochromocytoma treated by posterior retroperitoneoscopic adrenalectomy. Int J Surg Case Rep. 2017;30:201–4.

Deng J, Li H. Advances in genetic research of pheochromocytoma/paraganglioma. CMJ. 2015;95(15):1193–5.

Deng J, Li H, et al. Clinical diagnosis and prognosis of metastatic pheochromocytoma/paraganglioma. Med J Peking Union Med College Hosp. 2019;10(06):654–9.

Diaz Perez JA, Duran Rodriguez-Hervada A. Feocromocitomas paragangliomas. Revisionesen Cancer (Madrid). 2002;16:12–20.

Diaz B, Elkbuli A, Ehrhardt JD Jr, McKenney M. Pheochromocytoma-related cardiomyopathy presenting as broken heart syndrome: case report and literature review. Int J Surg Case Rep. 2019;55:7–10.

Ding L, Fang L, Zhu W, et al. Cardiovascular manifestations of pheochromocytoma. Chinese Cardiovasc J. 2013;18(02):65–7.

Ding L, Fang L, Zhu W, et al. Clinical significance of left ventricular hypertrophy in patients with pheochromocytoma and paraganglioma. Chinese J Cardiovasc Diseases. 2014;42(12):1029–34.

Dong D, Li H. Diagnosis and treatment of pheochromocytoma during pregnancy. J Matern Fetal Neonatal Med. 2014;27(18):1930–4.

Dong D, Li H, Ji Z, et al. Clinical diagnosis and treatment of pregnancy complicated with Pheochromocytoma (report of 4 cases). J Clin Urol. 2015;30(02):127–9.

Edo N, Yamamoto T, Takahashi S, et al. Optimizing hemodynamics with Transcatheter arterial embolization in adrenal Pheochromocytoma rupture. Intern Med. 2018;57:1873–8.

Erlic Z, Neumann HP. Diagnosing patients with hereditary paraganglial tumours. Lancet Oncol. 2009;10:741.

Fan H, Li H, Ji Z, et al. Analysis of clinical features of blood pressure surge during pheochromocytoma/paraganglioma surgery (report of 219 cases in a single center). Chinese J Urol. 2019;04:267–71.

Favier J, Amar L, Gimenez-Roqueplo AP. Paraganglioma and phaeochromocytoma: from genetics to personalized medicine. Nat Rev. Endocrinol. 2015;11:101–11.

Feral CC, Tissot FS, Tosello L, et al. 18F-fluorodihydroxyphenylalanine PET/CT in pheochromocytoma and paraganglioma: relation to genotype and amino acid transport system L. Eur J Nucl Med Mol Imaging. 2017;44:812–21..

Frayssinet C, Vezzosi D, Huyghe E, et al. Retroperitoneal laparoscopic adrenalectomy in a pregnant woman presenting MEN2a with a pheochromocytoma: case report and review of the literature. Ann Endocrinol. 2008;69(1):53–7.

Gill AJ, Benn DE, Chou A, et al. Immunohistochemistry for SDHB triages genetic testing of SDHB, SDHC, and SDHD in paraganglioma-pheochromocytoma syndromes. Hum Pathol. 2010;41:805–14.

Gruber LM, Young WF Jr, Bancos I. Pheochromocytoma and Paraganglioma in pregnancy: a new era. Curr Cardiol Rep. 2021;23(6):60.

Haddad S, Al-Raiy B, Madkhali A, et al. Cardiorespiratory crisis at the end of pregnancy: a case of pheochromocytoma. Middle East J Anaesthesiol. 2013;22(2):195–202.

Hamidi O, Young WF Jr, Gruber L, et al. Outcomes of patients with metastatic phaeochromocytoma and paraganglioma: a systematic review and meta-analysis. Clin Endocrinol. 2017;87:440–50.

Jategaonkar SR, Butz T, Burchert W, et al. Echocardiac features simulating hypertrophic obstructive cardiomyopathy in a patient with pheochromocytoma. Clin Res Cardiol. 2009;98(3):195–8.

Jayarajah U, Herath KB, Fernando MH. Phaeochromocytoma of the urinary bladder presenting with malignant hypertension and hypertensive retinopathy. Asian J Urol. 2020 Jan;7(1):70–2.

Jiang YJ, Sun ZX, Gong DX, et al. The comparison between static pheochromacytoma and non-static pheochromacytoma. J Clin Urol. 2003;18:212–3.

Jin C, Shao Y, Zeng Z, et al. Analysis of clinical efficacy of 131I-meta-iodobenzylguanidine in the treatment of malignant pheochromocytoma/paraganglioma. Chinese J Urol. 2015;36(01):24–8.

Kota SK, Kota SK, Panda S, et al. Pheochromocytoma: an uncommon presentation of an asymptomatic and biochemically silent adrenal incidentaloma. Malays J Med Sci. 2012;19:86–91.

Langton K, Tufton N, Akker S. Pregnancy and phaeochromocytoma/paraganglioma: clinical clues affecting diagnosis and outcome—a systematic review. BJOG. 2021;128(8):1264–72. https://doi.org/10.1111/1471-0528.

Lee T, Sywotzkyl C, Lavelle M, et al. Cystic pheochromocytoma. Radiographics. 2002;22:935–40.

Lee C, Walz M, Park S, et al. A comparative study of the transperitoneal and posterior retroperitoneal approaches for laparoscopic adrenalectomy for adrenal tumors. Ann Surg Oncol. 2012;19:2629–34.

Lee M, Minaskan N, Wiedemann T, et al. Targeting PI3K/mTOR signaling exerts potent antitumor activity in pheochromocytoma in vivo. Endocr Relat Cancer. 2017;24:1–15.

Li C, Chen Y, Wang W, et al. A case of clinically silent giant right pheochromocytoma and review of literature. Can Urol Assoc J. 2012;6:E267–9.

Lian P, Ding L, Zhang X, et al. Perioperative treatment of 5 cases of pheochromocytoma with severe catecholamine cardiomyopathy. J Peking Univ (Med Edn). 2013;45(04):605–8.

Limberg J, Stefanova D, Ullmann TM, Zarnegar R, Fahey TJ 3rd, Beninato T. Not all laparoscopic adrenalectomies are equal: analysis of postoperative outcomes based on tumor functionality. Surg Endosc. 2020;35:2601–6. https://doi.org/10.1007/s00464-020-07678-2.

Liu G, Weifeng X, Xie Y, et al. Diagnosis and treatment of microbladder paraganglioma. Basic Medicine and Clinical. 2017;37(11):1615–9.

Liu H, Li B, Yu X, et al. Perioperative management during laparoscopic resection of large pheochromocytomas: a single-institution retrospective study. J Surg Oncol. 2018;118:709–15.

Łubińska M, Hoffmann M, Jendrzejewski J. Successful surgical treatment of pheochromocytoma during pregnancy. Pol Arch Intern Med. 2018;128(5):322–3.

Maharaj R, Parbhu S, Ramcharan W, et al. Giant cystic pheochromocytoma with low risk of malignancy: a case report and literature review. Case Rep Oncol Med. 2017;2017:4638608.

Mannelli M, Dralle H, Lenders JW. Perioperative management of pheochromocytoma/paraganglioma: is there a state of the art? Horm Metab Res. 2012;44(5):373–8.

Mannelli M, Lenders JW, Pacak K, et al. Subclinical phae-242.

Martins D, Rodrigues D, Melo M, et al. Laparoscopic adrenalectomy as an effective approach to massive bilateral pheochromocytomas. BMJ Case Rep. 2017;2017:bcr2017221009.

Meune C, BertheraT J, Dousset B, et al. Reduced myocardial contractility assessed by tissue Doppler echocardiography is associated with increased risk during adrenal surgery of patients with pheochromocytoma: report of a preliminary study. J Am Soc Echocardiogr. 2006;19(12):1466–70.

Mishra A, Agarwal G, Agarwal A, et al. Laparoscopic adrenalectomy of large cystic pheochromocytoma. Surg Endosc. 2001;15: 220.30:201–4.

Miura M, Kawano H, Yoshida T, et al. The histological features of a myocardial biopsy specimen in a patient in the acute phase of reversible catecholamine-induced cardiomyopathy due to Pheochromocytoma. Intern Med (Tokyo, Japan). 2017;56(6):665–71.

Moretti A, Minuto M, Berti P, et al. Unusual association of adrenal pheochromocytoma and Para-aortic neurofibroma in pregnancy. J Endocrinol Investig. 2006;29(8):738–41.

Nakamoto R, Nakamoto Y, Ishimori T, et al. Clinical significance of quantitative 123 I-MIBG SPECT/CT analysis of pheochromocytoma and paraganglioma. Clin Nucl Med. 2016;41:e465–72.

Nakatani T, Hayama T, Uchida J, et al. Diagnostic localization of extra-adrenal pheochromocytoma: comparison of (123) I-MIBG imaging and (131) I-MIBG imaging. Oncol Rep. 2002;9:1225–7.

Nieman LK. Approach to the patient with an adrenal incidentaloma. J Clin Endocrinol Metab. 2010;95:4106–13.

Noto RB, Pryma DA, Jensen J. Phase 1 study of high-specific-activity I-131 MIBG for metastatic and/or recurrent pheochromocytoma or paraganglioma. J Clin Endocrinol Metab. 2018;103:213–20.

Otusanya O, Goraya H, Iyer P, et al. A vicious cycle of acute catecholamine cardiomyopathy and circulatory collapse secondary to pheochromocytoma. Oxf Med Case Rep. 2015a;2015(10):343–5.

Otusanya O, Goraya H, Iyer P, Landi K. A vicious cycle of acute catecholamine cardiomyopathy and circulatory collapse secondary to pheochromocytoma. Oxf Med Case Rep. 2015b;27:343–5.

Pacak K, Eisenhofer G, Carrasquillo JA, et al. 6-[18F] fluorodopamine positron emission tomographic (PET) scanning for diagnostic localization of pheochromocytomas. Hpertension. 2001;38:6–8.

Pace DE, Chiasson PM, Schlachta CM, et al. Minimally invasive adrenalectomy for pheochromocytoma during pregnancy. Surg Laparosc Endosc Percutan Tech. 2002;12(2):122–5.

Pan DL, Li HZ, Zeng ZP, et al. Twenty-six patients with nonfunctional pheochromocytomas. Chin Med J. 2005;118:866–8.

Pang Y, Liu Y, Pacak K, et al. Pheochromocytomas and paragangliomas: from genetic diversity to targeted therapies. Cancers (Basel). 2019;11:E436.

Parisien-La Salle S, Provençal M, Bourdeau I. Chromogranin a in a cohort of Pheochromocytomas and Paragangliomas: usefulness at diagnosis and as an early biomarker of recurrence. Endocr Pract. 2021;27(4):318–25.

Park M, Hryniewicz K, Setaro JF. Pheochromocytoma presenting with myocardial infarction, cardiomyopathy, renal failure, pulmonary hemorrhage, and cyclic hypotension: case report and review of unusual presentations of pheochromocytoma. J Clin Hypertens (Greenwich). 2009;11(2):74–80.

Phupong V, Witoonpanich P, Snabboon T, et al. Bilateral pheochromocytoma during pregnancy. Arch Gynecol Obstet. 2005;271(3):276–9.

Rong S, et al. Progress in diagnosis and treatment of bladder paraganglioma. Chinese J Clin (Electr Edn). 2012;6(13):3492–4.

Rufini V, Treglia G, Castaldi P, et al. Comparison of metaiodobenzyl-guanidine scintigraphy with positron emission tomography in the diagnostic work-up of pheochromocytoma and paraganglioma: a systematic review. Q J Nucl Med Mol Imaging. 2013;57:122–33.

Safford SD. ^{131}I-MIBG treatment in pheochromocytomas and paraganglioma. J Nucl Med. 2004;45:57.

Samejima M, Taguchi S, Miyagawa S, et al. Acute hypotension induced by suction of cystic fluid containing extremely high concentrations of catecholamines during resection of giant pheochromocytoma. IJU Case Rep. 2019;2:218–20.

Sarveswara V, Kumar S, Kumar A, et al. A giant cystic pheochromocytoma mimicking liver abscess an unusual presentation—a case report. Clin Case Rep. 2015;3:64–8.

Shen WT, Grogan R, Vriens M, et al. One hundred two patients with pheochromocytoma treated at a single institution since the introduction of laparoscopic adrenalectomy. Arch Surg. 2010;145:893–7.

Siatelis A, Konstantinidis C, Volannis D, et al. Pheochromocytoma of the urinary bladder: report of 2 cases and review of literature. Minerva Urol Nefrol. 2008;60:137–40.

Song Y, Li H, Ma L, et al. Four cases of late pregnancy complicated with pheochromocytoma treated by cesarean section and pheochromocytoma resection. Chinese J Obstetr Gynecol. 2014;15(01):84–5.

Tanriver Y, Betz MJ, Nibbe L, et al. Sepsis and cardiomyopathy as rare clinical manifestations of pheochromocytoma—two case report studies. Exp Clin Endocrinol Diabetes. 2010;118(10):747–53.

Thekekara J, Gunasekharan A, Kwon Y. Catecholamine-induced cardiomyopathy and multiple organ failure in pheochromocytoma. J Community Hosp Intern Med Perspect. 2020;10(5):480–2.

Urabe F, Miki J, Kimura T. Combination of unblock transurethral resection with laparoscopic partial cystectomy for paraganglioma of the bladder. IJU Case Rep. 2019;4:283–6.

van Nederveen FH, Gaal J, Favier J, et al. An immunohistochemical procedure to detect patients with paraganglioma and pheochromocytoma with germline SDHB, SDHC, or SDHD gene mutations: a retrospective and prospective analysis. Lancet Oncol. 2009;10:764–71.

Wang H, Sun B, Xu Z, et al. Undiagnosed giant cystic pheochromocytoma: a case report. Oncol Lett. 2015;10:1444–6.

Weifeng X, Li H, Yan W, et al. Transurethral resection of bladder paraganglioma: report of 11 cases. Chinese J Urol. 2014;35(10):753–6.

Wen J, Li H, Ji Z, et al. Clinical study of 3D laparoscopic surgery for adrenal pheochromocytoma/paraganglioma. Chinese J Urol. 2015;36(07):511–3.

Wu D, Tischler AS, Lloyd RV, et al. Observer variation in the application of the Pheochromocytoma of the adrenal gland scaled score. Am J Surg Pathol. 2009;33:599–608.

Yoo KH, Choi T, Lee HL. Aggressive Paraganglioma of the urinary bladder with local recurrence and pelvic metastasis. Pathol Oncol Res. 2020;26(4):2827–9.

Zelinka T, Widimsky J, Weisserov J. Diminished circadian blood pressure rhythm in patients with asymptomatic normotensive pheochromocytoma. Physiol Res. 2001;50:631–4.

Zhai H, Ma X, Nie W. Paraganglioma of the urinary bladder: a series of 22 cases in a single center. Clin Genitourin Cancer. 2017;15(5):e765–71.

Zhang Y, Chen L, Li F, et al. 131I-MIBG imaging in the diagnosis of pheochromocytoma. Chinese Med Imaging Technol. 2009;25:1283–5.

Zhao X, Weifeng X, Li H, et al. Analysis of prognostic factors in malignant pheochromocytoma/malignant paraganglioma. Chinese J Urol. 2012;11:847–50.

Zhou Z, Li H, Shi B, et al. Clinical analysis of 29 cases of functionally quiescent pheochromocytoma. Basic Med Clin Practice. 2014;34(02):240–3.

3 Surgical Treatment of Pheochromocytoma and Retroperitoneal Paraganglioma

Yu Shi Zhang, Zi Xing Ye, Jin Wen, Yuzhi Zuo, Jie Dong, Juan Sun, Yi Qiao, Chang Liu, Ying Jie Li, and Yong Huang

3.1 Section 1: Preoperative Localization of Pheochromocytoma/Retroperitoneal Paraganglioma

The location of PPGL varies greatly. Preoperative localization and diagnosis are particularly important. Not only the location of the tumor but also its size and its relationship with the surrounding anatomical structures should be understood. Some scholars reviewed 519 cases of PPGL and pointed out that 416 cases occurred in the adrenal gland. Most of common PPGL in other parts are located next to the abdominal aorta. The study concluded that PPGL was characterized by abundant blood supply and that most of them were located next to the renal artery, aorta, and vena cava with serious adhesions to surrounding tissues. At present, the commonly used imaging localization methods include CT, MRI, 131I-MIBG radionuclide imaging, PET-CT, and so on. Accurate preoperative localization has important clinical significance for tumor resectability assessment, treatment selection, and prognosis. In recent years, with the advancement of anatomical imaging examinations, especially with the application of 3D reconstruction and 3D printing technology, the adjoining relationship between the tumor and surrounding tissues, as well as the distribution of the arteries supplying the tumor, can be more clearly displayed. Scenarios provide important information as references.

The main treatment for PPGL is surgical resection. Abdominal PPGL, especially PPGL located in the abdominal adrenal glands or above the adrenal glands, can be managed by transperitoneal laparoscopic surgery. The type of surgery depends on the size and location of the individual tumor. Due to the variability of its location, treatment can be difficult. Imaging can assist in intra-abdominal localization of tumors. However, we still need information of relationship between body surface positions to help make decisions such as surgical approaches during surgery.

The current abdominal partitioning mostly adopts the four-zone and nine-zone method. However, for PPGL that requires precise positioning, it is still unable to guide the treatment. For example, for a mass located in the lower abdomen according to the nine-zone method, the

Zi Xing Ye and Yu Shi Zhang contributed equally to this work.

Y. S. Zhang · Z. X. Ye · J. Wen (✉) · Y. Zuo · J. Dong · J. Sun · Y. Qiao · C. Liu · Y. J. Li
Department of Urology, Peking Union Medical College Hospital, Beijing, China

Y. Huang
Animation School of Beijing Film Academy, Beijing, China

J. Wen (ed.), *Surgical Management of Pheochromocytoma and Retroperitoneal Paraganglioma*, https://doi.org/10.1007/978-981-99-8421-3_3

mass can be located at multiple sites such as the upper, left, right, and middle sections of the lower abdomen. In the meantime, the left and upper-/lower-right portions of the abdomen referred to by the four-zone method are different from those referred by the nine-zone method. The content of the abdomen is quite different between the left and right upper (lower) abdomen referred to by the nine-zone method.

Based on previous research reports and the characteristics of PPGL, a new method of abdominal partitioning and imaging-assisted localization can be used to assist in the surgical treatment of PPGL. PPGL mostly occurs next to the abdominal aorta and beside the renal arteries. According to the course of the arteries, the descending aorta migrates to the abdominal aorta at the aortic hiatus that penetrates the diaphragm at the height of the 12th thoracic vertebra and immediately below the renal artery, celiac trunk, and superior mesenteric artery. The inferior mesenteric artery originates from the abdominal aorta at the level of the third lumbar vertebra. Therefore, PPGL is mostly found in the abdominal cavity from below the xiphoid process to the upper umbilicus, which can be identified as the upper abdominal vascular area. Other common areas running along the blood vessels can be divided into renal vascular area and iliac vascular area.

The editor believes that PPGL can be classified according to the three dimensions of tumor size, location, and relationship with the main branches of the artery. The classification is:

1. Adrenal pheochromocytoma
2. Upper abdominal vascular area paraganglioma (celiac trunk and superior mesenteric artery)
3. Paraganglioma in the renal vascular area (next to the renal artery)
4. Paraganglioma in the lower abdominal vascular area (inferior mesenteric artery and iliac vessels)
5. Pelvic paraganglioma (including bladder paraganglia, tumor, vaginal paraganglioma, etc.)

For PPGL located in different vascular regions, different surgical approaches and treatment strategies are used to achieve the best therapeutic effect.

3.2 Section 2: Surgical Approach to Pheochromocytoma/Retroperitoneal Paraganglioma

Surgical resection is the basic treatment method of PPGL. The principle of surgical treatment is a complete tumor removal, a prevention of tumor rupture, spillage and residue, a gentle operation, and a complete hemostasis. Since Gagner et al. used laparoscopy to perform adrenal tumor resection in 1992, laparoscopic surgery has gradually replaced open surgery as the most commonly used surgical method, thanks to its advantages of small trauma, less bleeding, less pain, small incision, fast postoperative recovery, and fewer surgical complications. Laparoscopic surgery has become the gold standard for the treatment of adrenal tumors. The indications have gradually expanded, constantly breaking through the tumor size limit. In addition, robot-assisted laparoscopic adrenal tumor resection has also been used in clinical practice. In recent years, more and more scholars believe that for giant pheochromocytoma with a diameter of 6 cm, laparoscopic surgical resection is also safe and effective. The size of adrenal tumors is no longer the determinant of surgical methods and routes.

There are a variety of options for surgical approach, mainly including transabdominal approach and retroperitoneal approach. The transabdominal approach is divided into anterior transabdomerital. Lateral transperitoneal, and transperitoneal approach. Retroperitoneal approach is divided into lateral retroperitoneal and posterior retroperitoneal approach. Current studies have shown that the two approaches are substantially similar in the processes of respiratory, circulatory, and stress response changes. In addition to strictly mastering the indications, the choice of approach should also be affected by the proficiency and operating habits of the operator. This section mainly introduces the main steps of laparoscopic transperitoneal approach and transperitoneal approach with their advantages and disadvantages.

3.2.1 Transperitoneal Laparoscopic Surgery

3.2.1.1 Paracolic Sulcus Route

The procedures of this route include general anesthesia tracheal intubation, routine venipuncture to monitor central venous pressure and arterial pressure, and indwelling gastric and urinary catheters. The patient is placed in a 70° recumbent position on the healthy side. A 5 mm trocar is placed under the xiphoid process in the right case to provoke the liver. The paracolic sulcus is opened. The colon is freed and pushed to the opposite side. The prerenal fascia was opened. The tumor is exposed freely in the gap between the prerenal fascia and the perirenal fat sac. The central vein of the right tumor returns to the inferior vena cava, and the central vein of the left tumor returns to the left renal vein. The central vein is double clipped and severed with Hem-o-lok. After complete tumor resection, the tumor is taken out in a specimen bag. A drainage tube was placed in the surgical field.

Advantages: Laparoscopic surgery has the longest time of development and is the most widely used. It has the advantages of large operating space, clear anatomical landmarks, clear vision, and simultaneous treatment of bilateral lesions.

Disadvantages: The abdominal organs interfere with the operation to a certain extent. The abdominal organs may be damaged during the operation, especially when operating on obese patients. When exposing the left spleen, pancreas, and right liver, it is troublesome to dissociate and stretch. It takes a certain amount of time for the recovery of intestinal function after operation. For patients with a history of abdominal surgery or infection, intra-abdominal adhesions will greatly increase the difficulty of surgery, prolong the operation time, and increase the probability of complications.

3.2.1.2 Mesenteric Route

The method of anesthesia is the same as above. The patient is in a flat supine position with a slight elevation on the affected side. Pneumoperitoneal needle puncture establishes CO_2 artificial pneumatic abdomen with an intraperitoneal pressure 12–14 mmHg. After the introduct escadronion of 10 mm Trocar and 30° laparoscopy to observe the abdominal organs without damage, 5 mm and 10 mm Trocars are punctured around the tumor body, respectively. The injury-free separation forceps and ultrasonic knife are introduced. After pushing open the intestinal tube, a huge tumor bulge can be seen in front of it.

The mesentery is very thin and even transparent. The vascular area is large, which is convenient for cutting the mesenteric membrane to fully expose the tumor for dissection and resection. Ultrasonic knife is used to cut the mesenteric membrane in avascular zone of the mesenteric bulge of the colon. Attention to protect the mesenteric vascular arch should be paid. The mesenteric membrane and posterior peritoneum are incised to expose the tumor. Gradual dissection of tumor envelope is continued by using the ultrasound knife with sharp and blunt combination. Thicker tumor blood vessels are pinched off with Hem-o-lok clip. Squeezing the tumor is avoided. When there is blood pressure fluctuations, surgery is paused for a moment. When blood pressure is stabilized, operation can be then proceeded. The tumor is completely removed. Tumor specimen is loaded. The wound is completely hemostatic. The mesenteric blood vessels and intestinal tubes are checked against damage. The color of the intestine is observed to be normal. The skin incision is enlarged to remove the specimen. The drainage tube is placed in the surgical field. The trocar is removed, and the incision is routinely sutured.

Advantages: This approach can avoid a wide range of unnecessary steps such as the dissection of colon. It directly exposes the lesion site, greatly shortens the operation time, and avoids the dissection and ligament removal of the colon, liver, and spleen. Therefore, it reduces the probability of intestinal injury and spleen injury, reduces the manipulation of the intestine, and helps restore postoperative intestinal function.

Disadvantages: The scope of mesenteric windowing is limited. The exposure range is not as good as the conventional colonic lateral pathway. Especially when some tumors are located behind the pancreas, the operation channel needs to be increased during surgery. The mesenteric membrane is provoked by a blunt manipulator to help expose. Sometimes, the mesenteric fat is thicker, and it is difficult to avoid damage to the mesenteric blood vessels through this route.

3.2.1.3 Retroperitoneal Laparoscopic Surgery (Semi-recumbent Position)

Main surgical procedures include general anesthesia for tracheal intubation, routine action venipuncture to detect central venous pressure and arterial pressure, 50–70° on the healthy side of the semi-lateral recumbent position (lateral tilt to the dorsal side 20–40°), and slightly elevated waist bridge. Along the front of the kidney in the outer peritoneum, the inner side of the adrenal pole is separated upward. The adrenal gland is found in the inner side of the adrenal pole. Along its envelope surface, the gland and tumor are separated. For obese patients, part of the adrenal gland fat can be removed because the texture of the adrenal tumor is more brittle. Less "grasp" action should be taken during the dissection and separation of tumor. The stimulation of the tumor is minimized. Clamping tumor body is avoided. It can cause bleeding that is not easy to control. The use of ultrasound knife for blunt and sharpening dissection allows safe management of adrenal artery branches. Dissecting the inner and lower parts of the adrenal pole is continued. The central adrenal vein is found and cut off after the double Hem-o-lok clamp. The rest of the adrenal arteries and veins are managed sequentially. Adrenal glands is dissected along the adrenal envelope. Tumor is resected. After careful examination for active bleeding, the tumor is removed by specimen bag. The drainage tube is routinely placed.

Advantages: The advantage of the retroperitoneal laparoscopic approach is that it directly reaches the targeted organ. The urological surgeon is familiar with the retroperitoneal anatomy. The operation is relatively safe, and the approach is not affected by abdominal adhesions, avoiding the interference of abdominal organs, reducing the chance of abdominal organ damage. Therefore, it is widely used.

Disadvantages: Mainly relatively difficult to expose and relatively narrow operating space are the disadvantages. Anatomical markers are not easy to be identified. Excessive obesity and a history of postperitoneal surgery are relative contraindications.

3.2.2 Efficacy Evaluation and Surgical Complications

The choice of transabdominal or retroperitoneal approach is still inconclusive. It depends on the experience of the surgeon, the size of the tumor, and the specific location. Some scholars believe that if the tumor is greater than 5 cm in diameter, it is more inclined to undergo the abdominal route. Andrew et al. retrospectively analyzed the clinical data of 153 patients with pheochromocytoma in three centers and found that compared with open surgery, patients in the laparoscopic treatment group were better than open surgery in terms of operation time and bleeding volume. Robotic surgery had similar effects to laparoscopic surgery. Lu Dingheng and others retrospectively analyzed the surgical process of 186 cases of pheochromocytoma. They found that the transabdominal group was better than the transperitoneal group in terms of operation time, postoperative resumption of feeding, and postoperative drainage fluid volume. Transabdominal robotic surgery group was better than the transperitoneal group in terms of operation time and the removal of large tumors.

As with open surgery, laparoscopic surgery inevitably has associated with complications, particularly when the tumor is touched during surgery, which can lead to the release of catecholamines that in turn can lead to transient increase in blood pressure and increased heart rate. The most common surgical complications of laparoscopic pheochromocytoma adrenectomy include pleural injury, vascular damage, wound bleeding, postoperative adrenal hypocortex function, and intraoperative hypertensive crisis.

Further Reading

Aygun N, Uludag M. Pheochromocytoma and paraganglioma: from treatment to follow-up. Sisli Etfal Hastan Tip Bul. 2020;54(4):391–8.

Bai Y, Wang L, Li D, et al. Clinical application value of SPECT/CT tomosynthesis in localization and diagnosis of pheochromocytoma. Modern Oncol. 2021;29(04):652–5.

Chang CA, Pattison DA, Tothill RW, et al. 68Ga-DOTATATE and 18F-FDG PET/CT in paraganglioma and pheochromocytoma: utility, patterns and heterogeneity. Cancer Imaging. 2016;16:22.

Deng J, et al. A clinical study of the anatomical distribution and functional characteristics of PPGL. In: The 17th national urology symposium. Xi'an, Shaanxi, China; 2010.

Dingheng L, Wang D, Li X, et al. Perioperative comparison of da Vinci robot and traditional laparoscopy with different approaches in adrenal pheochromocytoma resection. J Clin Urol. 2021;36(03):197–200.

Expert consensus on diagnosis and treatment of PPGL (2020 edition). Chinese J Endocrinol Metab. 2020;36(09):737–50.

Fang AM, Rosen J, Saidian A, et al. Perioperative outcomes of laparoscopic, robotic, and open approaches to pheochromocytoma. J Robot Surg. 2020;14(6):849–54.

Fonte JS, Robles JF, Chen CC, et al. False-negative ^{123}I-MIBG SPECT is most commonly found in SDHB-related pheochromocytoma or paraganglioma with high frequency to develop metastatic disease. Endocr Relat Cancer. 2012;19(1):83–93.

Hao Y, et al. Difficulties in imaging localization of upper abdominal retroperitoneal and abdominal tumors. Chinese J Med Ultrasound (Electr Edn). 2010;7(09):1428–9.

Hwang I, Jung SI, Yu SH, et al. Is larger tumor size a contraindication to retroperitoneal laparoscopic adrenalectomy? World J Urol. 2014;32(3):723–8.

Janssen I, Blanchet EM, Adams K, et al. Superiority of 68Ga-DOTATATE PET/CT to other functional imaging modalities in the localization of SDHB-associated metastatic Pheochromocytoma and Paraganglioma. Clin Cancer Res. 2015;21(17):3888–95.

Li H, Zhang Y, et al. Perioperative management of pheochromocytoma/paraganglioma. Modern J Urol. 2012;17(04):329–32.

Li W, Li Z, Huang H, et al. Comparison of the effect of laparoscopic resection of larger adrenal tumors in lateral and hemilateral positions. Guangdong Med. 2013;34(16):2486–8.

Liu X, Jiang B, et al. New progress in minimally invasive surgical treatment of adrenal disease. J Modern Genitourin Oncol. 2012;4(03):129–31.

Miura K, Kobayashi N, Satomi H. Surgical resection of a middle mediastinal paraganglioma that caused diabetes. Surg Case Rep. 2020;6(1):241.

Shank J, Prescott JD, Mathur A. Surgical approach to endocrine hypertension in patients with adrenal disorders. Endocrinol Metab Clin N Am. 2019;48(4):875–85.

Smith JA Jr, et al. Hinman's atlas of urologic surgery. Netherlands: Elsevier Inc; 2018. p. 257–68.

Vorselaars W, Postma EL, Mirallie E, et al. Hemodynamic instability during surgery for pheochromocytoma: comparing the transperitoneal and retroperitoneal approach in a multicenter analysis of 341 patients. Surgery. 2018;163(1):176–18.

Wang B, Zhou N, Zhai H, et al. The value of ultrasonography and MRI in the diagnosis of adrenal pheochromocytoma. Chinese Med Equip J. 2017;14(08):69–72.

Wen J, Li H, Ji Z, et al. Clinical study of 3D laparoscopic surgery for adrenal pheochromocytoma/paraganglioma. Chinese J Urol. 2015;36(07):511–3.

Wen J, Li H, Ji Z, et al. Analysis of 35 cases of adrenal pheochromocytoma/paraganglioma with 3D laparoscopic surgery. Basic Med Clin Practice. 2016;36(07):1014–6.

Zhang H, Liang W, Zhao X, et al. Clinical application of two approaches for laparoscopic adrenal pheochromocytoma resection. J Laparosc Surg. 2017;22(07):490–3.

4 Multidisciplinary Treatment of Adrenal Pheochromocytoma

Wei Gang Yan, Dong Wang, Jin Wen, Zhong Ming Huang, Hou Feng Huang, Yi Xie, and De Xin Dong

4.1 Case 4.1

Patient: Male, 71 years old

4.1.1 Chief Complaint

Examinations revealed a tumor of the left adrenal gland for more than 4 months.

4.1.2 History of Present Illness

Four months ago, the patient underwent ultrasonography in a local hospital because of dysuria. The examination shows a cystic and solid mass between the spleen and kidney. The mass likely originated from the kidney. Further enhanced CT shows that the mass was from the left adrenal with 8.4 × 7.4 cm in size. The scan shows no obvious enhancement for the low-density areas in the middle part.

Wei Gang Yan and Dong Wang contributed equally to this work.

W. G. Yan · D. Wang · J. Wen (✉) · Z. M. Huang · H. F. Huang · Y. Xie · D. X. Dong
Department of Urology, Peking Union Medical College Hospital, Beijing, China

4.1.3 Past History

Patient has a diabetes mellitus for 15 years. Blood sugar is well controlled. Patient has a history of subclinical hypothyroidism for 2 months, now under treatment with levothyroxine sodium.

4.1.4 Examination

Adrenal enhancement CT + 3D reconstruction + CTA (Figs. 4.1, 4.2, and 4.3): The normal structure of the left adrenal gland disappears. In the left adrenal region, a large irregular cystic solid mass can be seen. In the lower part, the small flaky high-density shadow is found. The enhanced scan shows that solid component and separation of the occupant are slightly strengthened. The cystic component can be seen in the liquid level with no obvious strengthening. The size is about 9.1 × 8.9 × 8.2 cm with the rough edge. The boundary with the pancreatic tail and the base of the stomach is not clear. The left kidney is stressed. The blood supple of mass is provided by the branches of the abdominal aorta and the artery trunk of the abdominal cavity.

Endocrine Examination

NMN 9.81 nmo1/L↑

MN 1.51 nmo1/L↑ (ten times higher than the normal upper limit)

J. Wen (ed.), *Surgical Management of Pheochromocytoma and Retroperitoneal Paraganglioma*,
https://doi.org/10.1007/978-981-99-8421-3_4

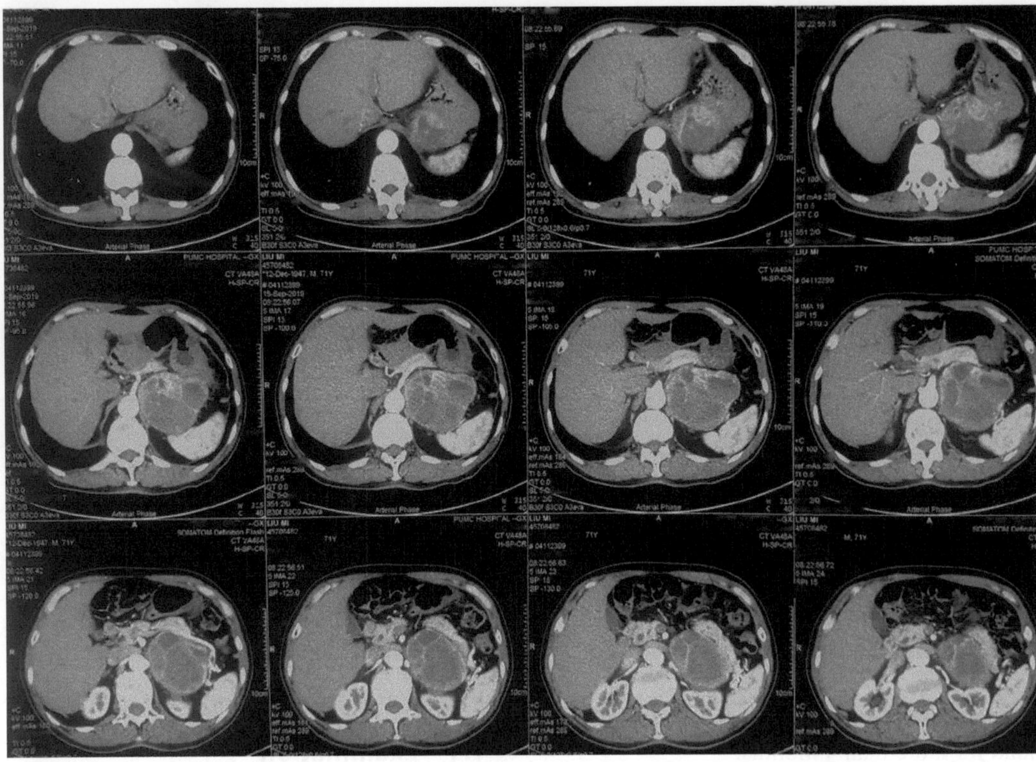

Fig. 4.1 Adrenal enhancement CT

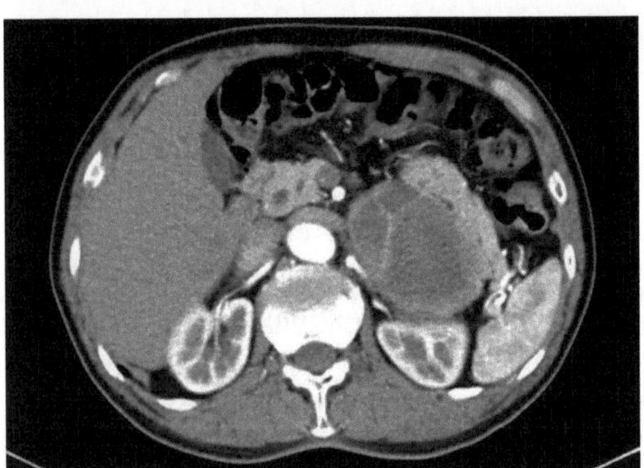

Fig. 4.2 Adrenal enhancement CT

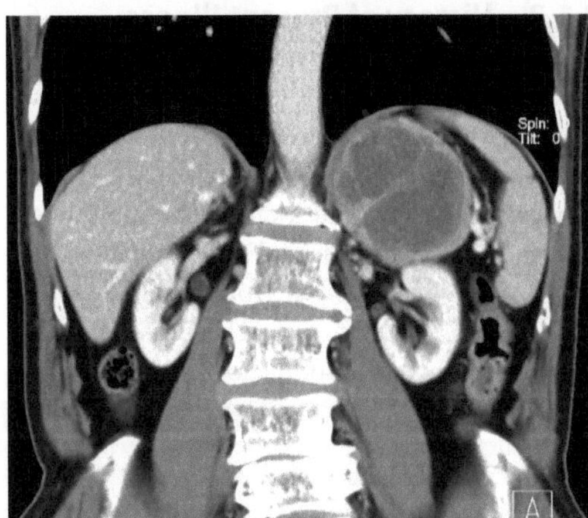

Fig. 4.3 Tumor coronary reconstruction

24 h Urinary catecholamines: NE 23.02 μg/24 h, E 2.62 μg/24 h, DA 211.01 μg/24 h
Somatostatin receptor imaging: negative
^{131}I-MIBG: positive

The normal structure of the left adrenal gland is lost, and in the left adrenal region, a large irregular cystic solid mass can be seen. A small flaky high-density shadow can be seen in the lower part, and the solid composition and separation of the mass can be slightly strengthened after enhancement. The size is about 9.1 × 8.9 × 8.2 cm

The cystic components inside the tumor are visible in the fluid level without a significant reinforcement.

The edge of the tumor is rough. The boundary with the tail of the pancreas and the base of the stomach is not clear, and the left kidney is under pressure

4.1.5 Current Diagnoses

Left adrenal pheochromocytoma

Type II diabetes

Hypothyroidism

4.1.6 MDT Discussion

4.1.6.1 Endocrinology

The following suggestions are provided: continue the treatment of phenol benzylamine 10 mg q12h; instruct patient to drink more water and maintain a daily intake of more than 3 L; monitor 24-h inflow; record day and night urine output; monitor blood pressure and heart rate in the recumbent position (at least two times a day); and monitor weight and HCT changes.

At present, the patient has no episodic blood pressure increase, no increased heart rate, and no obvious orthostatic hypotension. HCT shows a downward trend. Blood pressure and blood sugar are normal, and defecation is normal. Preoperative drug preparation can be considered and can be selected for surgical treatment. Anesthesiology and ICU are consulted before surgery to assess surgical risks, and vital signs are monitored closely during the perioperative period.

If the condition allows, the fundal and aortic ultrasound, echocardiogram, etc. are taken to evaluate for complications.

Screening for calcitonin, serum calcium, phosphorus, PTH, insulin, and anterior pituitary function is completed to exclude the possibility of MEN1.

The use of drugs such as gastric reassurance, morphine, and Betaloc are avoided. Squeezing the abdomen is prohibited, and be wary of pheochromocytoma crises.

4.1.6.2 Department of Anesthesiology

It belongs to American Society of Anesthesiologists (ASA) grade III. It is recommended to improve lung function and myocardial enzymes + NT-proBNP. The patient is anesthetized according to the routine preparation of pheochromocytoma. Arterial and venous passages are established. Vasoactive drugs are prepared. The monitoring of vital signs during the operation is strengthened. The balance of myocardial oxygen supply and oxygen consumption is maintained. The perfusion of important organs is ensured. Fully explain the risk of cardiovascular and cerebrovascular accidents and major bleeding in the perioperative period. Pay attention to blood sugar fluctuations. It is important to maintain water and electrolyte balance and to fully prepare blood transfusion. It is recommended to monitor patient in the ICU after surgery.

4.1.6.3 Department of Critical Care Medicine

The recommendations are fully explain the surgical risks and related perioperative complications; closely monitor blood pressure and hemodynamic stability; ensure perioperative blood pressure stability; ensure the perfusion of important organs such as the heart, brain, and kidneys; monitor and maintain the stability of electrolytes and internal environment; and determine the date of surgery. Patient can be monitored in the ICU after surgery.

4.1.6.4 Urology

In a 71-year-old male patient, a mass was found to occupy the left renal area after the examination for the symptom of difficulty in urination 4 months ago. Further enhanced CT suggested a left adrenal mass. Outpatient examination of NMN and MN 1.51 nmol/L showed all ten times higher than the upper limit of normal values. Somatostatin receptor imaging was negative. 131I-MIBG was positive. Adrenal enhancement CT could see a huge cystic solid mass in the left adrenal region. The strengthening was not obvious after enhancement. The size was about 9.1 cm × 8.9 cm × 8.2 cm, and the boundary between the pancreatic caudal and gastric base was not clear. The patient had taken phenol benzylamine 10 mg q12h to prepare for 8 weeks and had plans to undergo surgery in the near future.

Based on the patient's symptoms, signs, and relevant adjunctive test results, the diagnosis of pheochromocytoma was basically clear. Due to the large size of the tumor, attention on careful dissection should be paid during the operation and the amount of bleeding after the tumor rupture. Preoperative preparation should be fully done.

Fully explain the risks to the patient before surgery, and obtain an informed consent. The operation may be more inclined for an open manner, but laparoscopic operation can be tried. The procedure should be determined according to the specific situation during the operation. Careful operation with close hemostasis should be implemented.

4.1.7 Surgical Modalities

3D laparoscopic left adrenal pheochromocytoma resection under general anesthesia (Fig. 4.4).

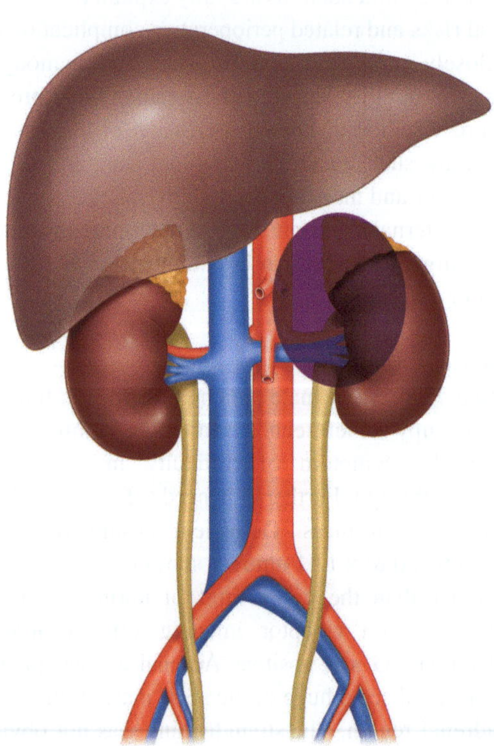

Fig. 4.4 Schematic diagram of the location of the mass

4.1.8 Postoperative Pathological Diagnosis

(Left adrenal gland) pheochromocytoma. Immunohistochemical results are Melan-A(−), AE1/AE3(−), CgA(+), Ki-67(index 2%), S-100(+), α-inhibin(−), and NeuN(−).

4.2 Case 4.2

Patient: Female, 43 years old

4.2.1 Complaints

Hypertension for more than 2 years; physical examination found a right adrenal gland mass for more than 3 months.

4.2.2 History of Present Illness

The patient's blood pressure was found to be elevated 2 years ago, with a maximum of about 170/100 mmHg. She received valsartan antihypertensive treatment, and the blood pressure was stabilized at 120/80 mmHg. During the physical examination 3 months ago, the B-ultrasound found a mass in the area of right adrenal gland. Enhanced CT of abdominal and pelvis (Fig. 4.5) showed an abnormal density mass of right adrenal gland, about 3.9 cm × 3.3 cm in size, obvious uneven enhancement, and irregular slightly low-density necrosis area in the center. A definitive diagnosis of pheochromocytoma was considered. The patient received phenoxybenzamine 5 mg twice a day in the outpatient clinic. After 3 weeks of treatment, she was admitted to our department on December 9, 2020. The dose of phenoxybenzamine was gradually adjusted to 10 mg three times a day. The drug was taken for 5 weeks. The current blood pressure control was 120–150/65–80 mmHg for supine blood pressure with a heart rate of 66–86 beats/min. Standing blood pressure was 115–145/61–77 mmHg with a heart rate of 70–96 beats/min. There was no significant change in body weight. The hemato-

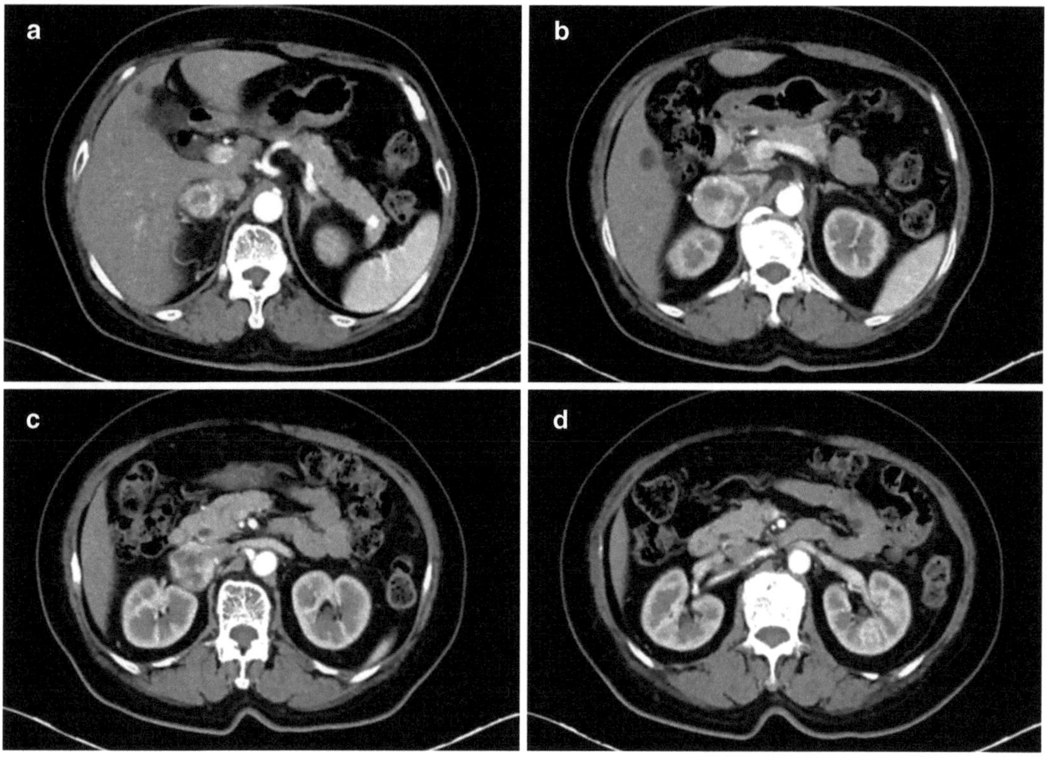

Fig. 4.5 Adrenal enhancement CT. (**a**–**d**) A mass of abnormal density in the right adrenal gland, about 3.9 × 3.3 cm in size, with significantly uneven intensifications and irregular slightly lower density necrosis areas visible in the center

crit HCT decreased from 42.7% to 38.0%. There was mild nasal congestion.

4.2.3 Past, Personal, Marriage and Childbirth, Family History

One year ago, she had two cerebral infarctions. High blood pressure and diabetes were found. She had undergone cholecystectomy. Personal, marital, and family histories were unremarkable.

4.2.4 Examination

Abdominal pelvic enhanced CT (Fig. 4.5): A mass of abnormal density in the right adrenal gland, about 3.9 × 3.3 cm in size, with significantly uneven intensifications and irregular slightly low-density necrosis areas visible in the center

Endocrine test: 24 h urinary catecholamines: NE 77.54 μg/24 h, E 1.92 μg/24 h, DA 126.00 μg/24 h, NMN 5.61 nmol/L, MN 0.09 nmol/L. 131I-MIBG is positive, and somatostatin receptor imaging is negative.

4.2.5 Current Diagnoses

Right adrenal pheochromocytoma
Hypertension
Type 2 diabetes
Past cerebral infarction

4.2.6 MDT Discussion

4.2.6.1 Endocrinology

It is recommended to increase the dosage of phenolic benzylamine. Blood calcium, phosphorus, ALP, thyroid ultrasound, and other related examinations are needed. In patients with cerebral infarctions, the risk of surgery is greater. Please consult the ICU and anesthesia department for the risks during surgery. Patients currently had no episodic symptoms with a well-controlled blood pressure. Nasal congestion and warm extremities were found. Preoperative preparation was basically sufficient. Surgical treatment could be considered. The risk of surgery was fully explained to patient. Follow up was continued.

4.2.6.2 Anesthesiology

The patient's current drug preparation was good. There was no anesthesia contraindication. Phenoxybenzamine was discontinued 1 day before and the morning of the operation, and it was recommended to return the patient to the ICU after the operation.

4.2.6.3 ICU

Agree to your diagnosis and treatment plan, and you can transfer to the ICU to continue treatment after surgery.

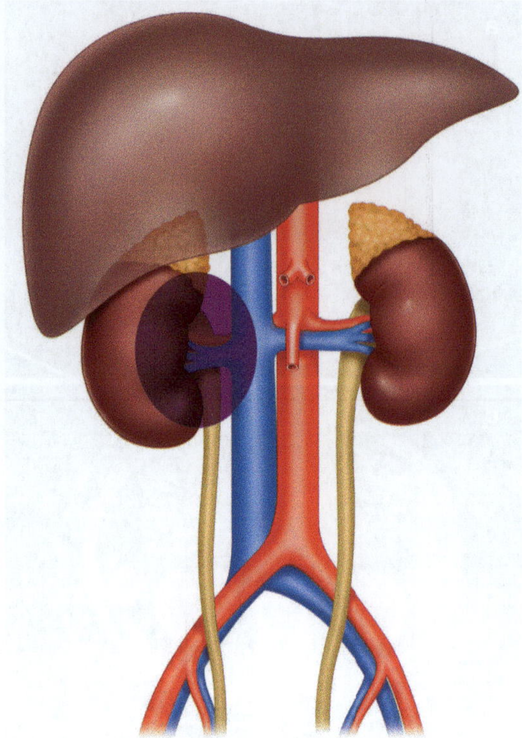

Fig. 4.6 Schematic diagram of the location of the mass

4.2.7 Surgical Modalities

Under general anesthesia, laparoscopic right adrenal pheochromocytoma resection was performed (Fig. 4.6).

4.2.8 Postoperative Pathology

Adrenal pheochromocytoma on the right side with adrenal tissue visible around it.

Immunohistochemical results were Melan-A(−), AE1/AE3(−), CgA(+), Ki-67(index 1%), S-100(+), α-inhibin(−), Syn(+), and SDHB(+).

4.3 Case 4.3

Patient: Male, 52 years old

4.3.1 Complaints

Hypertension for 20 years; tumor found in the right adrenal gland 2 months ago

4.3.2 History of Present Illness

An increase in blood pressure was found 20 years ago. The specific cause is unknown. It was not taken seriously and not treated. The blood pressure was not monitored. Symptoms of bloating and vomiting presented twice in 20 years. Hypertension was considered, but blood pressure was untested at the time of the attack. Symptoms improved after hydration. Eight years ago, physical examination suggested a blood pressure of 170/100 mmHg, and he began to take 1 qd of compound reserpine regularly. Self-monitored blood pressure was at 150/90 mmHg. Blood pressure is not monitored regularly. In September 2020, the B ultrasound found during the physical examination of our hospital a low echo mass of the right adrenal gland with 4.4 × 3.6 × 3.1 cm. Abdominal pelvis enhancement CT showed a slightly less dense nodule in right adrenal oval, about 3.9 × 3.0 cm.

The patient was hospitalized in the endocrinology department on November 2, 2020, and preparation of α-receptor blockers with phenol benzylamine 10 mg q12h began. According to the blood pressure situation, the dose of phenolic benzylamine was adjusted, and the current supine blood pressure is controlled at 35–152/82–95 mmHg, heart rate 57–95 beats/min, and standing blood pressure 94–125/62–92 mmHg, heart rate 94–125 beats/min. Body weight increased in the past month with 3.5 kg. The hematocrit HCT decreased from 43.9% to 40.9%. On December 14, 2020, he was transferred to our department for further treatment. Test results of admission suggested blood type A. RHD was negative, and yu test results were not special.

4.3.3 Past, Personal, Marriage and Childbirth, Family History

Gout, vitiligo, etc.; nothing special for the rest. Personal history, marital history, and family history are unremarkable.

4.3.4 Accessory Examination

Ventral enhancement CT (Fig. 4.7): slightly less dense nodules in the right adrenal ovoid, about 3.9 × 3.0 cm. The boundary is clear. The enhancement scan shows significant uneven strengthening. The edges are significantly strengthened. Patchy without/low-strength foci can be seen in the center.

Endocrine test: 24-h urinary catecholamines: NE 27.41 μg/24 h, E 4.09 μg/24 h, DA 209.00 μg/24 h. 131I-MIBG is to complete. Somatostatin receptor imaging and other tests are positive. Pheochromocytoma is likely considered.

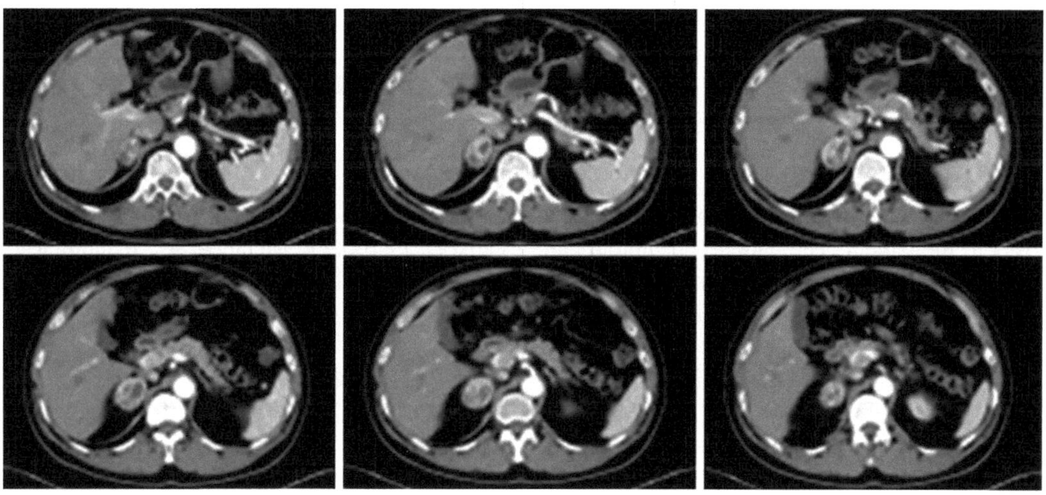

Fig. 4.7 Adrenal enhancement CT. (**a**–**f**) Right adrenal ovoid is occupied by a slightly less dense nodule, about 3.9 cm × 3.0 cm. The boundary is clear. The enhanced scan shows significantly uneven strengthening. The edges are significantly strengthened. Patchy without/low-strength foci can be seen in the center

4.3.5 Current Diagnoses

Right adrenal pheochromocytoma
- Hypertension
- Hyperuricemia
- Vitiligo
- Lipoma removed

4.3.6 MDT Discussion

4.3.6.1 Ophthalmology

Binocular lens density is increased. The remaining anterior segment is (−). The optic disc boundary is clear. The retinal vascular direction is correct. A-V = 1:3 A-V cross signs can be seen. No exudation and bleeding are seen. Impression of diagnosis: arteriosclerosis of the retina of both eyes and amblyopia in the left eye

4.3.6.2 General Surgery

It is recommended to perform the ultrasound of the gallbladder. If necessary, the abdominal pelvis by enhanced CT is applied. Close attention is paid to changes in abdominal symptoms and signs.

4.3.6.3 Stomatology

Swollen and painful gums in the upper-right posterior teeth has lasted for 3 days. Recurrence often occurred in the past. Anti-inflammatory treatment is recommended with Baxin 0.25G bid + tinidazole tablets 1.0G qd po + cetylpyridinium Chloride 20 mL three times a day as mouthwash. If an abscess forms, incision and drainage are required.

4.3.6.4 Urology

Fully explain the treatment options and surgical risks to the patient. The patient's symptoms are not obvious. The physical examination finds that the adrenal gland area is occupied. The decrease of postoperative blood pressure is not obvious. The current preoperative preparation is continued. The stability of the blood pressure in the recumbent position is to be controlled.

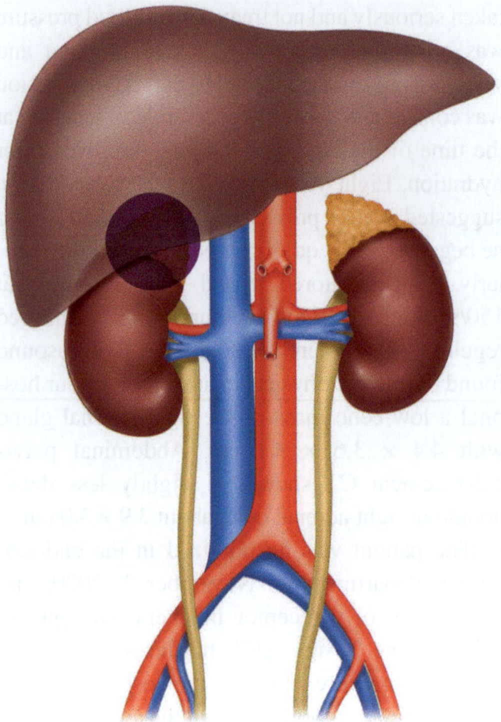

Fig. 4.8 Schematic diagram of the location of the mass

4.3.7 Diagnosis and Treatment

Laparoscopic right adrenal pheochromocytoma resection under general anesthesia (Fig. 4.8)

4.3.8 Postoperative Pathology

Right adrenal mass is consistent with pheochromocytoma.

Immunohistochemical results: Syn(+), CgA(+), S-100(+), Melan-A(−), α-inhibin(−), AE1/AE3(−), SDHB(+), Ki-67(index 1%).

4.4 Case 4.4

Patient: Female, 35 years old

4.4.1 Complaints

Right adrenal mass found for more than 5 years and left adrenal nodule found 2 months ago

4.4.2 History of Present Illness

In 2015, a physical examination revealed a right adrenal mass, which was about 2.8 cm in size. It was not accompanied by hypertension, palpitations, headache, sweating, and other discomforts. The tumor gradually grew. During the physical examination in our hospital 2 months ago, it was found that the right adrenal gland was seen as a circular isodense shadow with a diameter of about 34 mm, and a similar nodular shadow was seen in the left adrenal body, with a size of about 11 mm × 9 mm. The possibility of pheochromocytoma was considered. The patient has been treated with phenoxybenzamine 10 mg bid for 4 weeks. Blood pressure is currently controlled between 110 and 130/60 and 90 mmHg, without nasal congestion, orthostatic hypotension, palpitations, and other discomforts. Now, for the surgical treatment, the patient is admitted to our department with a right adrenal tumor. At present, blood pressure in the supine position is 110–130/60–75 mmHg, and the heart rate is 64–80 beats/min. Standing blood pressure is 100–130/60–73 mmHg with a heart rate 100–120 beats/min. After admission, body weight increased by 1 kg. The hematocrit was 34.7%. Slight dizziness and nasal congestion were present.

4.4.3 Past, Personal, Marital and Childbearing, Family History

No history of hypertension. The patient underwent caesarean section 4 years ago.

4.4.4 Accessory Examination

Abdominal pelvis enhanced CT: right adrenal hypertrophic mass with blood supply, approximately 34 mm in diameter (Fig. 4.9).

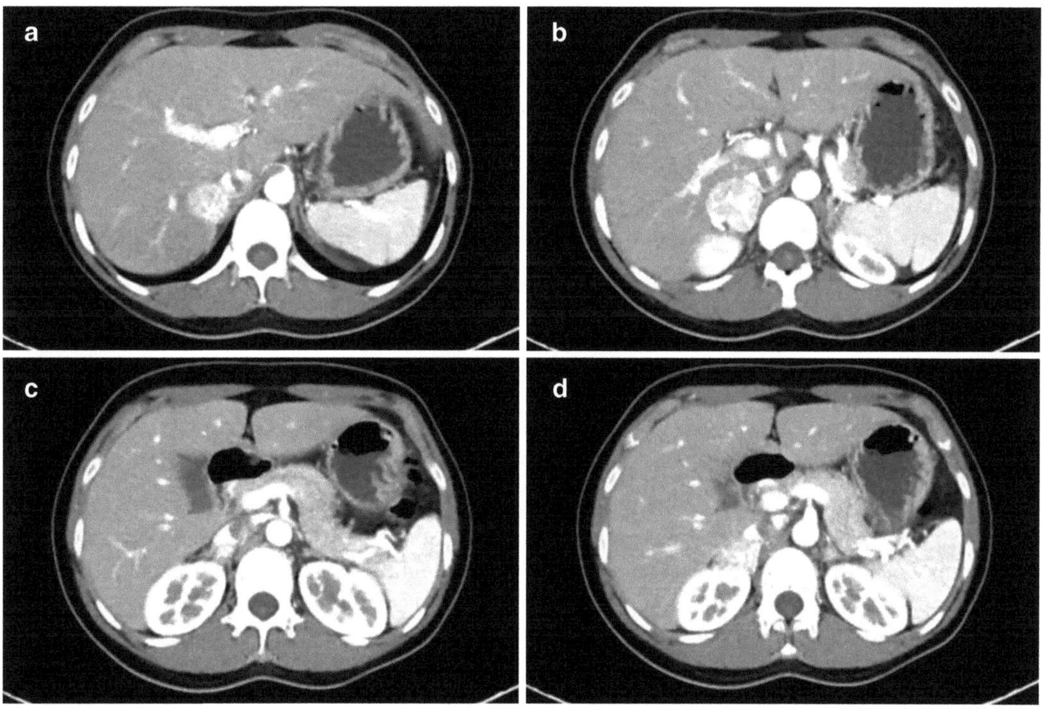

Fig. 4.9 Adrenal enhancement CT. (**a–d**) Right adrenal gland is occupied by a mass rich of blood, about 34 mm in diameter. A similar nodular shadow is seen in the left adrenal gland, about 11 mm in size×9 mm in size. Pheochromocytoma is considered

Endocrine test: 24 h NE 614.71 μg/24 h, 24 h DA 345.37 μg/24 h, residual ACTH, cortisol, aldosterone, renin and angiotensin (−)

Somatostatin receptor imaging: soft tissue nodules can be seen in both sides of the carotid artery at the upper corner level of the hyoid bone, with a size of 1.9 × 1.5 cm and 2.8 × 1.6 cm. Possibility of paraganglioma is considered. The high expression of somatostatin receptors in the right adrenal region about 3.5 × 3.4 × 3.1 cm in size is found, suggesting the possibility of pheochromocytoma.

4.4.5 Current Diagnoses

Bilateral adrenal pheochromocytoma

Double cervical paraganglioma

Past caesarean section

4.4.6 MDT Discussion

4.4.6.1 Endocrinology

Patient currently have no episodic blood pressure increase, no increased heart rate, and no obvious orthostatic hypotension. HCT shows a downward trend. Preoperative drug preparation is considered. Patient can be electively operated on. If the condition allows the assessment of complications such as involving the fundus, aortic ultrasound and echocardiography are performed. Screening for calcitonin, serum calcium, phosphorus, PTH, insulin, and anterior pituitary function is also considered.

4.4.6.2 Anesthesiology

During the operation, the patient is anesthetized according to the routine preparation of pheochromocytoma. Procedures such as establishment of arteriovenous veins, preparation of vasoactive drugs, monitoring of changes in vital signs, maintenance of the balance of myocardial oxygen supply and oxygen consumption, and perfusion of important organs are routine measures. Fully explain the risk of perioperative cardiovascular and cerebrovascular accidents and major bleeding. Pay attention to blood glucose fluctuations, and maintain water-electrolyte balance.

4.4.6.3 ICU

Closely monitor blood pressure and hemodynamic stability, ensure perioperative blood pressure stability, ensure the perfusion of the heart, brain, kidney, and other important organs, and monitor and maintain the stability of electrolytes and internal environment.

4.4.6.4 Urology

Based on the patient's symptoms, signs, and relevant adjunctive test results, the diagnosis of bilateral pheochromocytoma is considered. Pay attention to fully explaining the risks to the patient before surgery, and obtain informed consent. The operation may be more inclined to an open manner, but a laparoscopic operation can be tried. The procedure should be determined according to the specific situation during the operation. Careful operation with close hemostasis should be performed.

4.4.7 Surgical Approach

Laparoscopic bilateral adrenal pheochromocytoma resection is performed under general anesthesia (Fig. 4.10)

4.4.8 Postoperative Pathology

Right adrenal tumor is consistent with pheochromocytoma.

Left adrenal tumor is consistent with pheochromocytoma.

Immunohistochemical Results

Wax blocks A1: Melan-A(−), Calretinin(−), CgA(+), Ki-67 (index 4%), Syn(+), Vimentin(+), α-inhibin (scattered in weak +), S-100 (scattered in +)

Wax blocks B2: Melan-A(−), Calretinin(−), CgA(+), Ki-67 (index 5%), Syn(+), Vimentin(+), α-inhibin (scattered in weak +), S-100 (scattered in +)

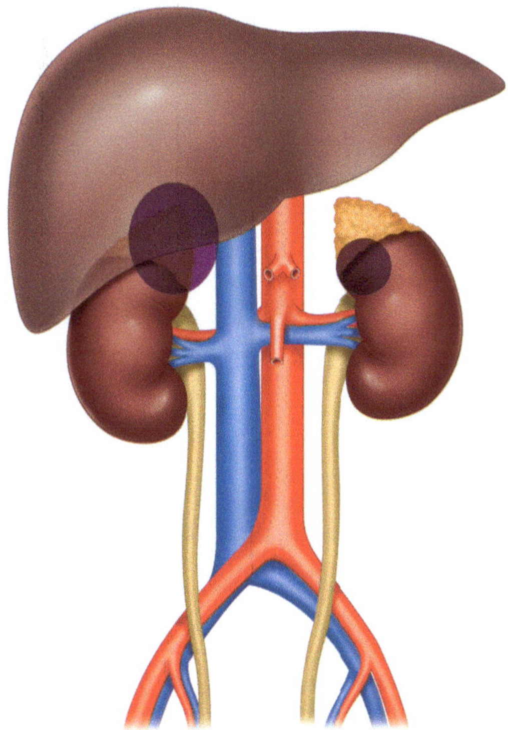

Fig. 4.10 Schematic diagram of the location of the mass

4.5 Case 4.5

Patient: Female, 43 years old.

4.5.1 Complaints

Physical examination revealed a left adrenal mass 2 months ago.

4.5.2 History of Present Illness

In October 2019, CT examination found a left adrenal gland mass with no palpitations, sweating, headache, limb numbness, fatigue, and other discomfort. Pelvic enhanced CT and adrenal thin scan (Fig. 4.11a–d) suggest a left adrenal mass, 68.8 mm × 62.4 mm. Pheochromocytoma may be considered. Multiple cysts of the liver were found; cystic lesions in the left adnexal area and large ovarian cyst may also exist. He was admitted to the clinic with a diagnosis of pheochromocytoma. Oral benzylamine therapy started on November 13, 2019, 10 mg twice daily for 1 week → 5 mg twice a day for 1 week → 10 mg twice a day for 2 weeks until December 14. From December 14 to present, the dose is 25 mg/day. Currently, patient complains of warm hands and feet and nasal congestion; there is absence of obvious fatigue and dizziness; patient had weight gain of 0.5 kg, with Hct 38.5% (November 11) → 35.1% (December 11).

4.5.3 Past, Personal, Family, Marital History

Allergic to mangoes.

4.5.4 Accessory Examination

Pelvic enhanced CT plus adrenal thin-spondy: left adrenal mass with a size of 68.8 mm × 62.4 mm. Pheochromocytoma may be considered.

Somatostatin receptor imaging: somatostatin receptor hyperexpression lesions in the left adrenal region. Combined with CT, the possibility of neuroendocrine tumors may be considered.

Endocrine examination: 24 h urinary catecholamines: E 28.64 μg/24 h (normal 1.74–6.42 μg/24 h). Plasma NMN: 2.91 nmol/L (normal: <0.9 nmol/L). MN: 7.45 nmol/L (Normal: <0.9 nmol/L). Renin activity (standing) PRA2: 0.01 ng/mL/h. 24 h-UFC, blood F, ACTH, DH and DHS sulfate: no significant abnormalities were seen.

Left adrenal mass, 68.8 × 62.4 mm. Pheochromocytoma may be considered.

4.5.5 Current Diagnosis

Left adrenal pheochromocytoma.

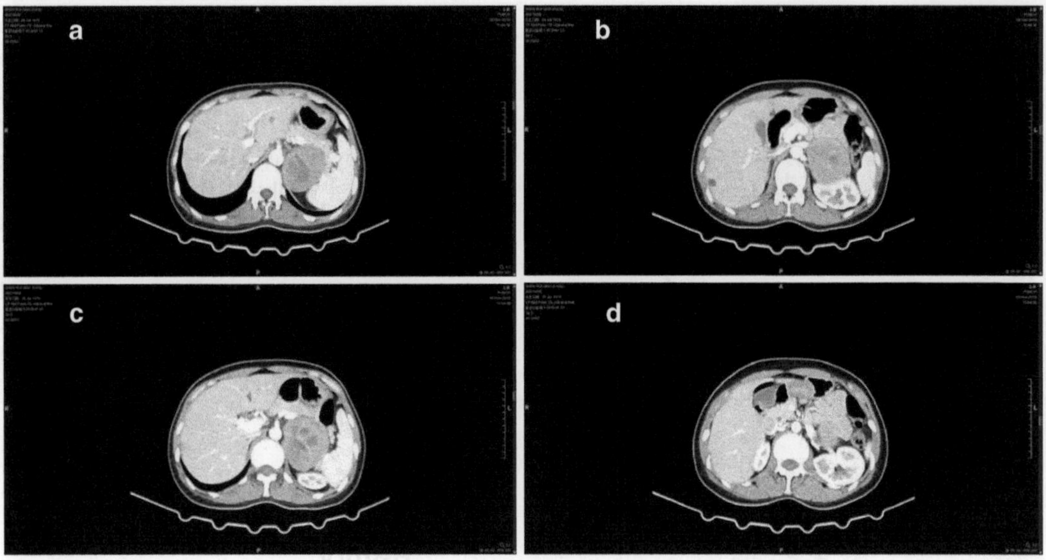

Fig. 4.11 Adrenal enhanced CT: (**a**–**d**) Left adrenal mass, 68.8 x 62.4mm, pheochromocytoma possible

4.5.6 MDT Discussion

4.5.6.1 Endocrinology

Monitor the 24-h inlet and outlet. Ensure that the daily intake is greater than 3-4 L. Monitor the weight, Hct, and blood pressure in the recumbent position. Surgical preparation should be sufficient. It can be selected for surgical treatment, except for the possibility of MEN.

4.5.6.2 Department of Anesthesiology

ASA Class I and elective surgery are considered. The risk of anesthesia for pheochromocytoma is high. The risk for hemodynamic fluctuations and cardiovascular and cerebrovascular events is explained. ICU is needed after surgery.

4.5.6.3 ICU

Fully explain the surgical risks and related perioperative complications. Monitor closely blood pressure and hemodynamic stability. Ensure perioperative blood pressure stability and cardio-cerebral, kidney, and other organ perfusion. Monitor and maintain the stability of the internal environment, and return to the ICU after surgery.

4.5.7 Surgical Approach

Laparoscopic left adrenal pheochromocytoma resection under general anesthesia (Fig. 4.12).

4.5.8 Postoperative Pathology

Left adrenal gland and mass consistent with pheochromocytoma. Immunohistochemical results: Melan-A(−), AE1/AE3(−), CgA(+), Ki-67 (index 1%), S-100 (scattered in +), α-inhibin(−), SDHB(+).

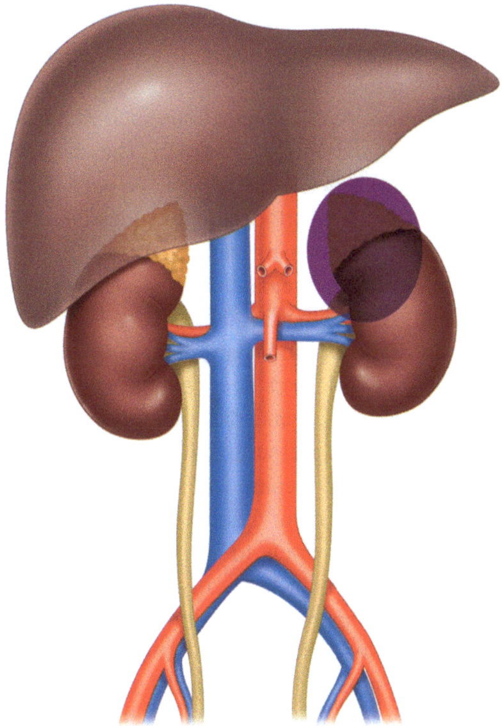

Fig. 4.12 Schematic diagram of the location of the mass

4.6 Case 4.6

Patient: Male, 47 years old.

4.6.1 Complaints

Left adrenal tumor had been found for 3 months.

4.6.2 History of Present Illness

In 2015, with no obvious cause, there was episodic dizziness, sweating, palpitation, abdominal pain, and vomiting. At that time, the blood pressure was not measured. The symptoms were relieved after about 20 min. No treatment was taken. Two years ago, a blood pressure with an unknown diastolic blood pressure (170–180/? mmHg) was measured. No treatment was taken. In December 2020, with no obvious precipitating cause, the above symptoms developed again.

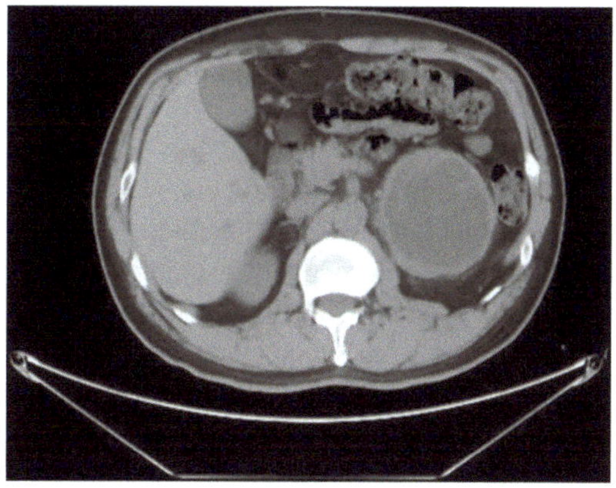

Fig. 4.13 Abdominal pelvic CT scan + adrenal thin scan

After about 20 min, the symptoms relieved on its own. Ultrasound and abdominal pelvic enhancement CT were performed in outpatient clinic of other hospital before March. It was found that the left adrenal gland was occupied by a tumor about 9 × 8 cm in size (Fig. 4.13). The possibility of pheochromocytoma was considered.

For further diagnosis and treatment, the patient was admitted to our outpatient clinic on December 24, 2020. The diagnosis of left adrenal pheochromocytoma was clearly considered in our outpatient clinic. There were indications for surgery. Patient was in full spirits, eating and sleeping normally, with normal stool and weight loss of 10 kg after the initiative to lose weight in the past month.

On January 15, 2021, phenol benzylamine 10 mg two times/day was taken. On January 26, 2021, phenol benzylamine was increased to 10 mg one time/8 h, Bai Xintong 30 mg one time/day, Betaloc 12.5 mg two times/day. Starting February 2, 2021, phenol benzylamine 15 mg one time/8 h + Betaloc 12.5 mg two times/day were taken. Starting February 10, phenol benzylamine 20 mg one time/8 h + Betaloc 12.5 mg three times/day were taken. A total of more than 40 days of drug preparation was performed.

A thick-wall and cystic low-density shadow is seen in the left adrenal region with a maximum cross-section of about 9.0 × 7.9 cm. A cord shadow is seen at the edge. The adjacent organs are pressed.

4.6.3 Past, Personal, Marital and Childbearing, Family History

In 2016, a high blood glucose was found. Diabetes mellitus was undiagnosed. FBG of 8.6 mmol/L was recently measured. Patient is now under treatment of miglitol with a FBG of 7–8 mmol/L. In 2015, he underwent varicose vein surgery on both calves (not specified). There is a history of allergy to penicillin and cephalosporins.

4.6.4 Accessory Examination

Enhanced CT of abdomen and pelvis: a thick-wall and cystic low-density shadow was seen in the left adrenal region with a maximum cross-section of about 9.0 × 7.9 cm.

^{131}I-MIBG and somatostatin receptor imaging were all positive.

Endocrine examinations: NMN 24.82 nmo1/L↑, MN 1.72 nmo1/L↑.

24 h urine catecholamines: NE 944.58 μg/24 h↑, E 26.99 μg/24 h↑, DA 295.18 μg/24 h.

Other endocrine examinations showed no obvious abnormality.

4.6.5 Current Diagnoses

Left adrenal pheochromocytoma.

Hypertension (grade 3, very high risk).

Bilateral carotid atherosclerosis.

Multiple micronodules in bilateral lungs.

Right hepatic lobe cyst.

Diabetes (this should be added).

Past surgery on double calf varicose.

4.6.6 MDT Discussion

4.6.6.1 Endocrinology

(1) High-sodium and high-protein diet; ensure that the amount is greater than 3000 mL; monitor intake and output and the weight; measure blood pressure and heart rate at least two to three times a day on recumbent position; and review Hct once a week. Avoid drastic postural changes, laborious bowel movements, agitation, exertion, and infection. Avoid medications such as gastric reassurance and morpholine. (2) The patient's current blood pressure control is acceptable. There is no serious orthostatic hypotension, nasal congestion, weight gain, and warm extremities. The preoperative preparation is basically sufficient. (3) Explain the risk during surgery, closely monitor vital signs and heart rate during the perioperative period, and be vigilant against the hypertensive crises and the alternation of high and low blood pressure. (4) Before surgery, please consult the Department of Anesthesiology and the Department of Critical Care Medicine to assist in the assessment to have a full account of surgical risks. (5) In terms of diabetes, monitor blood glucose spectrum, and control targeted levels: fasting blood glucose 4–7 mmol/L, postprandial blood glucose less than 10 mmol/L, and HbA1c less than 7%. If the blood glucose is not up to the standard, insulin can be given for a hypoglycemic therapy.

4.6.6.2 Department of Anesthesiology

(1) Follow the advice of the endocrine department for blood glucose control. (2) At present, it is acceptable to consider the preparation of phenol benzylamine. (3) Pheochromocytoma resection is a high-risk operation. The risk of perioperative pheochromophoposis and cardiovascular and cerebrovascular events is high. It should be fully explained to the patient. (4) The tumor is large and close to the pancreas, making surgery difficult. There is a risk for major bleeding. Please contact the blood bank to prepare for blood transfusion. Our department provides an invasive arteriovenous monitoring, the preparation of vasoactive drugs, and, if necessary, the preparation of blood recovery devices. (5) Return the patient to the ICU after surgery.

General surgery: (1) The left adrenal mass is closely related to the pancreas. The condition of splenectomy of or partial resection of the pancreas may be needed. Risks and possible complications should be explained to the patient. (2) Preoperative intestinal preparation is needed.

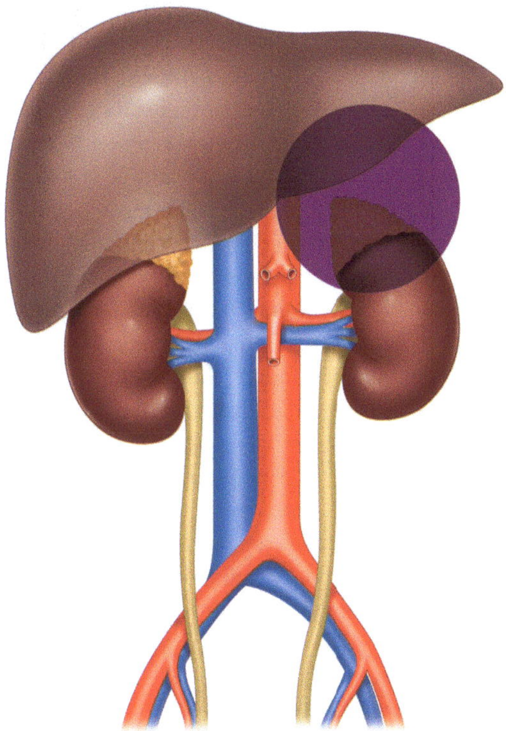

Fig. 4.14 Schematic diagram of the location of the mass

4.6.6.3 ICU

(1) Blood pressure fluctuations during operation and high risk of bleeding are fully explained. (2) If the patient returns to the ICU after surgery, contact our department before surgery.

4.6.7 Surgical Approach

Transabdominal 3D laparoscopic resection of left adrenal pheochromocytoma (Fig. 4.14).

4.6.8 Postoperative Pathology

Left adrenal pheochromocytoma.

4.7 Case 4.7

Patient: Male, 27 years old.

4.7.1 Complaints

Blood pressure increase and right adrenal mass found 4 months ago.

4.7.2 History of Present Illness

On May 23, 2020, myeloid to C2 spinal cord angioblastoma resection was performed in other hospital. Intraoperative systolic blood pressure up to 170 mmHg was found and followed by a sustained increase in blood pressure to 130–150/80–90 mmHg after surgery. After oral nifedipine two to three times/day, blood pressure was controlled at 130–140/80–90 mmHg with occasional dizziness, headache, and other discomfort. Abdominal pelvic enhancement CT shows that a 94 mm × 75 mm × 71 mm tumor is visible in the right adrenal gland. Pheochromocytoma was considered. Because pancreas and renal multiple cystic changes were found, VHL syndrome was considered. The outpatient diagnosis of the right adrenal tumor was clear, and the possibility of pheochromocytoma was high. Therefore, he was admitted to the hospital.

The patient began preoperative preparation for pheochromocytoma on August 11, 2020. Phenol benzylamine 10 mg once per 12 h was given in terms of drug preparation. The patient was in good condition after taking the drug. He complained of occasional nasal congestion but no other discomfort. Blood pressure control was feasible, and no orthostatic hypotension occurred. Now drug preparation had been for more than 2 weeks with a nasal congestion during the drug treatment, blood pressure of 140/90 mmHg, recumbent position pressure difference within 30 mmHg, easy palpitations when standing, HR of 100–120 bmp, and no dizziness, headache, abdominal pain, and other symptoms.

4.7.3 Past, Personal, Marital and Childbearing, Family History

The father was suspected for the VHL syndrome.

4.7.4 Accessory Examination

Flat peritoneal CT scan + thin adrenal scan and 3D visualization reconstruction (Figs. 4.15 and 4.16).

94 × 75 × 71 mm mass can be seen in the right adrenal gland, with clear boundaries and obvious strengthening during the enhancement phase

4.7.5 Endocrine Examination

24 h urinary catecholamines: NE 495.80 μg/24 h ↑, E 7.14 μg/24 h, DA 333.86 μg/24 h.

Blood catecholamines and metabolites: NMN20.85 nmo1/L↑, MN0.24 nmo1/L↑.

Somatostatin receptor imaging: (+); MIBG(+).

4.7.6 Current Diagnoses

Right adrenal giant pheochromocytoma.

4.7.7 MDT Discussion

4.7.7.1 Department of Anesthesiology

Pheochromocytoma patient with phenol benzylamine preparation. Dizziness and panic symptoms still occurred after the position was changed. It is recommended to continue to expand infusion if necessary. Patient is to take phenol benzylamine until the morning of surgery according to the advice of the endocrinology department. Ensure adequate daily intake control. Control lying blood pressure below 140/90 mmHg. If necessary, ask the endocrine consultation again to adjust the current medication to assess whether the preparation of phenol benzylamine is perfect. Explain to patient that intraoperative hemodynamic fluctuations may occur violently, which may result in myocardial ischemia heart failure, malignant arrhythmias, cerebral infarction, cerebral hemorrhage, fundal hemorrhage, and risk of circulatory failure. Intraoperative monitoring is strengthened. Preparation of vasoactive drugs to maintain the balance of myocardial oxygen supply and consumption, adequate blood preparation, and intraoperative monitoring of coagulation function are needed. If necessary, timely correction of coagulation disorders is performed. Postoperative return to the ICU is planned.

4.7.7.2 Endocrinology

Monitor inflow and weight at least twice a day, measure blood pressure and heart rate in the recumbent position, and repeat Hct once a week. Avoid drastic postural changes, defecation effort, emotional exertion, and infection. Avoid the use of gastric reassurance and morphine and other drugs. The patient has no episodic symptoms. The supine blood pressure and heart rate are basically normal. Phenol benzylamine Q12H treatment can be maintained, but the patient has orthostatic hypotension. The difference of blood pressure in current recum-

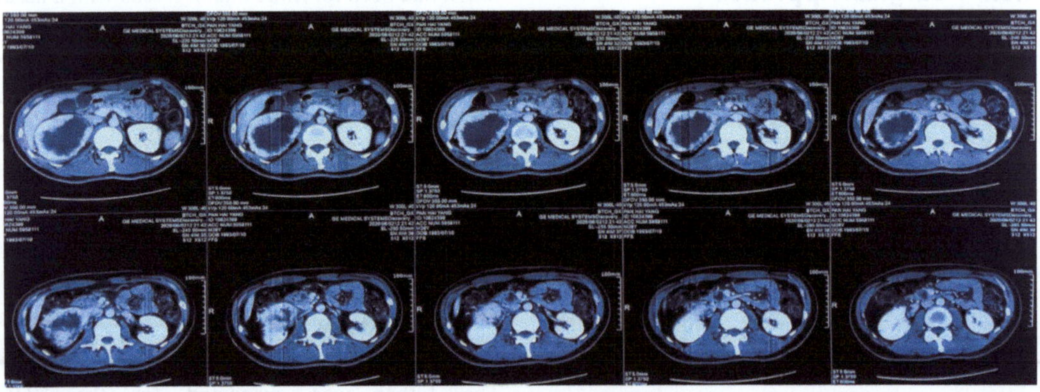

Fig. 4.15 Abdominal pelvic CT scan + adrenal thin scan

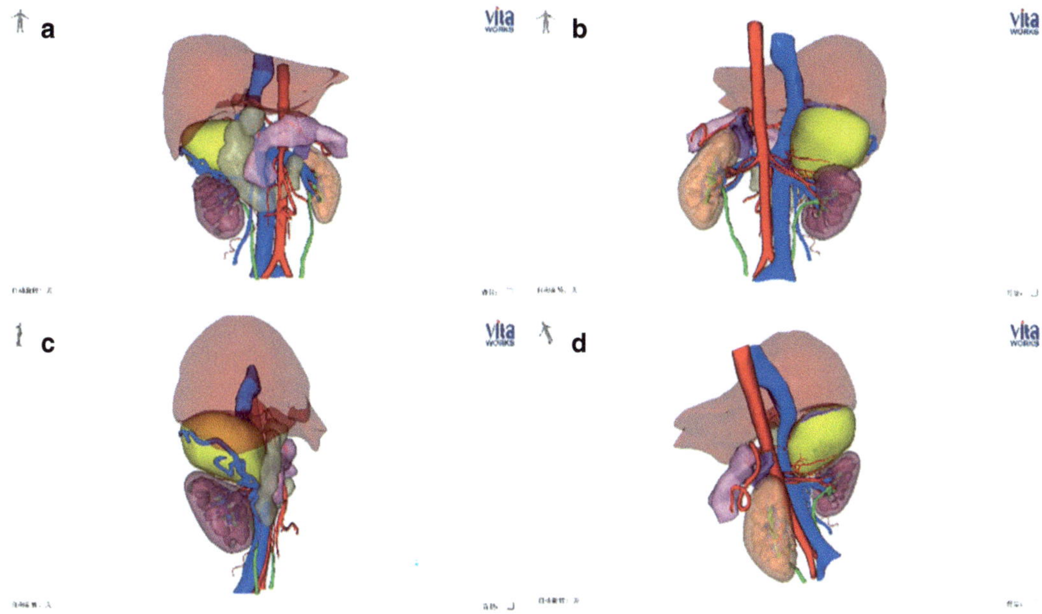

Fig. 4.16 (**a**–**d**) 3D visualization reconstruction

bent position is obvious. Upon standing, heart rate is faster, which suggests an insufficient intake. Patient is asked to increase drinking water to 3–4 L/day. If necessary, intravenous infusion is needed. Check again blood routine, Liver and kidney function, improved parathyroid hormone, calcitonin, nail work, thyroid ultrasound, and other examinations. Please consult with the ophthalmologist, and follow up with the endocrinology clinic to conduct a genetic screening.

4.7.8 Surgical Approach

Transabdominal 3D laparoscopic resection of giant pheochromocytoma of the right adrenal gland (Fig. 4.17).

4.7.9 Postoperative Pathology

(Right adrenal pheochromocytoma) Adrenal pheochromocytoma; large areas of degenerative necrosis may be seen.

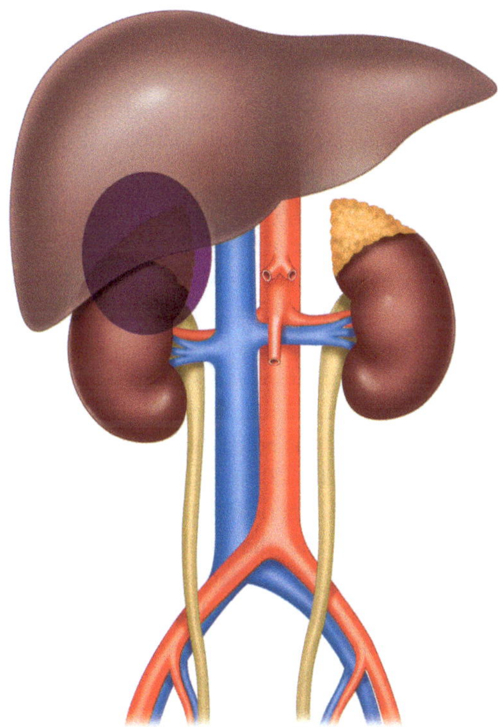

Fig. 4.17 Schematic diagram of the location of the mass

Immunohistochemical results: Melan-A(−), Calretinin(−), CgA(+), Ki-67(index 1%), Syn(+), Vimentin(+), α-inhibin(弱+), S-100(+), SDHB(+).

4.8 Case 4.8

Patient: Male, 51 years old.

4.8.1 Complaints

Blood pressure has been elevated for 20 years, and neck pain has been felt for more than 1 year.

4.8.2 History of Present Illness

The patient's blood pressure was found to be elevated during the physical examination in 2000, BP 150/90 mmHg, and the local hospital gave him an oral valsartan 80 mg qd. The blood pressure remained normal without other special treatment.

In June of 2019, the patient had a pinprick sensation in the left neck with no obvious trigger and was admitted to the local hospital.

Carotid artery CTA suggested a mass in left common carotid artery bifurcation place, about 23 × 21 mm in size. It was diagnosed with "carotid body tumor." On January 3, 2020, left carotid aneurysm surgery was performed. Postoperative pathology was the paraganglioma of medium differentiation. Self-reported stability of blood pressure was noted during surgery.

On February 4,2020, a follow-up of pet/CT found (1) a tumor in pericardial area (between the ascending aorta and the aortic artery), about 3.0 × 2.8 cm, and (2) a hypermetabolic nodule in the right adrenal gland, about 1.8 cm. On February 7, the examinations were checked: E 47.73 pg/mL, NE 1002.09 pg/mL (0–600.00 pg/mL), and DA 92.20 pg/mL. The diagnosis by other hospital was "pheochromocytoma paraganglioma, multiple metastases."

The first and second courses of chemotherapy of TP regimen were administered, respectively, on February 10 and March 7 of 2020 specifically with paclitaxel 240 mg iv d1 and nedaplatin 60 mg iv d1–2.

On August 5, 2020, the patient's reexamination of abdominal enhancement CT suggested a tumor in the right adrenal gland with the size about 15 mm × 18 mm. The boundary was still clear. The paraganglioma was considered.

Echocardiography suggested an intrapericardial mass, located between the root of the aorta and the right ventricular outflow and aortic pulmonary artery. The size was about 36 mm × 22 mm. The cardiac contractility and diastolic function were normal. So he was admitted to the Department of Cardiac Surgery of our hospital.

During hospitalization, the patient was reexamined for blood NMN 4.07↑nmol/L, blood MN 0.13nmol/L; 24 h urinary catecholamines (urine volume 2100 mL): NE 161.18 μg↑, E 2.91 μg, and DA 260.37 μg. Phenol benzyl tablet 5 mg qd → 20 mg q8h was given to control blood pressure (total course of treatment 28 days) after admission, except for contraindications. Cardiac paraganglioma resection was performed on October 16, 2020. The operation was successful. Pathological diagnosis was lesions conforming to paragangliomas, and enveloping invasion may be seen. After surgery, the patient discontinued phenolic benzylamine. The MAP could be maintained at 90–107 mmHg. On October 21, 2020, reexamination was done: blood NMN 0.89 nmol/L and blood MN 0.10 nmol/L. 24 h urinary catecholamines: NE 77.57 μg/24 h, E 3.15 μg/24 h, DA 231.56 μg/24 h.

After the last discharge, the patient continued oral antihypertensive valsartan 80 mg qd. Self-reported blood pressure fluctuated between 120 and 140/80 and 90 mmHg. Occasionally, measured blood pressure increased up to 150/90 mmHg with no sweating, palpitations, and headache. In order to further diagnose and treat adrenal lesions, patient was admitted to the endocrinology department of our hospital. After completing the relevant examinations, he was transferred to our ward on January 10, 2021. Currently, oral phenolic benzylamine (10–10–5 mg) was taken.

4.8.3 Past, Personal, Marital and Childbearing, Family History

Nothing special.

4.8.4 Accessory Examination

CTA tips (Figs. 4.18, 4.19, and 4.20): A tumor is found at the bifurcation of the left common carotid artery. The size is about 23 × 21 mm. The pericardial area (between the ascending aorta and the aortic artery) is about 3.0 × 2.8 cm. A hyperbolic nodules about 1.8 cm in diameter in the right adrenal gland is seen.

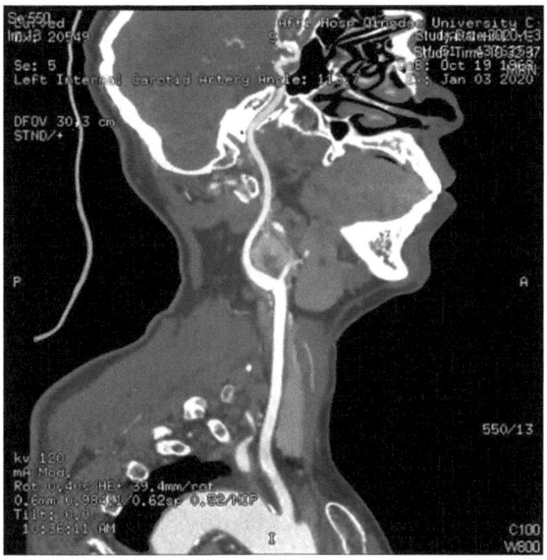

Fig. 4.18 Carotid CTA A tumor at the bifurcation of right common carotid artery, about 23 × 21 mm in size

Somatostatin receptor imaging: approximately a 3.1 cm × 2.1 cm tumor in place of anterior to the proximal ascending aorta, which may conform to paraganglioma. A tumor in right adrenal gland is found. The size is about 1.8 cm × 1.5 cm. Pheochromocytoma may be considered.

MIBG imaging: somatostatin receptors in the anterior of proximal segment of the ascending aortic are highly expressed and may be consistent with paragangliomas. The right adrenal nodules are mildly expressed, excluding the possibility of pheochromocytoma.

On August 20, 2020, Blood NMN was 2.95 nmol/L, blood MN 0.12 nmol/L; 24 h urine catecholamines (urine volume 1200 mL): NE 5.16 μg, E 0.67 μg, DA 25.78 μg.

The right adrenal gland is occupied by a tumor, about 15 × 18 mm in size. The border is still clear. Paraganglioma is considered.

4.8.5 Current Diagnoses

Multiple pheochromocytoma and paraganglioma; right adrenal pheochromocytoma; cardiac paraganglioma; left carotid paraganglioma after

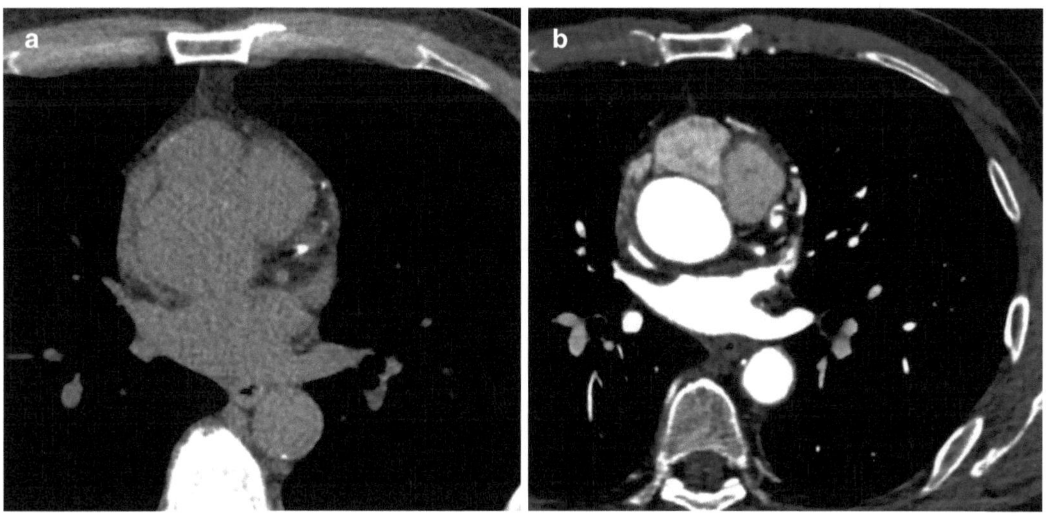

Fig. 4.19 (**a**, **b**) Cardiac CTA: A tumor about 3.0 × 2.8 cm in the pericardial area (between the ascending aorta and the aortic artery).

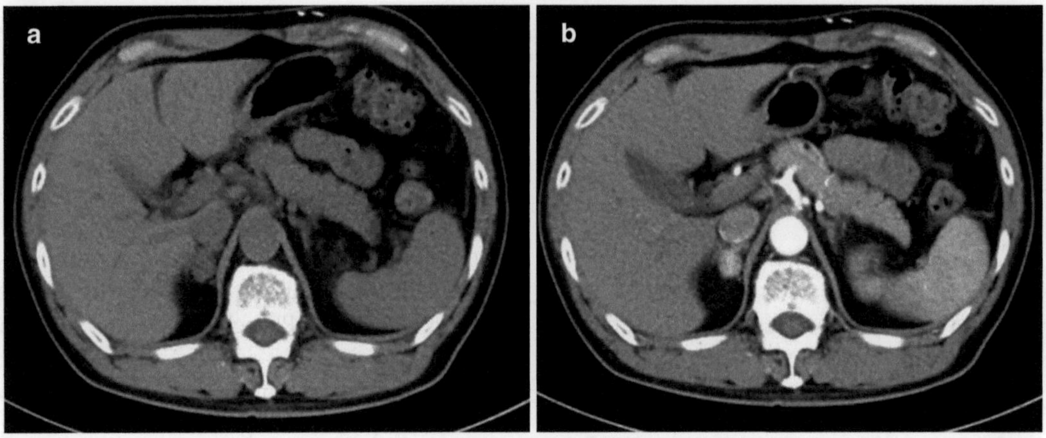

Fig. 4.20 (a, b) Abdominal enhancement CT.

cardiac paraganglioma resection; left carotid aneurysm after resection; possible right lateral carotid paraganglioma; hypertensive retinopathy (grade II); past 2 courses of TP chemotherapy; hyperlipidemia; hyperuricemia; systemic atherosclerosis (bilateral carotid arteries, right subclavian artery, arteries of both lower extremities); severe stenosis at the beginning of the celiac trunk; fatty liver; vitamin D deficiency; compressive fracture of the thoracic 12 vertebral body.

4.8.6 MDT Discussion

4.8.6.1 Vascular Surgery

During the patient's follow-up, there was no significant increase in the right neck mass. Somatostatin receptor imaging and I131-MIBG imaging did not suggest obvious abnormalities of radiological uptake of the right neck mass. The head CTA and carotid artery BUS could be regularly reviewed to assess the changes in the right neck mass and to further evaluate the indications for surgery. For the peritoneal stenosis, the current CTA suggested that the morphology of superior mesenteric artery could be correct. The collateral branch circulation was formed, and there was no indication for intervention.

4.8.6.2 Department of Anesthesiology

Continue preoperative preparation. Fully explain the risks to the patient, and recommend to be monitored in the ICU after surgery.

4.8.6.3 Ophthalmology

For binocular hypertensive retinopathy (grade II), treatment of primary disease and control of blood pressure were necessary.

4.8.6.4 Urology

Right adrenal mass is more likely to be pheochromocytoma. Surgical treatment can be considered. Preoperative preparation can be continued to improve. Maintain stable blood pressure. Consultation of the Department of Anesthesiology is necessary to assess the risk during adrenal surgery.

4.8.6.5 Cardiac Surgery

At present, the cardiac function is stable. There is no orthostatic hypotension, and there are no contraindications to surgery.

4.8.6.6 ICU

The patient has a clear diagnosis of chromophilus and should be returned to the ICU after surgery.

4.8.7 Treatment (Fig. 4.21)

Laparoscopic resection of right adrenal pheochromocytoma.

4.8.8 Postoperative Pathology

Right adrenal eosinophilic tumor.

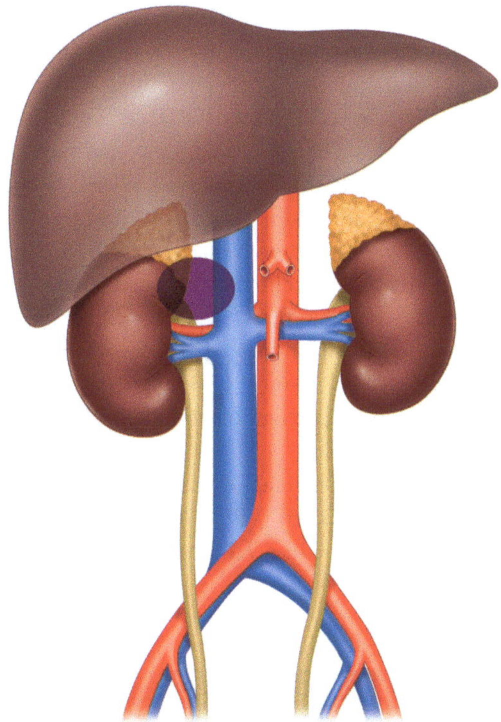

Fig. 4.21 Schematic diagram of the location of the mass

Immunohistochemical results: Melan-A (−), Calretinin (−), CgA (+), Ki-67 (index 1%), Syn (+), Vimentin (+), and α-inhibin (focal+).

4.9 Case 4.9

Patient: Female, 48 years old.

4.9.1 Complaints

Paroxysmal hypertension over 6 years.

4.9.2 History of Present Illness

Increase in blood pressure for over 6 years, up to 140/100 mmHg, with no obvious discomfort. One year ago, patient experienced blood pressure of 200/100 mmHg with dizziness, palpitation, nausea, and heavy sweating occasionally. Symptom relieved by itself 1 or 2 min later. In February of 2020, increased frequency of attacks (one time/week → two to three times/week) and increased blood pressure level (250/139 mmHg) were noticed. In April of 2020, CT by local hospital showed a tumor of 10 cm in the left adrenal gland. From May 2020 to June 2020, patient was examined in endocrinology and urology outpatient clinics in our hospital. She was admitted by our hospital with a "left pheochromocytoma."

On June 9,2020, patient started drug preparation with an antihypertensive drug regimen: phenolic benzylamine 10 mg q8h + bisoprolol 5 mg qd. From June 16, dosage of drug changed: phenolic benzylamine 20 mg q8h + bisoprolol 5 mg qd. Blood pressure was controlled within 120–140/70–90 mmHg and heart rate within 70–85 bpm, Blood pressure occasionally increased to 160/100 mmHg, higher in the morning and evening. Patient experienced no headache, no dizziness, no palpitations, and no postural dizziness after treatment of the drug. Dry mouth, no nasal congestion, and dry stool were noticed. More than 3000 mL/day intake was recorded with a weight stabilization at 72 kg. On July 28, according to the opinion of endocrinology consultation, the drug was adjusted as follows: phenol benzylamine 25-15-25 mg q8h + bisoprolol 5 mg qd.

4.9.3 Past, Personal, Marital and Childbearing, Family History

In 2013, the diagnosis of myocardial infarction was established by another hospital. Aspirin 100 mg qd (discontinued on July 4, 2020) + atorvastatin 20 mg qn were given with no stent. On November 2019, coronary CTA was performed in a local hospital and did not find a definitive coronary stenosis.

In May 2020, our hospital finding for fasting blood glucose read 7.1 mmol/L, and HbA1c was 5.1%. Monitoring after hospitalization found a FBG of 5.8–6.4 mmol/L and a PBG of 6.4–9.3 mmol/L.

4.9.4 Accessory Examination

CTU (Figs. 4.22 and 4.23): Cystic mass in the left adrenal region with internal septum, clearly demarcated, local compression to the superior pole of left kidney, about 8.3 cm × 10.4 cm × 8.5 cm in size.

Somatostatin receptor imaging: left adrenal hyperexpression foci of somatostatin receptor. Pheochromocytoma with organic necrosis is more likely.

Systemic imaging of adrenal medullary: a larger ring-shaped area with abnormally concentrated radiation is found at the equal level to the left adrenal gland. Reduction of radiation is noticed in the center. Pheochromocytoma is more likely considered with the possibility of partial organization.

Urinary ultrasound: bilateral renal pelvis and ureteral distension are not found. The superior pole of left kidney is occupied by a tumor of extremely low echo, 8.9 × 8.3 cm, with the smooth border. The echo is uniform, and there is no echo found in the internal part. CDFI: Blood flow signals are visible inside the tumor. The bladder is well filled with the light wall, and no clear stones and placeholders are seen inside.

Renal blood flow chart: right kidney = 36.00 mL/min · 1.73 m^2, left kidney = 29.87 mL/min · 1.73 m^2. Blood flow perfusion and function of double kidney are slightly affected.

Blood biochemical examinations: HGB 117 g/L, HCT 37.6%, PLT 433 × 10^9/L ↑ K 4.1 mmol/L, Glu 7.1 mmol/L ↑, UA 380 μmol/L ↑.

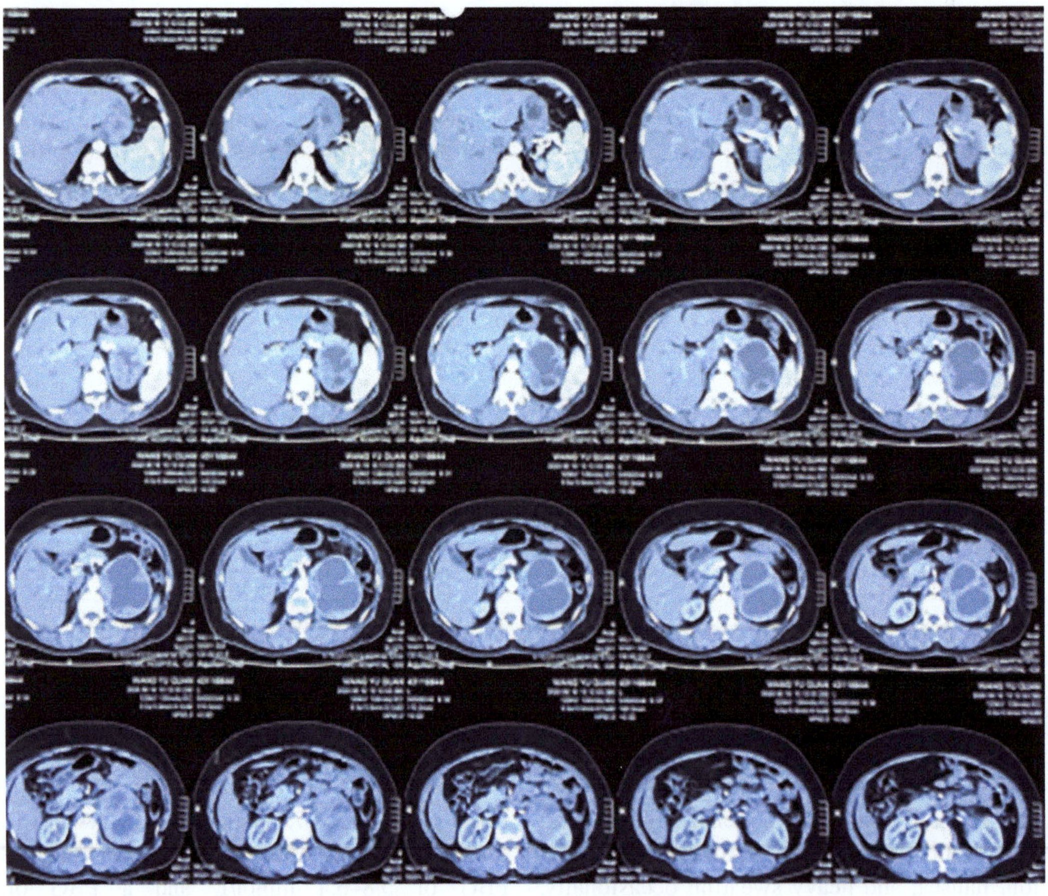

Fig. 4.22 Abdominal pelvic enhancement CT

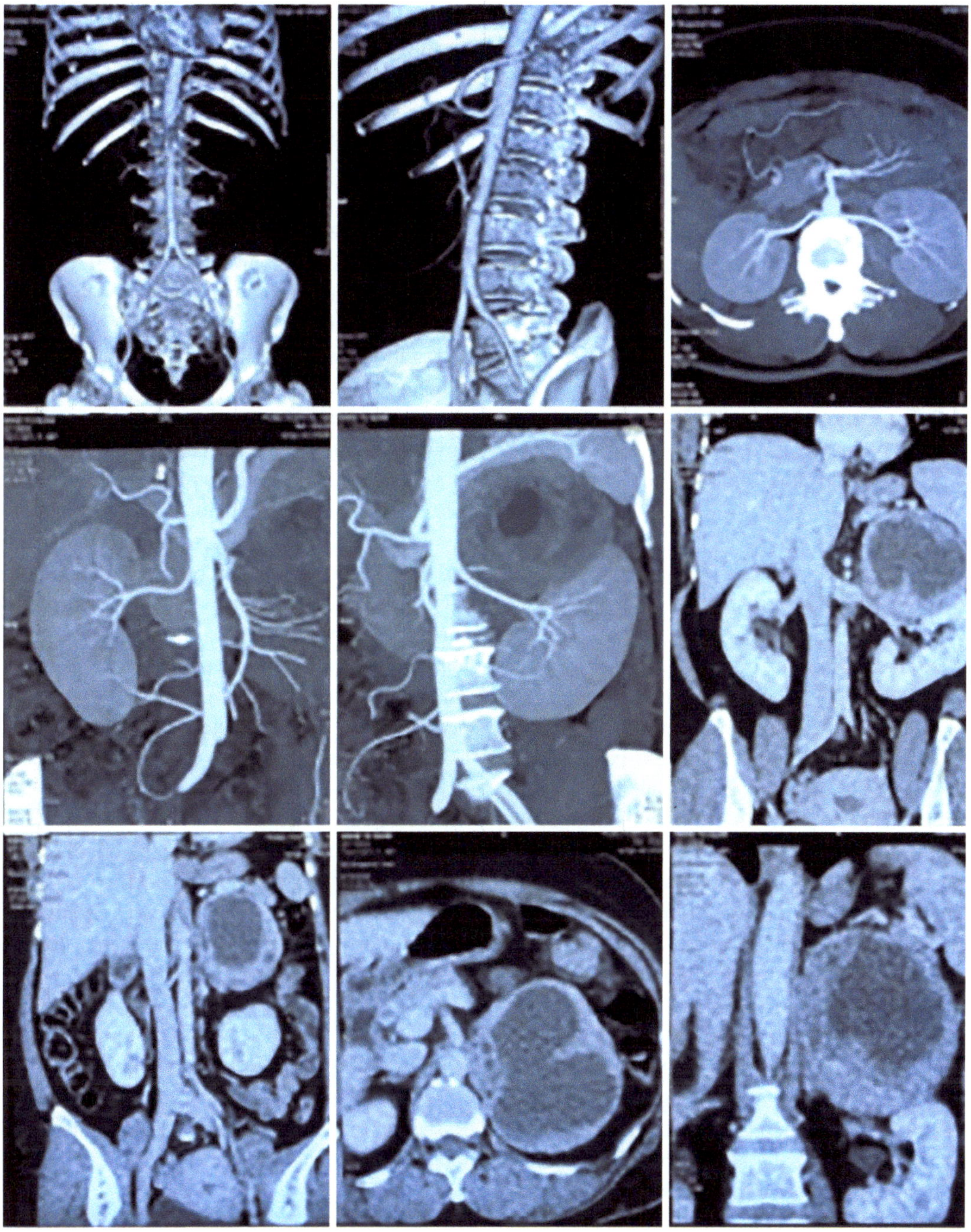

Fig. 4.23 Abdominal pelvis enhancement CTA

24 h urinary catecholamines: NE 153.13 μg/24 h↑(17–41), E 324.48 μg/24 h↑(1.74 ~ 6.42), DA 525.00 μg/24 h↑(121~331).

Plasma catecholamines and their metabolites: NMN 4.32 nmo1/L↑(<0.9), MN 14.90 nmo1/L(<0.5), residual RAAS, cortisol, sex hormone-related screening (−).

A cystic solid mass is seen in the left adrenal area, internally separated, clearly bordered, local compression of superior pole of the left kidney, about 8.3 cm × 10.4 cm × 8.5 cm. After the enhanced scan, the sac wall, the septum, and solid components show a mild-to-moderate strengthening. The cystic components are not strengthened.

The aorta and right renal arteries are involved in blood supply. There are no obvious abnormalities in the veins of both kidneys. Nodules are seen in the anterior of right kidney with the soft tissue density by ordinary scan (7im49). Enhanced scans show moderate intensification.

4.9.5 Current Diagnosis

Giant pheochromocytoma of the left adrenal gland.

4.9.6 MDT Discussion

4.9.6.1 Endocrinology

(1) Add up to monitor the recumbent blood pressure and heart rate at 8–10 pm in the evening. Re-check HCT every week. Pay attention to cardiovascular symptoms and stool conditions. Instruct patient to avoid defecation effort, emotional agitation, fatigue, infection, severe postural changes, and compression of the abdomen, as well as the use of morphine, gastric reassurance, and other drugs. (2) According to the patient's current recumbent blood pressure, it is recommended to adjust the treatment of phenol benzyl to 6 am 25 mg, 2 pm 15 mg, and 8 pm 25 mg. Please re-check the 24 h ambulatory blood pressure monitoring. Continue bisoprolol 5 mg qd. Increase the daily water intake to nearly 4 L. If the supine blood pressure is still high, the treatment of Baixintong 30 mg qd can be added. The goal is as follows: there is no paroxysmal hypertension attack; the supine blood pressure is controlled within 140/90, and there is no obvious orthostatic hypotension. (3) Please consider consultations with the anesthesiology and intensive care departments to assess perioperative risk. (4) The patient's outpatient calcitonin level is slightly elevated. Please re-check the thyroid ultrasound. (5) Patient was screened for vitamin D deficiency and mildly elevated parathyroid hormone levels on an outpatient basis. It is required to re-check PTH, serum calcium, and 25-hydroxyvitamin D. If necessary, regular vitamin D3800–1000 U qd orally is to be given.

4.9.6.2 Department of Anesthesiology

(1) Middle-aged woman, ASA grade III, elective surgery. (2) Pheochromocytoma with a history of coronary heart disease. Phenol benzylamine preparation can be taken. Please instruct the patient to take phenol benzylamine until the morning of surgery, according to the endocrinology consultation opinion. Ensure that the daily intake is sufficient. Fully explain the intraoperative hemodynamic fluctuations leading to myocardial ischemia, heart failure, malignant arrhythmia, cerebral infarction, cerebral infarction, cerebral hemorrhage, fundal hemorrhage, and circulatory failure risk. Strengthen monitoring during surgery, and prepare vasoactive drugs. Maintain the balance of myocardial oxygen supply and oxygen consumption. (3) Return patient to the ICU after surgery.

4.9.6.3 ICU

(1) The diagnosis of pheochromocytoma is clear, and the risk of perioperative pheochromocytoma is explained. (2) The risk of stress cardiomyopathy and arrhythmia is explained. (3) Return patient to ICU after operation.

4.9.7 Surgical Approach

Resection of left retroperitoneal giant pheochromocytoma by laparotomy (Fig. 4.24).

4.9.8 Postoperative Pathology

Lesions consistent with pheochromocytomas of the adrenal glands; intravessel tumor plugs may be seen.

Immunohistochemical results: Melan-A(−), AE1/AE3(−), CgA(+), Ki-67(index 1%), S-100(+), α-inhibin(−), CD34(+).

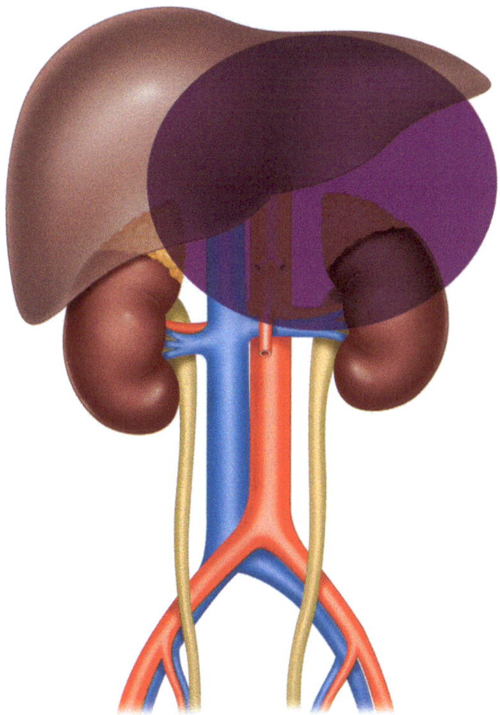

Fig. 4.24 Schematic diagram of the location of the mass

4.10 Case 4.10

Patient: Male, 39 years old.

4.10.1 Complaints

A tumor of the right adrenal gland had been found for more than 1 year.

4.10.2 History of Present Illness

In July 2019, a CT of the abdomen was performed after physical examination, which found a strong echoic nodule in the right adrenal region of 30 mm × 29 mm. Irregular measurements of blood pressure were taken in the past. A high Bp of 160/100 mmHg was found without treatment. In September 2019, he was admitted to the local urological surgery clinic and diagnosed with "adrenal adenoma without function." A laparoscopic surgery was performed. Intraoperative systolic blood pressure went up to 260 mmHg. The operation was discontinued.

In December 2019, he was admitted to the Urology Department of our hospital, and the diagnosis of right adrenal tumor was clear. The possibility of pheochromocytoma was high. In January 2020, the drug was prepared (phenolic benzylamine 10 mg once/12 h). The drug was stopped by the patient himself midway due to the pandemic. In April 2020, he began to take the drug again for nearly three weeks. The treatment changed to phenol benzylamine 20 mg once/12 h + Betaloc 12.5 mg. During the medical treatment, occasional dizziness and nasal congestion were found. Blood pressure was controlled at 120–130/70–90 mmHg.

4.10.3 Past, Personal, Marital and Childbearing, Family History

Liver dysfunction had been found for more than a year. Polyene phosphatidylcholine and ursodeoxycholic acid were orally administered.

4.10.4 Accessory Examination

Abdominal pelvic CT with enhancement + adrenal thin sweep (Fig. 4.25): A dense shadow like a round soft tissue is seen in the right adrenal region. The boundary is clear. The size is about 3.8 cm × 3.1 cm. After the enhancement of scan, the cortical medulla and parenchymal phase are unevenly and mildly strengthened. Mass' blood supply is provided by the adrenal branch of the abdominal aorta.

Somatostatin receptor imaging: (+).

Endocrine examination: 24 h Urinary catecholamines: NE 358.97 μg/24 h ↑, E 107.69 μg/24 h ↑, DA 92.31 μg/24 h ↑.

Blood catecholamines and metabolites: NMN 6.25 nmol/L ↑, MN 1.60 nmol/L↑.

(a) A shadow of density equal to the quasi-circular soft tissue is seen in the right adrenal region, with clear boundaries. The size is about 3.8 cm × 3.1 cm.
(b) After the enhancement of scan, the cortical medulla and parenchymal phase are unevenly and mildly strengthened. The blood supply of the mass is provided by the adrenal branch of the abdominal aorta.

4.10.5 Current Diagnosis

Right adrenal pheochromocytoma.

4.10.6 MDT Discussion

4.10.6.1 Endocrinology

(1) Increase the amount of liquid intake (greater than 3000 mL/day) with high-sodium

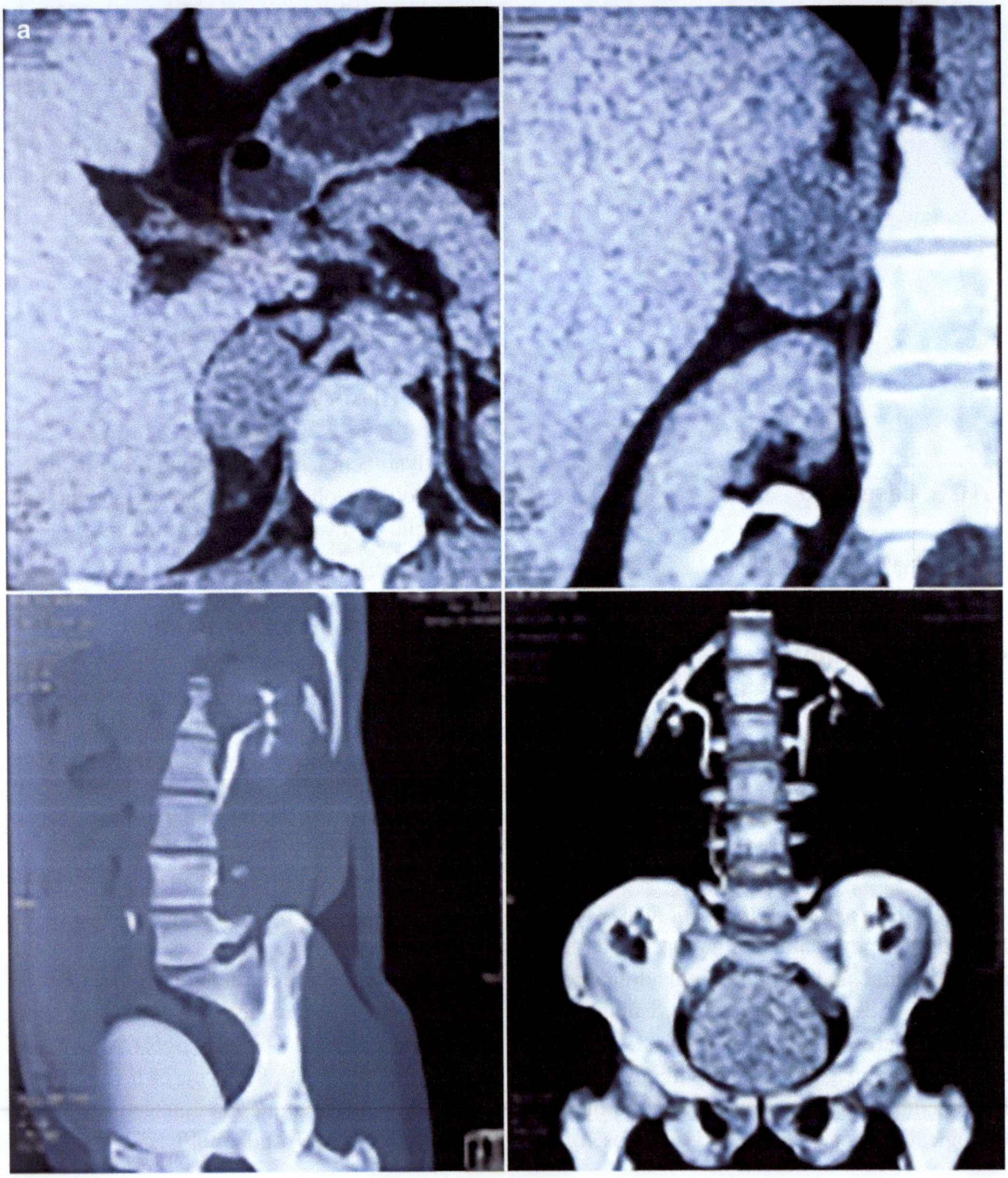

Fig. 4.25 (**a, b**) Abdominal pelvic CT with enhancement + adrenal thin scan

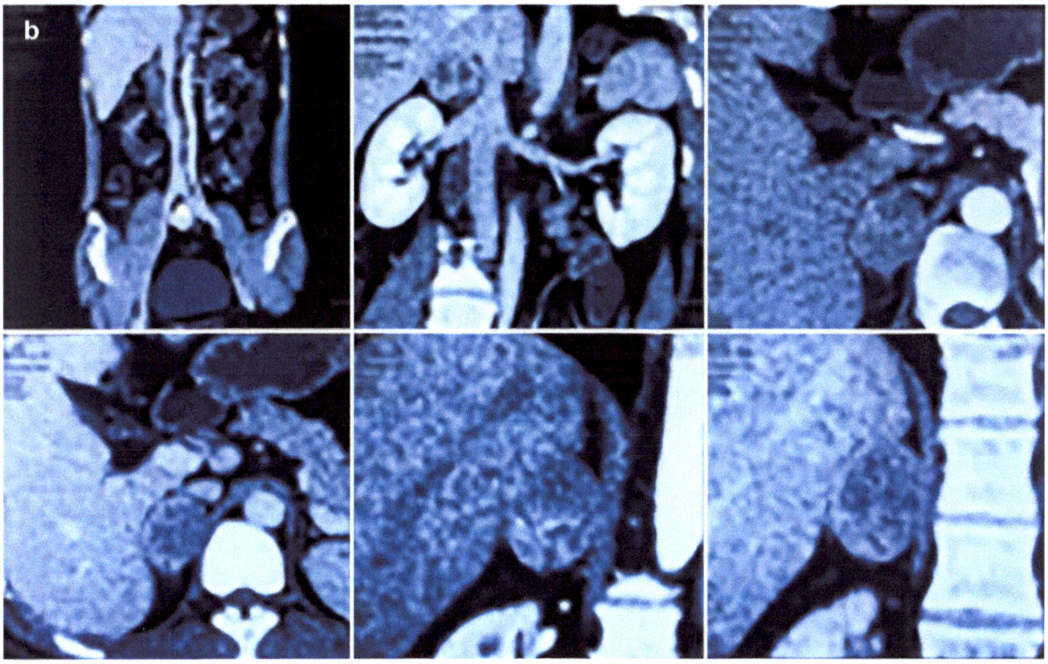

Fig. 4.25 (continued)

and high-protein diet. Monitor closely the intake and output, weight, Hct, and stool. Monitor at least two times the recumbent blood pressure and heart rate during every examination. Advise patient to avoid increasing abdominal pressure and caution with morphine, gastric reassurance, and other drugs. (2) The patient's right adrenal pheochromocytoma is probable. He has taken phenol benzylamine for more than half a year. He has no recent episodic symptoms. Blood pressure is well controlled. No obvious manifestations of orthostatic hypotension are noticed. The current preoperative preparation is adequate. A recent surgical treatment can be proposed. Patient is of greater risk during surgery. Fully explain the surgical risk to the patient and the family. Closely monitor the amount of intake and output, weight, recumbent blood pressure, electrolytes, and Hct during the perioperative period. Ask for consultations from anesthesiology department and ICU. Re-check 24-h urinary catecholamines and blood catecholamine results. Complete the following exams: thyroid function, calcitonin, CEA, thyroid ultrasound, blood calcium, phosphorus, PTH, gastrin, glucagon, insulin, GH, IGF1, and PRL to exclude MEN. (3) Follow-up by outpatient endocrinology.

4.10.6.2 Department of Anesthesiology

(1) Middle-aged men, ASA grade III, elective surgery. (2) It is recommended to perform an echography, excluding myocardial lesions. Patient still complains of high blood pressure. It is recommended to closely monitor the blood pressure in the recumbent position. Demand endocrinology consultation to assess whether preoperative preparation is adequate, and clarify the timing of surgery. (3) For pheochromocytoma, please ask the patient to take phenol benzylamine until the morning of the operation according to the opinions of endocrinology consultation. Ensure that the daily intake is sufficient, and communicate with the patient regarding risk of myocardial ischemia, heart failure, malignant arrhythmia, cerebral infarction, cerebral hemorrhage, fundal hemorrhage, and circulatory failure during the operation. (4) Difficulty in respiration may be encountered. Visible laryngoscopy and fibrous intubation are prepared. (5) Return patient

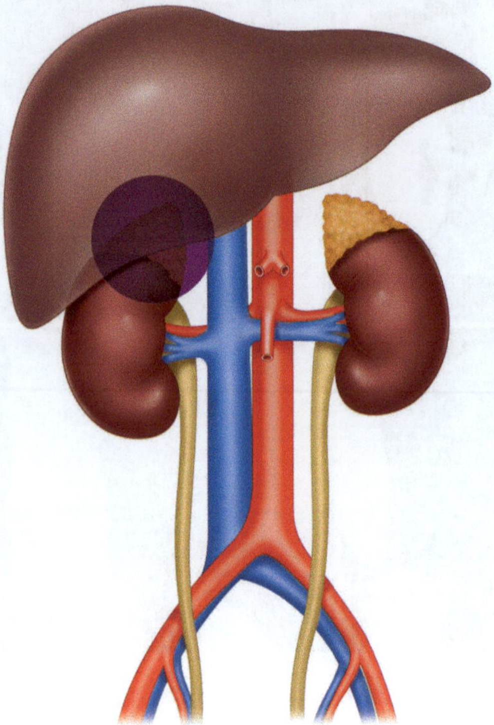

Fig. 4.26 Schematic diagram of the location of the mass

to the ICU after surgery, and follow-up with our department.

4.10.6.3 ICU

ICU consultation fully explain the possibility of perioperative chromophilic crisis due to stress, which may cause the risk of cardiovascular and cerebrovascular events. Postoperative return to ICU is a must.

4.10.7 Surgical Approach

Laparoscopic resection of right adrenal pheochromocytoma (Fig. 4.26).

4.10.8 Postoperative Pathology

It conforms to the right adrenal pheochromocytoma.

4.11 Case 4.11

Patient: Female, 53 years old.

4.11.1 Complaints

Increased blood pressure for 9 years and a tumor occupying the left adrenal gland found for a period of 4 months.

4.11.2 History of Present Illness

In 2009, the patient experienced dizziness during activity with no obvious cause, which could be relieved after rest. There was no headache, nausea, vomiting, palpitation, sweating, and other discomforts. The blood pressure was up to 140/90 mmHg measured in the local health center. Oral treatment of one reserpine tablet was given one time/day. Blood pressure could be controlled at 130/80 mmHg, and the symptoms of dizziness disappeared. In April 2018, the patient was injured in a car accident. In Handan People's Hospital, abdominal CT examination was performed and found "left adrenal mass" (specification unavailable). Patient was recommended to go to a higher-level hospital for further diagnosis and treatment. In May 2018, the patient was admitted to the Urology Department of our hospital. The abdominal pelvic enhancement CT + three-dimensional reconstruction suggested the following: left adrenal mass, with probable pheochromocytoma; retroperitoneal lesion at the level of the left renal hilum, paraganglioma more likely. Somatostatin receptor imaging suggested high expression of somatostatin receptors in the left adrenal region, considering the possibility of neuroendocrine tumors, with the possibility of partial necrosis. Considering the diagnosis of pheochromocytoma is basically clear, patient was instructed to stop reserpine and to take an oral treatment of phenol benzylamine 10 mg one time/12 h. Blood pressure was controlled at 120–130/80–90 mmHg, with a heart rate of about 80 times/min after patient had taken the drug so far. Patient had warm limbs, with no nasal congestion, dizziness, and other discomfort. The patient is now under further diagnosis and treatment at our department.

During the course of the disease, the spirit and appetite remained good, patient had poor sleep and normal stool, and there is no significant change in weight recently.

4.11.3 Past, Personal, Marital and Childbearing, Family History

Patient had a three-year history of lumbar spondylolisthesis and suffered from car accident injury 4 months ago, resulting in left clavicle fracture, left multiple rib fractures, and left shoulder blade fracture. Nothing special for personal history and family history.

4.11.4 Accessory Examination

On June 6, 2018, abdominal pelvic CT with enhancement (Fig. 4.27) found a left adrenal mass. Pheochromocytoma is probable after combining results with clinical manifestations. A retroperitoneal lesion is found at left renal portal level. Please combine clinical manifestations to establish if paraganglioma is more probable. Atherosclerotic changes of abdominal aorta and its branches appeared.

On May 30, 2018, somatostatin receptor imaging found hyperexpression lesions of somatostatin receptor in the adrenal region, which suggests the possibility of neuroendocrine tumor with the possibility of partial necrosis.

24 h urinary catecholamines: NE 35.56 μg/24 h, E 1.82 μg/24 h, DA 230.83 μg/24 h.

Aldosterone (cubic): ALD2 11.80 ng/dL.

Angiotensin II + renin activity (standing): PRA2 0.31 ng/mL/h, AT-II2 60.51 pg/mL.

Total renal: K4.3mmol/L, ACTH 17.9 pg/mL.

Total blood cortisol: F 10.76 μg/dL.

24-h uricosol: UFC 82.45 μg/24 h.

Left adrenal mass: pheochromocytoma is more probable. Retroperitoneal lesions at left hilar level: paraganglioma is more probable.

4.11.5 Current Diagnoses

Left adrenal pheochromocytes.

Retroperitoneal paraganglioma at left hilar level.

Large alveoli in the lower lobe of the left lung.

Spondylolisthesis.

Obsolete fracture of the left clavicle.

Multiple obsolete fractures of the left ribs.

Obsolete fracture of left scapula.

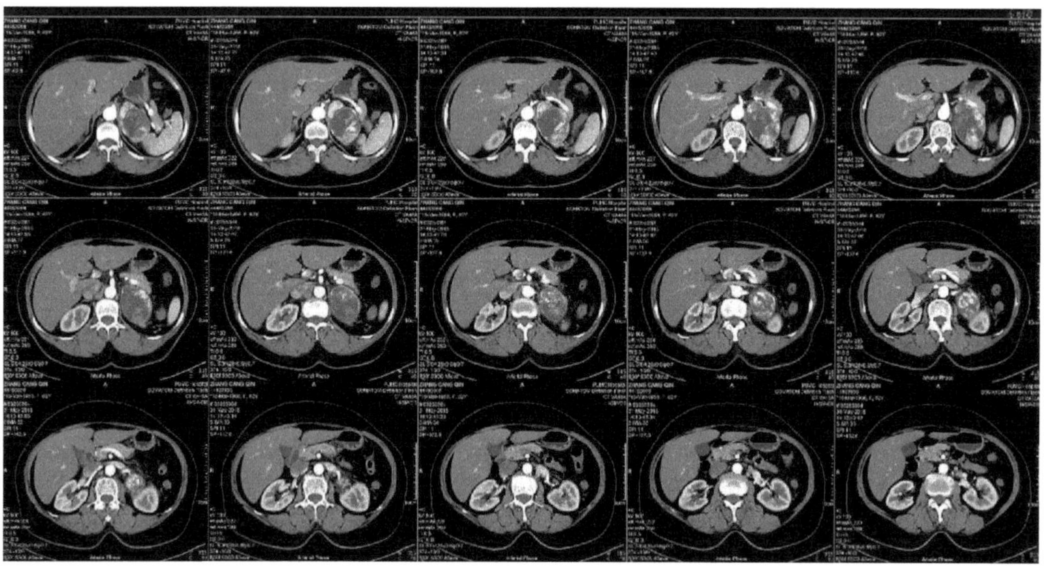

Fig. 4.27 Abdominal pelvic enhancement CT

4.11.6 MDT Discussion

4.11.6.1 ICU

Pheochromocytoma cannot be excluded. Explain to the patient the large fluctuations and the risk of cardiovascular and cerebrovascular events during the perioperative period. Patient can return to our department after surgery.

4.11.6.2 Endocrinology

(1) Re-check MIBG imaging and 24-h urinary catecholamines to help confirm the diagnosis. (2) Currently, blood pressure is still high. When there is a change in position, the blood pressure decreases, and the heart rate accelerates. It is recommended to continue the current phenol benzylamine treatment. If the blood pressure is not up to standard, phenol benzylamine can be slowly increased (10–10–5 mg). Instruct the patient to increase the amount of water (mainly light saline). Adequate indicators of preoperative preparation are as follows: blood pressure < 140/90 mmHg, no episodic hypertension and related symptoms, no postural hypotension, weight gain, HCT decline, and no high metabolic performance. (3) Re-check echocardiography, myocardial enzymes, fundus, aortic ultrasound, and ACR to assess for complications. If necessary, consult with relevant departments. Demand from the anesthesiology department assessment of perioperative risks before surgery. Monitor blood pressure in the supine position and blood glucose. (4) Re-check PTH, iCa, 24-h urinary calcium, nail work, calcitonin, and thyroid ultrasound to exclude MEN.

4.11.6.3 Department of Anesthesiology

(1) Elective surgery; (2) demand endocrine consultation to assist in the assessment of risks. Complete adequate preoperative preparations. Closely monitor BP. (3) Fully account for perioperative myocardial infarction, heart failure, stroke, arrhythmias, atelectasis, pneumothorax, lung infection, and the possibility of major bleeding. (4) Postoperative return to ICU is a must.

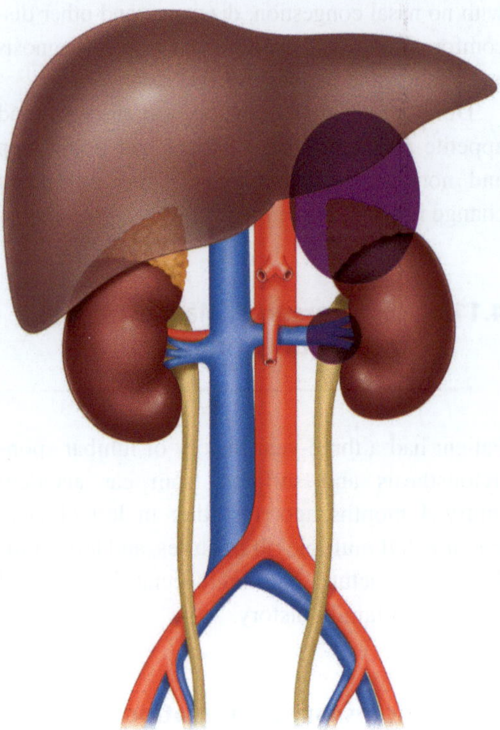

Fig. 4.28 Schematic diagram of the location of the mass

4.11.6.4 General Surgery

(1) Our department is willing to assist in diagnosis and treatment. If the date of surgery is determined, please contact our department. (2) Full gastrointestinal preparation before surgery must be done. (3) Follow-up with our department.

4.11.7 Surgical Approach

Laparoscopic resection of left retroperitoneal mass (Fig. 4.28).

4.11.8 Postoperative Pathology

(Mass I, II) Pheochromocytoma. Adrenal tissue can be seen around the mass (mass I).

Immunohistochemical results: Melan-A(−), AE1/AE3(±), CgA(+), Ki-67(index 2%), S-100(+), α-inhibin(−), Syn(+).

4.12 Case 4.12

Patient: Male, 64 years old.

4.12.1 Complaints

Hypertension for 20 years; mass in the left adrenal gland found 8 months ago.

4.12.2 History of Present Illness

Twenty years ago, it was found that the patient's blood pressure was increased. Oral nifedipine 30 mg qd was taken. Symptomatic antihypertensive effect was not obvious. In December 2019, he was admitted to the hospital for "episodic dizziness and palpitations." Measured blood pressure was 180/100 mmHg. A mass in the left adrenal gland was found by a chest CT scan (no report was seen). In January 2020, he was admitted to our hospital with a blood pressure of 155/101 mmHg. Drug preparation began in January 2020: phenol benzylamine 10 mg three times/day. Oropharyngeal discomfort caused to stop the drug. In the past 2 months, he regularly took nifedipine 30 mg, one time/day and enalapril 0.5 tablet, one time/12 h. Blood pressure was controlled at 140/90 mmHg.

4.12.3 Past, Personal, Marital and Childbearing, Family History

Nothing special.

4.12.4 Accessory Examination

Peritoneal enhanced CT + adrenal thin scan (Fig. 4.29): a nodule of soft tissue density is seen in the left adrenal junction. The density in the central part is reduced. The size is about 2.0 cm × 1.5 cm. The significant enhancement is noticed gradually and unevenly. Imaging corresponds to the possibility of pheochromocytoma with central necrosis.

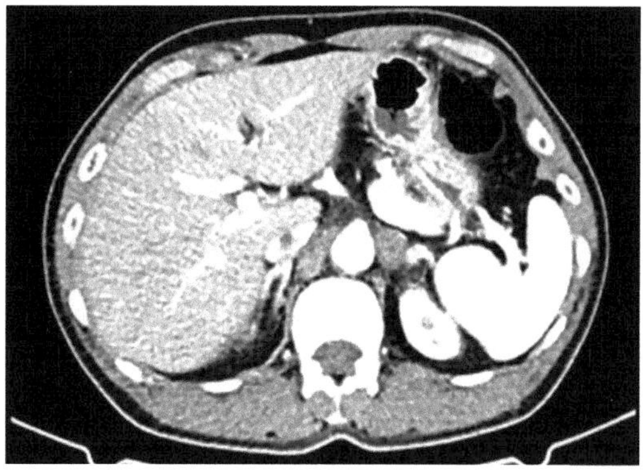

Fig. 4.29 Abdominal pelvic enhancement CT

Somatostatin receptor imaging: negative.

Endocrine examination: 24 h urinary catecholamines: NE 15.64 μg/24 h↓ E 1.04 μg/24 h ↓ DA 123.71 μg/24 h.

Blood catecholamines and metabolites: NMN: 0.57 nmol/L, MN 0.19 nmol/L.

AT-II2/PRA-2/UFC/ALD2 (−)K+ 4.1 mmol/L.

A nodule of soft tissue density is seen in the left adrenal junction. The density in the central part is reduced. The size is about 2.0 cm × 1.5 cm. Significant enhancement is noticed gradually and unevenly. Imaging corresponds to the possibility of pheochromocytoma with central necrosis.

4.12.5 MDT Discussion

4.12.5.1 Endocrinology

(1) At least measure the blood pressure and heart rate of the patient in recumbent position every day. Monitor intake and output and weight. Re-check HCT once a week. (2) The supine blood pressure is still high, so phenol

benzylamine and codohua have been added. The change in blood pressure in the recumbent position is to be observed. If it is still poorly controlled, the amount of nifedipine can be increased to 30 mg q12 and daily drinking water to 2–3 L. (3) Goals of adequate preoperative preparations are no episodic symptoms, stable blood pressure, smooth stools, and decreased HCT.

4.12.5.2 Department of Anesthesiology

Agree with endocrinology. Prepare according to preoperative standards, and avoid the risks of severe hypotension, hypertension, pheochromocytoma crisis, cerebral hemorrhage, shock, sudden death, etc.

4.12.5.3 ICU

Patient has a high risk for surgery. We are willing to prepare a bed. Blood type O RhD (+); already contacted with the blood bank (4 U red blood cells are currently available).

4.12.6 Current Diagnoses

Left retroperitoneal paraganglioma.

Hypertension.

Prostatic hyperplasia.

4.12.7 Surgical Approach

Laparoscopic removal of left pheochromocytoma (Fig. 4.30).

4.12.8 Postoperative Pathology

Left adrenal pheochromocytoma.

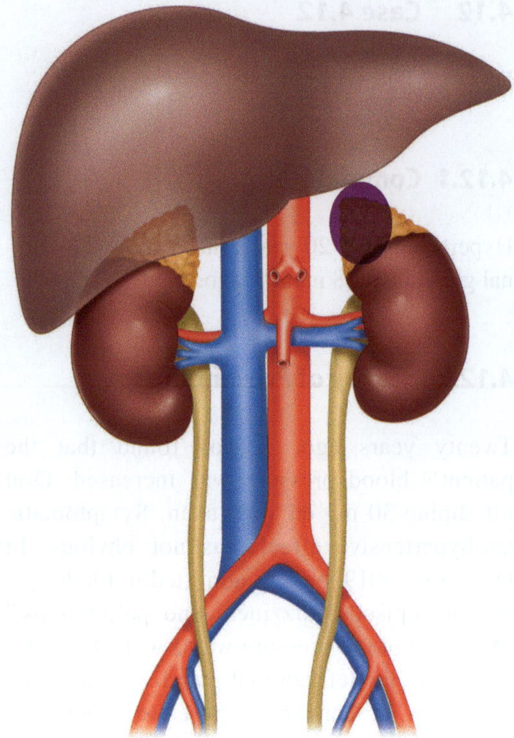

Fig. 4.30 Schematic diagram of the location of the mass

4.13 Case 4.13

Patient: Male, 40 years old.

4.13.1 Complaints

Episodic headache for more than 2 years. A tumor was found to occupy the right adrenal gland 9 months ago.

4.13.2 History of Present Illness

In November 2017, he developed headache with palpitations, a feeling of imminent death, and pallor in the face during a laborious defecation. The symptoms lasted about 1 1/2 min and then subsided. Since 2018, patient has had recurrent episodic headaches. He feels that the degree of pain has intensified, the frequency of attacks has increased, and the duration has prolonged, but the headache resolves on its own. Blood pressure and heart rate have not been measured. He has not paid attention to diagnosis and treatment.

In October 2019, the Department of Stomatology accidentally found in him an increased blood pressure of 220/150 mmHg. Nifedipine extended-release tablets and diltiazem extended-release capsules were successively given to control blood pressure. The effect was not obvious. In November 2019, he visited the China-Japan Friendship Hospital, and his adrenal gland was scanned. An isometric mass in the right adrenal gland of 42 mm × 43 mm with calcification was found.

Further endocrine tests were done.

24-h urinary catecholamines: 24 h Urine methoxephrine 4313 nmol/24 h↑ (<216), methoxy-norepinephrodine glands 3298 nmol/24 h↑(<312), 3-methoxytyramine 480 nmol/24 h↑ (<382).

24-h urine output: 1450 mL.

Blood methoxyephrine 3.31 nmol/L↑ (≤0.5), methoxy-norepinephrodine glands 6.33 nmol/L↑ (≤0.90).

"Trazosin 1 mg qn + diltiazem 90 mg bid" were given to control blood pressure. Blood pressure was controlled at 150–180/90–100 mmHg. Heart rate fluctuated in 60–105 times/min. Self-conscious headache, dizziness, and pain have improved.

In December of 2019, I-MIBG imaging in our hospital suggested a hypertrophic lesion of abnormal radiation in the right adrenal region. Pheochromocytoma is highly probable. The drug was changed to phenol benzylamine 10 mg three times/day for oral preparation before surgery. In July of 2020, he again visited our hospital and was admitted to undergo surgical treatment. Endocrine assessment indicated that he was not yet fully prepared, so he was discharged from the hospital to make endocrinologic adjustments. In October of 2020, he was hospitalized in endocrinology for 1 month, and treatment was gradually adjusted to phenol benzylamine 20 mg qid and nifedipine 30 mg bid. He was transferred to our department for surgery.

4.13.3 Past, Personal, Marital and Childbearing, Family History

Nothing special.

4.13.4 Accessory Examination

Abdominal pelvic enhanced CT + adrenal thin scan (Fig. 4.31): Adrenal CT shows an isometric mass in the edge of the right adrenal of 42 mm × 43 mm with calcification foci. The enhanced scan shows an uneven strengthening of the tumor.

3D visualization reconstruction (Fig. 4.32a–d): a 42 mm × 43 mm mass of the right adrenal gland, which is closely related to the surrounding organs and blood vessels.

Renal function of blood flow imaging: right kidney = 31.26 mL/min · 1.73 m^2, left kidney = 34.25 mL/min · 1.73 m^2.

Echocardiography: ejection fraction of 64%, widening of the ascending aorta, thickening of the aortic valve, and mild aortic valve insufficiency.

Blood: HGB 152 g/L, HCT 44.9%, PLT 248 × 109/L, WBC 5.92 × 109/L, NEUT% 65.3%.

Glucose fasting: 8–9 mmol/L, about 9–10 mmol/L after meals (metformin 0.5 g three times/day), myocardial enzyme profile (−).

A 42 mm × 43 mm mass in the right adrenal gland, which is closely related to the surrounding organs and blood vessels.

4.13.5 Current Diagnoses

Right adrenal pheochromocytoma.

Hypertension (grade 3, very high risk).

Diabetes.

Gallbladder stones.

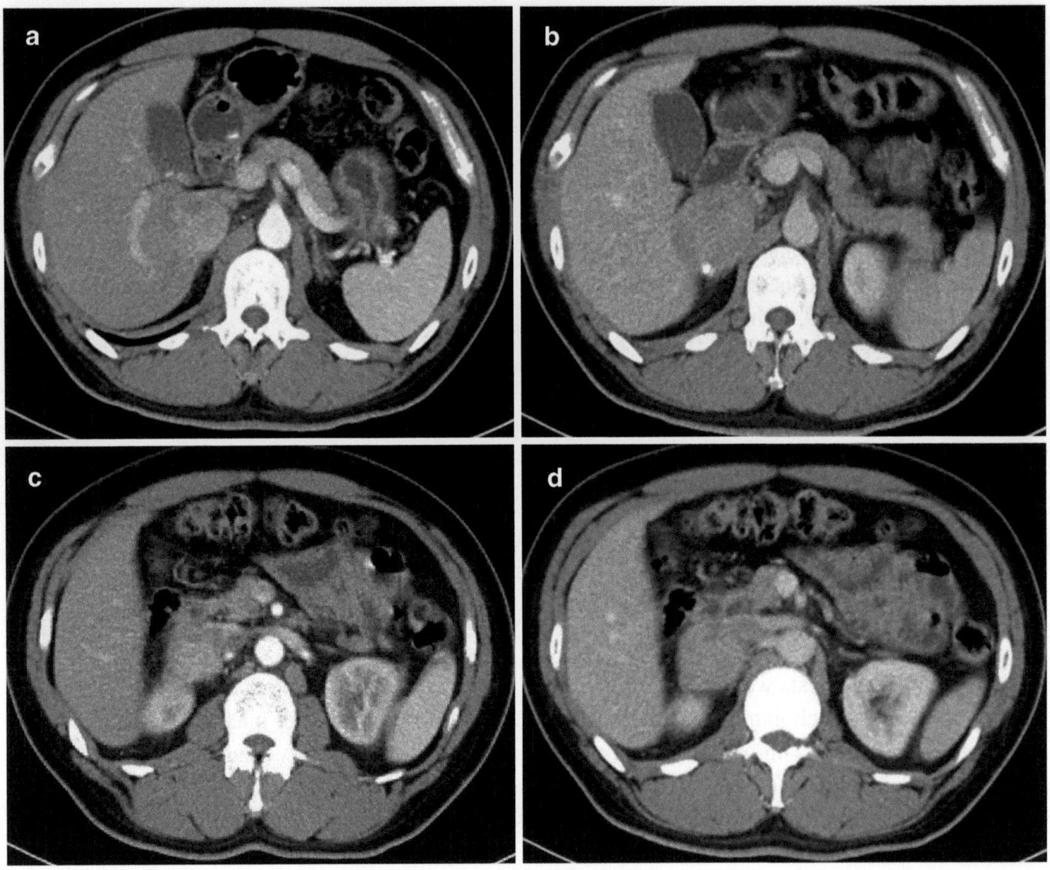

Fig. 4.31 Abdominal pelvis enhanced CT. (**a–d**) Adrenal CT shows an isometric mass of 42 mmx43 mm with calcification foci in the edge of the right adrenal gland. The enhanced scan shows an uneven strengthening of the tumor

4.13.6 MDT Discussion

4.13.6.1 Ophthalmology

No obvious abnormalities are seen in the fundus, and follow-up consultation is recommended.

4.13.6.2 Urology

(1) Patient complains of previous allergies to crabs but did not have obvious allergy symptoms from recent intake of river crabs, sea crabs, and seafood. It is recommended to re-check the abdominal pelvis enhanced CT + adrenal thin scan to further evaluate the lesions. (2) Continue to prepare for pheochromocytoma surgery; (3) follow up in our department.

4.13.6.3 Clinical Nutrition

Patient found that blood glucose increased last year. Lifestyle intervention was taken. High blood glucose on fasting was noticed. Blood glucose was acceptable after meals. At the end of August, patient began oral metformin to control blood glucose. FBG was 6.3–9.2 mmol/L. 2hPBG was 7.0–16.5 mmol/L. Diet adjustments were proposed. Diet review: basically follow the principle of low GI diet. Due to high blood pressure and palpitations, human activity was mainly walking. Patient's height was 184 cm, weight 89.5 kg, and BMI 26.4 kg/m^2. Weight loss of 1–2 kg was found after admission.

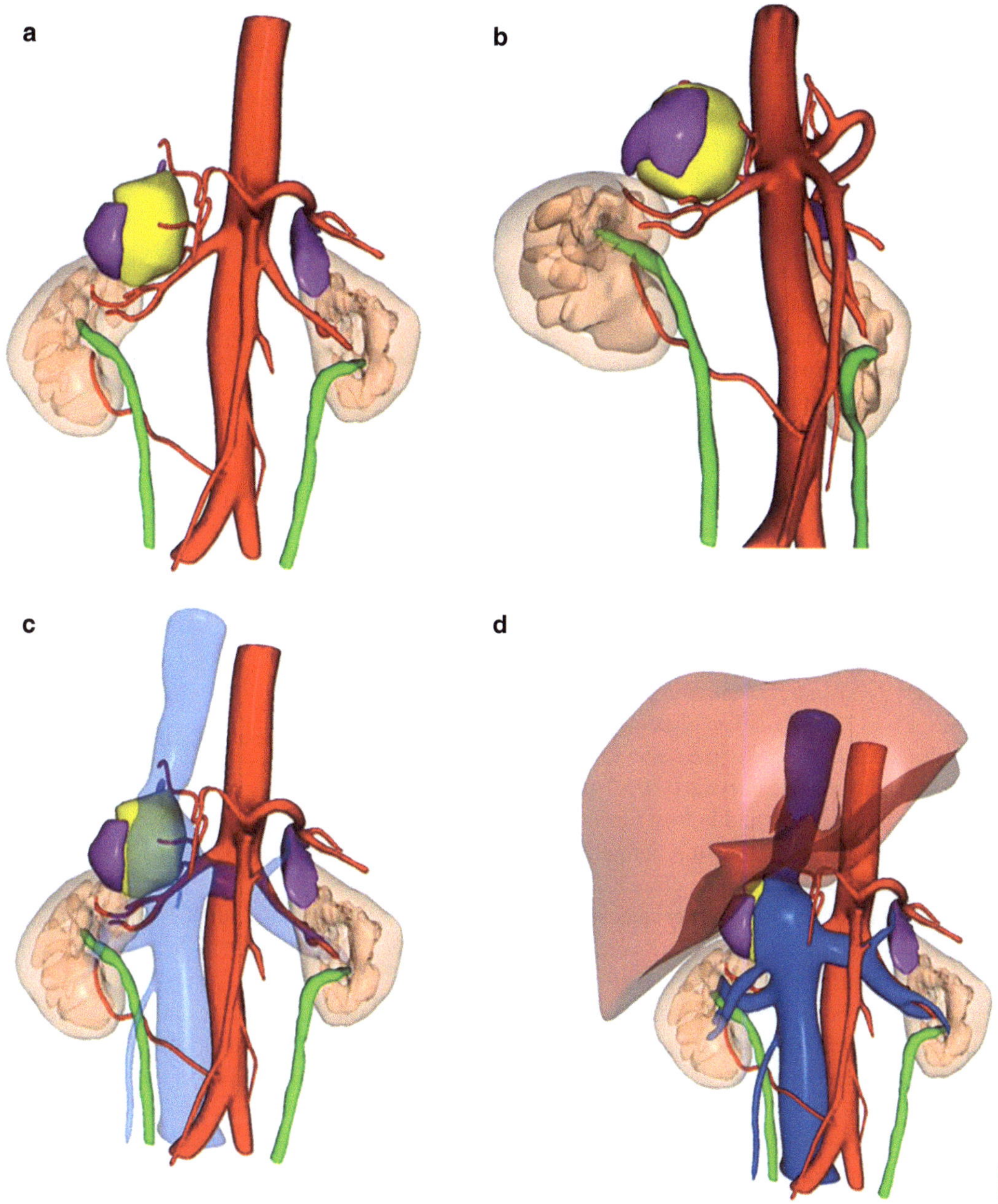

Fig. 4.32 3D visualization reconstruction. (**a**–**d**) A 42mm x 43mm mass in the right adrenal gland, closely related to surrounding organs and blood vessels

Recommendations: (1) Besides education, small amount of multiple meals is preferred, as well as appropriate weight loss up to 85 kg, low GI diet, and daily energy 2200 kcal. Daily staple food: 200 g (raw weight). Do not eat oiled staple food and stuffing staple food. Do not take porridge. Daily meat: 250 g (raw weight). Do not eat fat meat and animal skin. Do not drink animal soup. Patient can only take one egg, low-fat or skim milk of 500 mL, and low-sugar low-fat yogurt of 150G as snacks. Vegetables of 500 g with mainly leaves are necessary. Eat melons and other fruits of 200 g between meals. Cooking oil of 30 g is consumed with vegetable oil based on unsaturated fatty acids. (2) The patient is advised to eat less of, or if possible avoid, the following:

sweets, drinks, animal offal, fried food, barbecue, spicy and hot food, etc. (3) Twenty minutes of sports after each meal are conducted with mainly walking. After blood pressure is stable, slight strenuous activities can be carried out. (4) Monitor blood sugar and weight. Record dietary diary, and adjust diet in our department after 2–3 months.

4.13.6.4 Department of Anesthesiology

(1) Young men, diabetes mellitus, metformin control, fasting blood glucose 7–10, postprandial 6–12. (2) The diagnosis of pheochromocytoma is clear (24-h urinary catecholamines NE/E/DA are significantly increased, mainly NE/E). Under phenol benzylamine preparation for more than 2 months, patient has no obvious orthostatic hypotension, supine blood pressure within 107–140/70–90 mmHg, standing blood pressure within 90–140/60–90 mmHg, and heart rate 70–90 bpm. Nasal congestion, warm extremities, and sweaty hands are present. Weight gain is not obvious. (3) ECG (−). Cardiac ultrasound: widening of the aorta, thickening of the aortic valve; high CK, residual myocardial enzyme (−), NT-proBNP (−). Blood routine: liver and kidney functions are generally normal. Lung function is normal.

Treatment: (1) Continue the current monitoring and treatment. (2) 24-h urinary catecholamine NE/E is significantly elevated. Perioperative catecholamine crisis is a high risk. Please fully communicate with the family. (3) Department should prepare for invasive arterial monitoring and placement of central venous catheters and vasoactive drugs to cope with hemodynamic fluctuations. (4) Because there is a risk for major bleeding, please contact the blood bank to prepare blood transfusion, and our department will prepare the device of blood return transfusion. (5) Return patient to the ICU after surgery.

4.13.7 Surgical Approach

3D laparoscopic resection of right adrenal pheochromocytoma (Fig. 4.33).

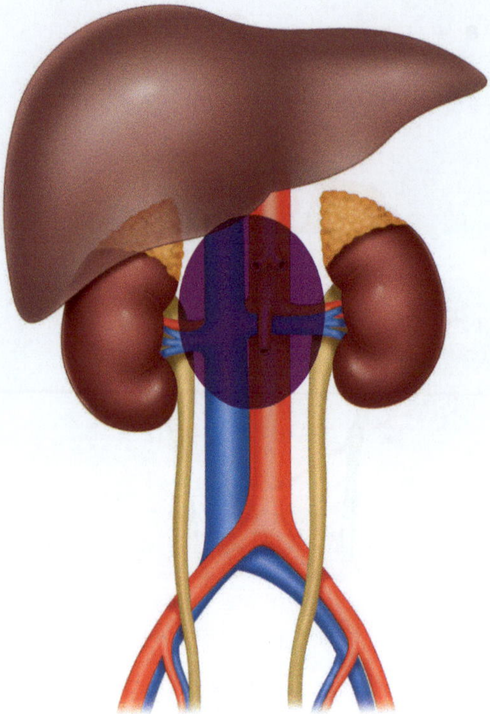

Fig. 4.33 Schematic diagram of the location of the mass

4.13.8 Postoperative Pathology

(Right adrenal tumor) adrenal pheochromocytoma. Calcification is seen in the peripheral adrenal gland.

Immunohistochemical results: Melan-A(−), AE1/AE3(weak+), CgA(+), Ki-67(index 5%), S-100(+), α-inhibin(−).

4.14 Case 4.14

Patient: Male, 36 years old.

4.14.1 Complaints

Physical examination revealed a mass in the left adrenal region more than 3 months ago.

4.14.2 History of Present Illness

On October 12, 2019, during the patient's physical examination, CT found a circular mass of moderate density in the left adrenal gland, about 6 cm in diameter, and a type of circular low-density lesions was seen inside. There were no previous episodic headaches, sweating, black haze, etc.

In November 2019, patient visited our hospital for endocrine examination, abdominal pelvic enhanced CT, somatostatin receptor imaging, and 24 h urinary catecholamine test. On November 18, 2019, NE was 56.93 μg/24 h↑ (16–40 μg/24 h). On December 9, 2019, results are the following: NE 41.41 μg/24 h↑. Blood catecholamine metabolites on November 13, 2019 showed the following: NMN 27.21 nmol/L↑ (<0.9). December 24, 2019: 20.20 nmol/L↑ (<0.9). CT of the abdominal pelvis found a round tumor with an uneven density found in the left adrenal region. The morphology is still regular, and the maximum cross-section of the lesion is about 75 mm × 65 mm. The outpatient department decided to admit him with left pheochromocytoma as diagnosis.

4.14.3 Past, Personal, Marital and Childbearing, Family History

Nothing special.

4.14.4 Accessory Examination

Abdominal pelvic enhanced CT (Fig. 4.34a, b): A mass of the uneven density can be seen in the left adrenal region. The morphology is still regular. The maximum cross-section of the lesion is about 75 mm × 65 mm. The enhanced scan is unevenly strengthened, and a circular lesion is visible inside. The pancreatic tail is pressed forward, and the spleen is adjacent to the lesion. Somatostatin receptor imaging: equivalent to masses of abnormally and unevenly elevated radioactive nuclide uptake in the left adrenal region. A neuroendocrine tumor is more probable.

4.14.5 Current Diagnosis

Left adrenal pheochromocytoma.

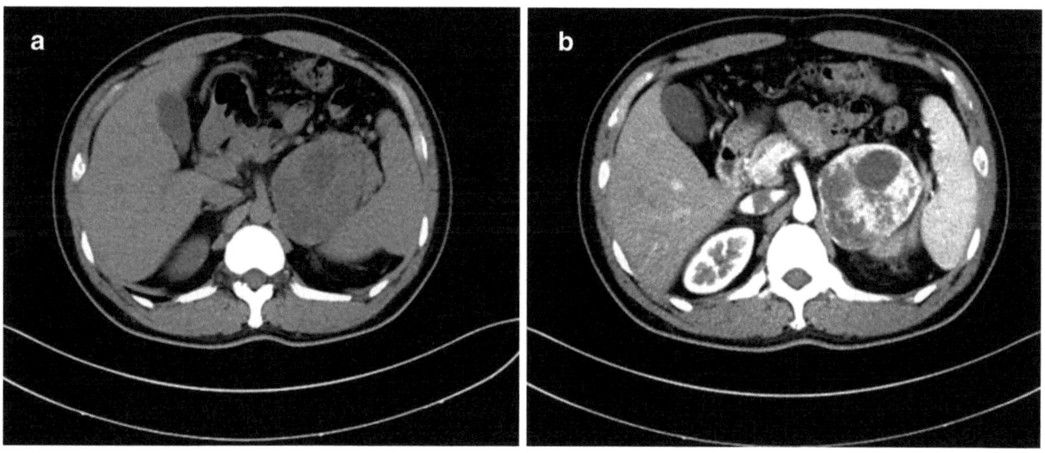

Fig. 4.34 Abdominal pelvic enhanced CT. (**a**, **b**) A mass of the uneven density can be seen in the left adrenal region. The morphology is still regular. The maximum cross-section of the lesion is about 75 mm × 65 mm. The enhanced scan is unevenly strengthened, and a circular lesion is visible inside. The pancreatic tail is pressed forward, and the spleen is adjacent to the lesion

4.14.6 MDT Discussion

4.14.6.1 Department of Critical Care Medicine

Male of 36 years old, due to left adrenal mass, is to undergo laparoscopic resection of left adrenal pheochromocytoma under general anesthesia. In the past, his physical health was good. There are no other chronic diseases such as coronary heart disease and diabetes. Recommendations: (1) Fully account for the surgical risks and related perioperative complications. (2) Closely monitor blood pressure and hemodynamic stability, ensure perioperative blood pressure stability, and ensure the perfusion of important organs such as the heart, brain, and kidneys. (3) Monitor and maintain electrolyte and internal environment stability. (4) Return the patient to the ICU after surgery.

4.14.6.2 Department of Anesthesiology

(1) Continue the current preparation of phenolic benzylamine, and please demand a consultation with endocrinology. (2) Closely monitor the risks for intraoperative hemodynamic fluctuations, major hemorrhage, cardiovascular and cerebrovascular events, etc. (3) Recommend returning to the ICU after surgery.

4.14.6.3 General Surgery

(1) Combining the patient's medical history, physical examination, and imaging, the left retroperitoneal mass is clear. Because the tumor is closely related to the pancreatic tail, the pressed push may be possible. There is also a possibility of invasion. (2) Preoperative explanation of the possibility of resection of pancreatic tail or splenectomy should be done.

4.14.6.4 Endocrinology

A thirty-six-year-old male patient was admitted to the hospital due to the discovery of an adrenal gland mass after a physical examination. The patient denied episodic headache, palpitations, and other discomforts but complained that the previous blood pressure measurement was normal. Three months ago, physical examination found that the left adrenal gland had a tumor with the size of about 6.8 cm × 5.7 cm. The abdominal pelvic enhanced CT suggested an uneven strengthening. Re-check the blood cortisol. RAAS assessment did not see obvious abnormalities. 24-h urinary catecholamines: NE 56.93 μg/24 h↑, E 5.69 μg/24 h, DA 290.07 μg/24 h. Plasma catecholamines and their metabolites: NMN 27.21 nmol/L↑, MN 0.17 nmol/L. On November 25, because of pheochromocytoma, phenol benzylamine 10 mg was added twice daily. On December 12, it was increased to 10 mg three times/day. On December 20, it was increased to 15 mg three times/day. After treatment of the drug, the patient experienced nasal congestion and increased sweating but no obvious headache and palpitations. The daily intake was 2–3 L. The stool was normal. The weight increase was about 2 kg. The lying blood pressure and heart rate were monitored after admission. The lying blood pressure was 111/57–62 mmHg, and the heart rate was 70–72 beats/min. The standing blood pressure was 106–115/59–69 mmHg, and the heart rate was 95–110 beats/min.

Management: (1) Monitor intake for 24 h, and ensure that the daily intake is greater than 3–4 L when allowed by cardiac function. Monitor weight, HCT, and stool. (2) The patient currently has no obvious orthostatic hypotension, but the difference in orthopedic heart rate is large, and HCT shows an upward trend. Because of the insufficient amount, instruct the patient to continue a high-sodium diet, increase the amount of fluid, and be vigilant against orthostatic hypotension. (3) Continue the current treatment of phenolic benzylamine. It is recommended to increase the amount of treatment after the recumbent heart rate is stable before the surgical treatment. (4) The patient's outpatient clinic has completed the screening of the MEN, and there is currently no evidence of MEN.

4.14.7 Surgical Approach

Laparoscopic resection of left adrenal pheochromocytoma under general anesthesia (Fig. 4.35).

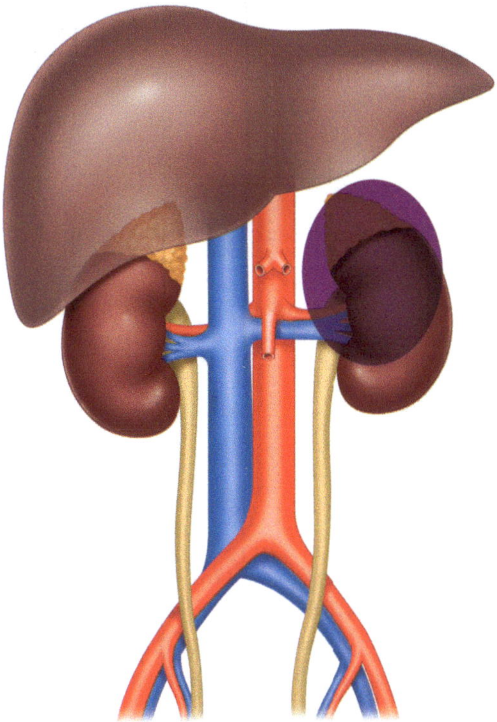

Fig. 4.35 Schematic diagram of the location of the mass

4.14.8 Postoperative Pathology

Lesions (left adrenal pheochromocytoma) are consistent with pheochromocytoma.

4.15 Case 4.15

Patient: Male, 12 years old.

4.15.1 Complaints

Elevated blood pressure had been found, accompanied by paroxysmal dizziness and palpitations for 2 years.

4.15.2 History of Present Illness

Two years ago, physical examination found that his blood pressure was increased to about 140/90 mmHg (the normal blood pressure of 12-year-old children is about 100/66 mmHg). There were episodic dizziness and palpitations. Symptoms were obvious when he changed in position, appearing two to three times a month. However, blood pressure and heart rate were not measured at the time of the attack. At the end of November 2020, ultrasound in the outer courtyard suggested a tumor in the right adrenal gland. On December 1, 2020, our hospital's results showed Blood NMN 14.74 nmol/L (15-fold increase), MN 0.18 nmol/L. 24 h urinary catecholamines: NE 208.16 μg/L/24 h, E 2.73 μg/L/24 h, DA 121.43 μg/L/24 h. Aldosterone, renin activity, angiotensin, ACTH, 24 h UFC, and DHEA sulfate were (−). Adrenal enhanced CT: a round mass of about 2.6 cm × 2 cm in size in the right adrenal region was found, which was significantly and unevenly strengthened. The enhancement started and disappeared quickly. The outpatient clinic decided to admit him with right pheochromocytoma.

4.15.3 Past, Personal, Marital and Childbearing, Family History (Fig. 4.36)

The patient's father, uncle, and cousin all suffer from pheochromocytoma. His father had a double adrenal pheochromocytoma, and the bilateral tumor was removed 10 years ago. He denies history of thyroid nodules and hypercalcemia.

4.15.4 Accessory Examination

Adrenal flat scan + enhanced CT (Fig. 4.37): A round mass of about 2.6 × 2 cm in size in the right adrenal region. MIBG: Mild elevation of radioactivity in the right adrenal region. Pheochromocytoma is considered.

A round mass of about 2.6 × 2 cm in size is found in the area of right adrenal gland. It is significantly strengthened. Local strengthening is uneven. Enhancement started and disappeared quickly.

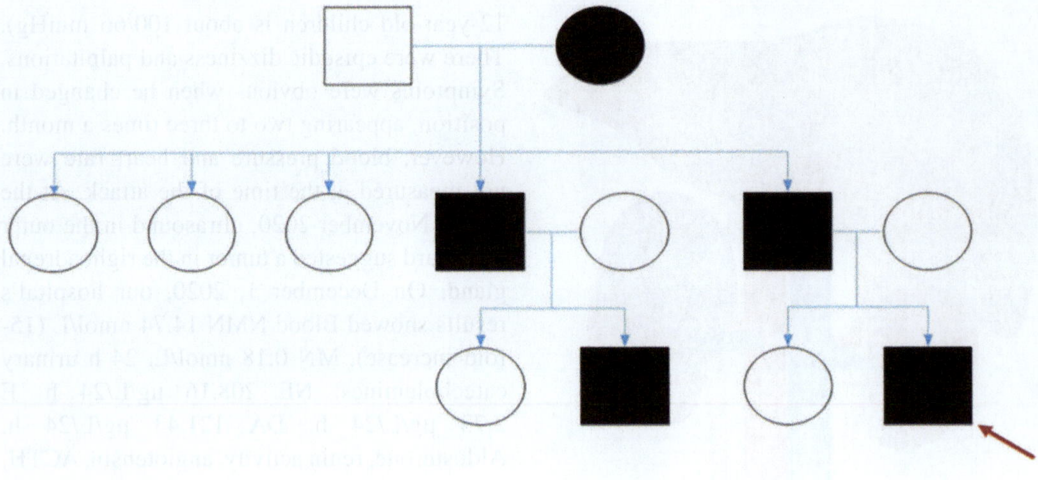

Fig. 4.36 Family history

4.15.5 Current Diagnoses

Right adrenal pheochromocytoma.

Hypertension.

Diabetes.

4.15.6 MDT Discussion

4.15.6.1 Intensive Care Medicine

Patient is a 12-year-old boy; due to increased blood pressure, a tumor was found in the right adrenal gland. He was hospitalized in January. Endocrine examination suggests pheochromocytoma. Currently under phenol benzylamine 5 mg bid × 9 days, 5 mg q8h × 9 days. After taking the drug, no episodic symptoms, mild nasal congestion, warm hands, weight gain of 1.5 kg, and HCT 41% → 38.7% were found. Supine blood pressure was 100–120/60–70 mmHg with a heart rate of 90–100 bpm. Standing blood pressure was 90–105/50–70 mmHg with a heart rate of 110–120 bpm. The resection of right adrenal pheochromocytoma is to be performed on Wednesday. He will return to the ICU after surgery.

4.15.6.2 Endocrinology

The patient's physical examination in 2019 found an increase in blood pressure, about 140/90 mmHg, with no further diagnosis and treatment. There was once a headache, palpitations, and sweating, which occurred during strenuous activity. Blood pressure was not measured. The symptoms were gradually relieved after the rest of about 1 h. The patient's physical examination in 2020 was checked again, and an increased blood pressure of 147/110 mmHg was found. HR was unknown. On November 11, 2020, in another hospital, abdominal ultrasound found a solid mass in right adrenal gland, which was about 30 × 22 mm in size. On December 1, 2020, patient was examined in our outpatient clinic. Blood examination: NMN 14.74 nmol/L, MN 18 nmol/L. 24 h urinary catecholamine: NE 208.16* urine volume (l) μg/24 h, E 2.73* μg/24 h, DA 121.43* μg/24 h. Abdominal/pelvic enhanced CT shows a round mass of soft tissue density in the right adrenal region with clear boundary, the larger section of 2.6 cm × 2.0 cm. It is significantly strengthened; local reinforcement is uneven. Fasting blood glucose is elevated (13.8 mmol/L). Because of the possibility of right adrenal pheochromocytoma, starting from December 18, 2020, to today, he takes phenolic benzylamine 5 mg bid, adjusted to phenol benzylamine 5 mg tid. Patient drinks about 2 L/day. Patient easts with a high-sodium and high-protein diet. He denies the following symptoms: episodic headache, palpitations, sweating, dizziness, palpitations, and blackout after position changes. No significant change in weight is found. Mild nasal congestion exists.

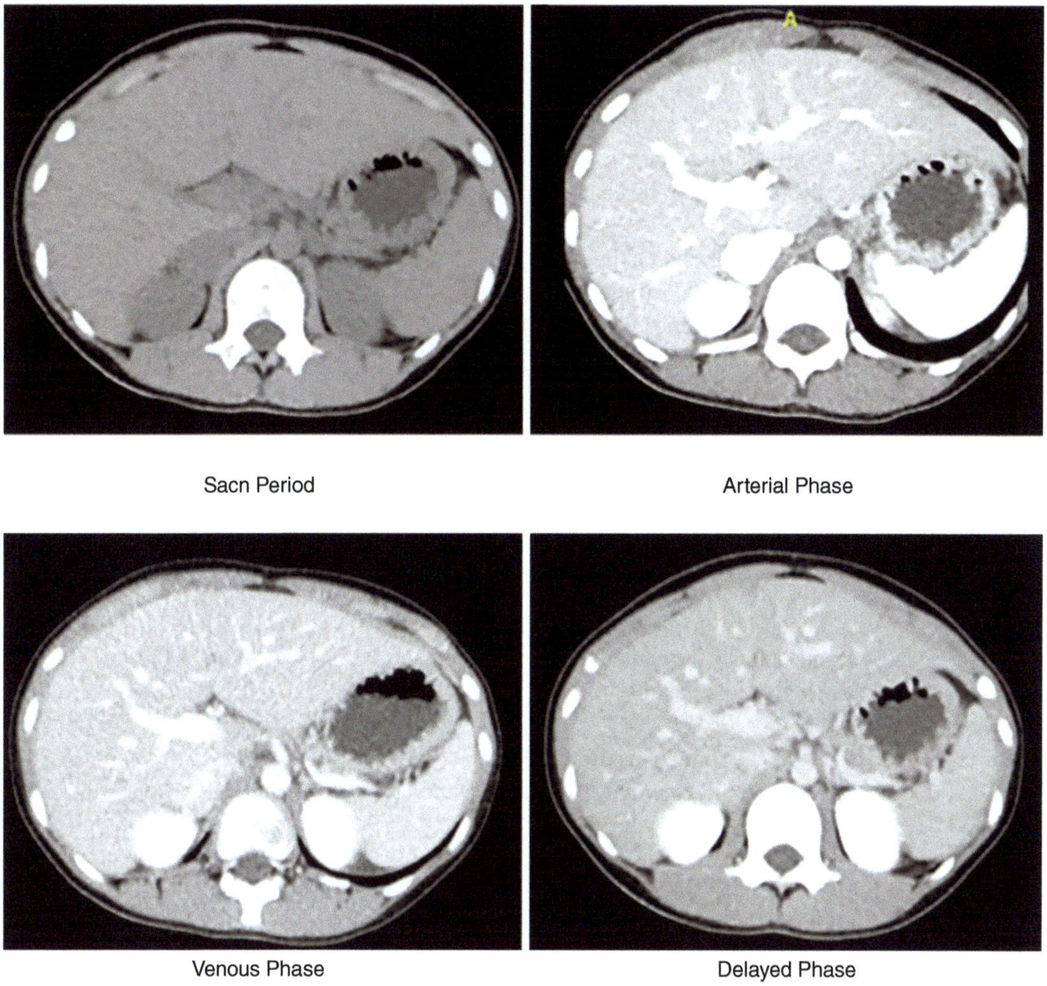

Fig. 4.37 Adrenal flat scan + enhanced CT

Patient denies a history of diabetes. He denies dry mouth, polyuria, and polydipsia. Elevated blood glucose was found after admission. Blood glucose spectrum was monitored: fasting 12.4–14.7 mmol/L and postprandial 19.3–21.4/9.9–18.2/18.8 mmol/L. He began to take ordinary insulin 6u tid from today.

Physical examination: Wt 35 kg, supine BP 110–125/65–76 mmHg, HR 103–116 bpm, standing BP 80–106/44–63 mmHg, HR 133–165 bpm, warm extremities, sweating, no swelling of the thyroid area, no milk coffee spots on the skin of the whole body. Accessory examination: HCT 41.0% ALT 25 U/L Cr(E) 40 μmol/L Glu 12.5 mmol/L Ca 2.48 mmol/L NT-proBNP 9 pg/mL. Urine routine: GLU 28 mmol/L, residual negative.

Management Opinions:

1. Ensure high-sodium and high-protein diet and the amount. If there is no contraindication, ensure that the daily dose is greater than 2000 mL. Monitor blood pressure and heart rate at least two times a day in the recumbent position; monitor intake and output, weight, and stool conditions every day, and measure HCT once a week. Avoid increasing abdominal pressure such as pressing the abdomen and straining stool, and avoid taking drugs such as for gastric reassurance and morphine.
2. Re-check 24-h urinary catecholamines. Patient currently has controlled blood pressure, but the heart rate is fast, and orthostatic hypotension is more obvious. Considering

that the preoperative preparation is insufficient, it is recommended to continue phenol benzylamine 5 mg q8h and to continue to strengthen volume. If necessary, saline or colloidal intravenous infusion can be given to improve volume. Closely monitor the changes in supine blood pressure.

3. In terms of diabetes, re-check the fasting and postprandial blood glucose, C-peptide, and type 1 diabetes-related antibody profile examination to further screen the cause of diabetes. In terms of treatment, ordinary insulin 6u tid ih can be continued with the addition of Novolin N 6u qn. Monitor the blood glucose spectrum. Control objectives are as follows: fasting 4–7 mmol/L, less than 10 mmol/L, and, after meals, HbA1c less than 7%. To avoid hypoglycemia, adjust the amount of ordinary insulin according to postprandial blood glucose, and adjust the amount of Novolin N according to fasting blood glucose.
4. Re-check PTH, blood calcium, phosphorus, 25-hydroxyvitamin D (rapid immunization method), calcitonin, CEA, thyroid ultrasound, glucagon, gastrin, prolactin, GH, IGF1, and thyroid function 1 to exclude MEN.
5. Demand consultations with the ICU and the Department of Anesthesiology for perioperative diagnosis and treatment.
6. The risk of surgery is extremely high, and the risk of surgery is fully explained to the patient.

4.15.7 Surgical Approach

Laparoscopic resection of right adrenal pheochromocytoma (Fig. 4.38).

4.15.8 Postoperative Pathology

(Right adrenal mass) adrenal pheochromocytoma is considered.

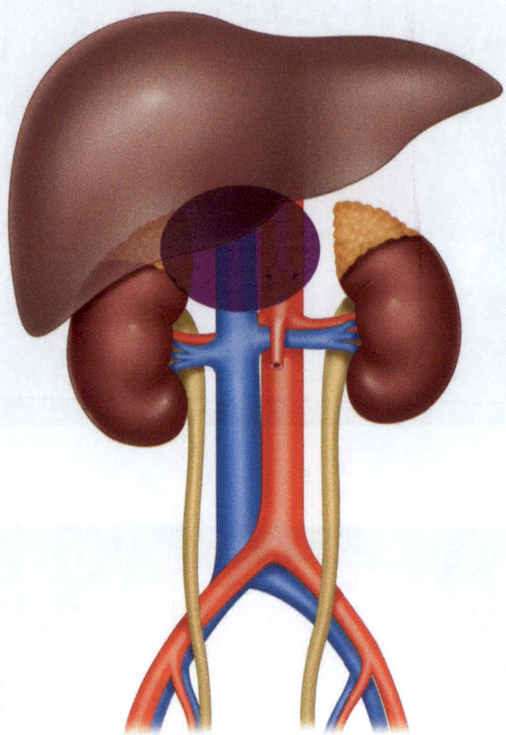

Fig. 4.38 Schematic diagram of the location of the mass

4.16 Case 4.16

Patient: Female, 61 years old.

4.16.1 Complaints

Examination has revealed a tumor of the left adrenal gland for 3 years.

4.16.2 History of Present Illness

The patient was found to have a tumor of the left adrenal gland in the outer hospital 3 years ago, with a size of about 1.7 cm, denying palpitations, sweating, dizziness, and headache and no limb weakness.

4.16.3 Past, Personal, Marital and Childbearing, Family History

Nothing special.

4.16.4 Accessory Examination

MRI in other hospital: a mass of 2.6 cm in the left adrenal gland area found.

Adrenal enhanced CT (Fig. 4.39): a circular mass of about 2.1 × 1.8 cm in size in the left adrenal gland area, which is significantly and unevenly strengthened. The enhancement appears and disappears quickly.

Endocrine examination: Blood NMN 1.01 nmol/L, MN 0.99 nmol/L. 24 h urinary catecholamines: NE 74.64 μg/L/24 h, E 4.88 μg/L/24 h, DA 188.93 μg/L/24 h. Aldosterone, renin activity, angiotensin, ACTH, 24 h UFC, DHEA sulfate are (−).

MIBG: elevated radioactivity in the left adrenal region. Pheochromocytoma is considered.

A round tumor of about 2.1 cm in size in the left adrenal gland, which is significantly and unevenly strengthened; the enhancement appears and disappears quickly.

4.16.5 Current Diagnosis

Left adrenal pheochromocytoma.

4.16.6 MDT Discussion

4.16.6.1 The Department of Critical Medicine

The fluctuations of perioperative blood pressure and high risk of bleeding are fully accounted for the patient. If she needs to return to the ICU after surgery, it is necessary to submit online the relevant information on epidemic

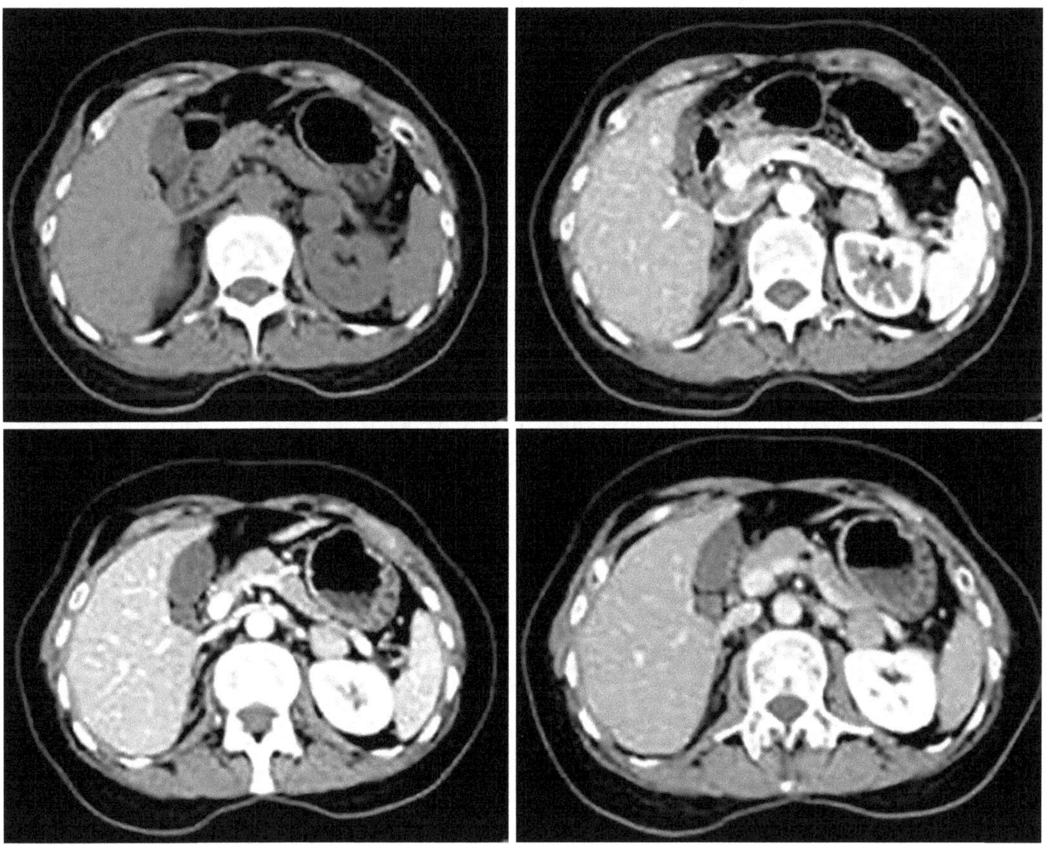

Fig. 4.39 Adrenal flat scan + enhanced CT

prevention and control in advance and to contact our department before surgery to reserve a bed.

4.16.6.2 Department of Anesthesiology

Elderly woman with left adrenal pheochromocytoma. Laparoscopic resection of left adrenal tumor resection is planned. Ordinarily healthy, she can walk for 2 km on flat road. She denies precordial discomfort, black syncope, and coughing up sputum and asthma. She is allergic to penicillin. To prepare for surgery, she has taken phenol benzylamine 5 mg two times/day for 11 days. The following are found: warm extremities, no significant change in weight, no nasal congestion; fluctuations of recumbent blood pressure at 123–98/75–56 mmHg with fluctuations of heart rate at 65–85 bpm, fluctuations of standing blood pressure at 134–86/75–60 mmHg with fluctuations of heart rate at 81–110 bpm; and denial of orthostatic hypotension. PE: Quick response to question with a clear conscience. Heart and lungs are normal. Accessory examination: ECG, 24 h urinary catecholamines, myocardial enzyme profile, NT-proBNP, and coagulation are normal. 3-NMN 0.99 (<0.9), 3-MN 1.01 (<0.5), Hct 34.5%, and Hb 114 g/L. The result of cardiac ultrasound has not been received.

Management opinion: There may be a pheochromopsis crisis during perioperative period, resulting in cardiovascular and cerebrovascular events including ACS, cardio-cerebral and renal hypoperfusion, malignant arrhythmias, heart failure, cerebral infarction, etc. Please fully explain with the patient and the family the risks during surgery. Depending on the intraoperative situation, she will return to the ICU after surgery.

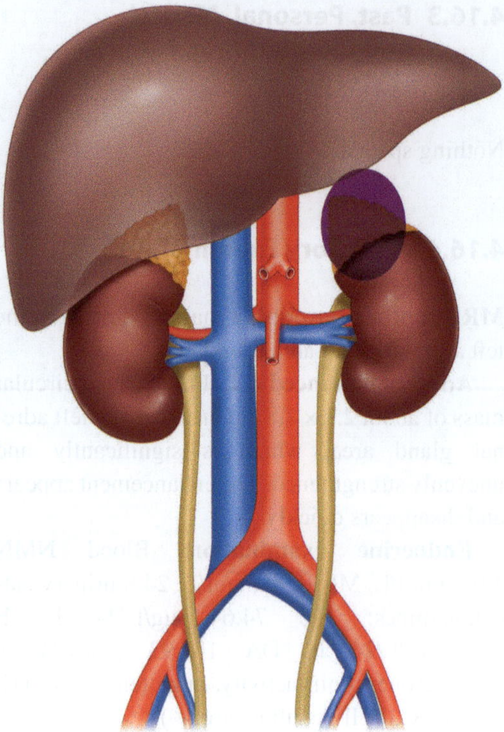

Fig. 4.40 Schematic diagram of tumor location

4.16.7 Surgical Approach

Laparoscopic resection of left adrenal pheochromocytoma under general anesthesia (Fig. 4.40).

4.16.8 Postoperative Pathology

Left adrenal pheochromocytoma.

Immunohistochemical results: Melan-A(−), AE1/AE3(−), CgA(+), Ki-67(index 1%), S-100(+), α-inhibin(−), Syn(+), SDHB(+).

Multidisciplinary Treatment of Paragangliomas in the Vascular Area of the Epigastric Region

5

Guang Hua Liu, Yi Zhao, Jin Wen, Zhi En Zhou, GuoYang Zheng, Yang Zhao, Ting Kai Yang, Xin Zhao, Wei Feng Xu, and Qing Zhen Wen

Guang Hua Liu and Yi Zhao contributed equally to this work.

5.1 Case 5.1

Patient: Female, 51 years old

5.1.1 Complaints

Paroxysmal palpitations and an increased blood pressure for 15 years and tumors in the left adrenal region found for 15 years

5.1.2 History of Present Illness

Fifteen years ago, with no obvious precipitating cause, patient suffered from paroxysmal palpitations and headache, accompanied by heavy sweating. The symptoms were more obvious when excited with emotional agitations. Blood pressure was increased at the time of the attack, up to 200/130 mmHg. Ultrasound in the outer hospital showed an abdominal mass (no report was seen). She did not take a further diagnosis and treatment. Ten years ago, the patient redeveloped the above symptoms when she was emotionally agitated and then experienced nausea, vomiting, and loss of consciousness. Ultrasonography showed a 10.0 cm × 9.7 cm cyst-solid mixed echo inside the spleen. She underwent laparotomy in the outer hospital. Because the patient's blood pressure and heart rate changed greatly when the tumor body was touched, no further resection of tumor was carried out. Two months ago, headache, palpitations, and hyperhidrosis worsened than before, and she came to our hospital.

5.1.3 Past, Personal, Marital and Childbearing, and Familial History

Diabetes mellitus for more than 6 years, history of surgery of caesarean section, history of laparotomic exploration surgery

5.1.4 Accessory Examination

Abdominal enhanced CT (Figs. 5.1, 5.2, and 5.3): A large mass shadow of uneven soft tissue in the left splenic-renal area and adrenal region. The

Guang Hua Liu and Yi Zhao contributed equally with all other contributors.

G. H. Liu · Y. Zhao · J. Wen (✉) · Z. E. Zhou · G. Zheng · Y. Zhao · T. K. Yang · X. Zhao · W. F. Xu · Q. Z. Wen
Department of Urology, Peking Union Medical College Hospital, Beijing, China

J. Wen (ed.), *Surgical Management of Pheochromocytoma and Retroperitoneal Paraganglioma*, https://doi.org/10.1007/978-981-99-8421-3_5

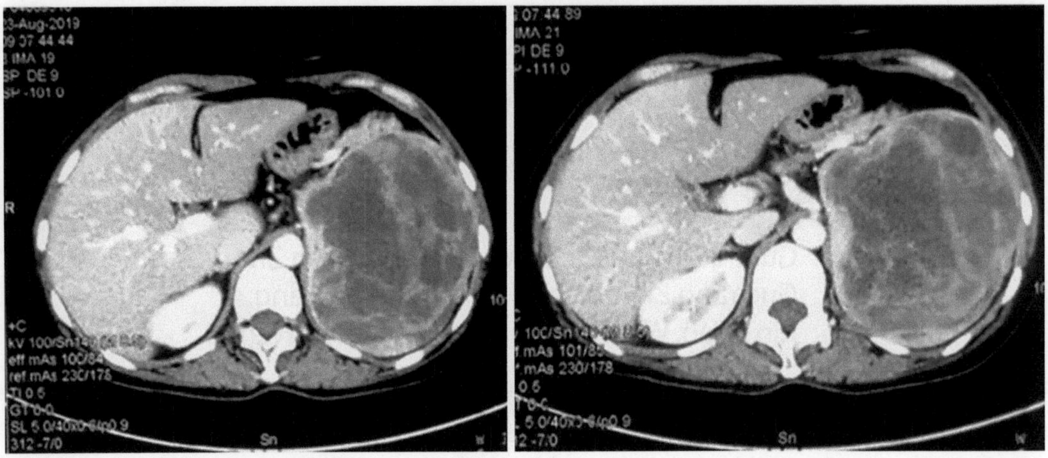

Fig. 5.1 Adrenal flat scan + enhanced CT

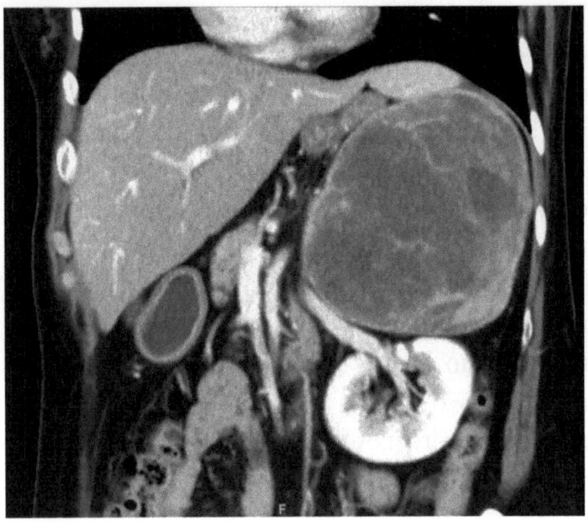

Fig. 5.2 CTA

scan finds multiple opacities of flocculent high density inside the tumor. The boundary is still clear. The left adrenal gland is not shown. The lesion ranges about 11.2 cm × 12.8 cm × 11.3 cm. The occupying effect is obvious, and the surrounding organs (pancreatic tail, spleen, and left kidney) are pressed and pushed. The tumor and the fat gap around the above organs are still visible. The tumor is unevenly strengthened after the enhancement. The internal multi-plaque patches are always weakly strengthened. CAT shows that the artery of peritoneal stem emits small branches into the tumor. The distal segment of the splenic artery is localized with a neoplastic protrusion. The edges are seen in arc calcification and crescent-shaped filling defects. The fish-hook-like changes are seen at the beginning of artery of the abdominal stem. The lumen is severely narrowed, and the distal main lumen is slightly expanded. Splenic vein is pushed and shifted.

Endocrine examination: Blood NMN 5.33 nmol/L↑, MN 19.84 nmol/L↑, 24-h urinary catecholamines/NE 55.89 μg/24 h↑, E 76.49 μg/24 h↑; somatostatin receptor imaging: lesions of high expression of somatostatin receptors in the left upper abdomen; 131I-MIBG: a giant mass of abnormal and unevenly increased radioemouption in the left mid-upper abdomen. Pheochromocytoma is considered.

A large mass shadow of uneven soft tissue in the left splenic-renal area and adrenal region. The scan finds multiple opacities of flocculent high-density inside the tumor. The boundary is still clear. The left adrenal gland is not shown. The lesion ranges about 11.2 cm × 12.8 cm × 11.3 cm. The occupying effect is obvious, and the surrounding organs (pancreatic tail, spleen, and left kidney) are pressed and pushed. The tumor and the fat gap around the above organs are still visible. The tumor is unevenly strengthened after the enhancement. The internal multi-plaque patches are always weakly strengthened.

CAT shows that the artery of peritoneal stem emits small branches into the tumor. The distal segment of the splenic artery is localized with a

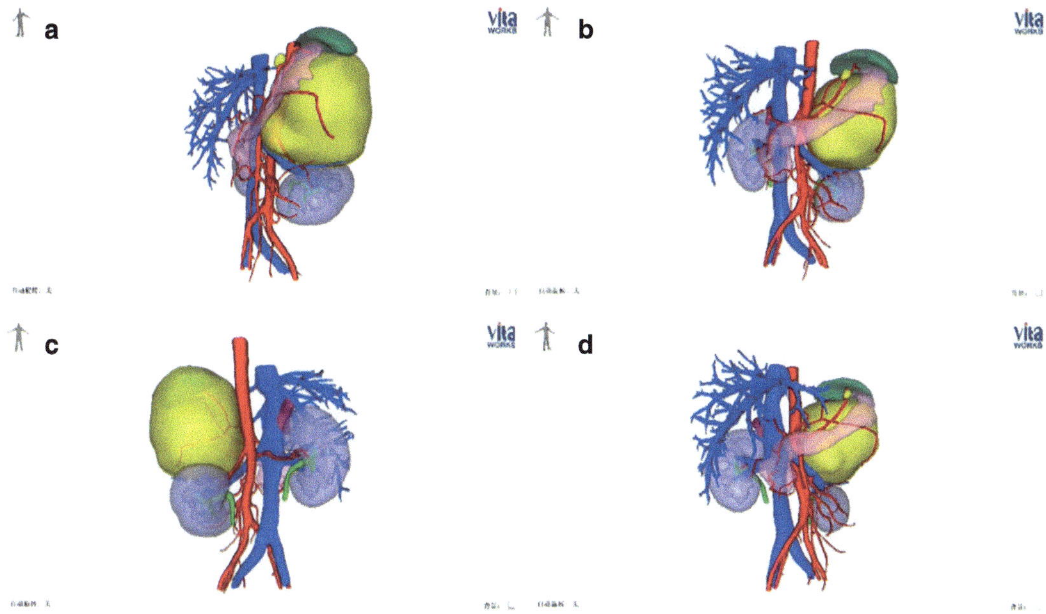

Fig. 5.3 3D visualization image of reconstruction (**a**–**d**)

neoplastic protrusion. The edges are seen in arc calcification and crescent-shaped filling defects. The fish-hook-like changes are seen at the beginning of artery of the abdominal stem. The lumen is severely narrowed, and the distal main lumen is slightly expanded. Splenic vein is pushed and shifted.

5.1.5 Current Diagnoses

Left adrenal pheochromocytoma
 Hypertension
 Type 2 Diabetes
 Past caesarean section
 Post-laparotomy

5.1.6 MDT Discussion

5.1.6.1 General Surgery

Account for the preoperative risk of surgery. The joint resection of intraoperative organ may be performed. If splenectomy is performed, postoperative fever, platelet elevation, and oral anticoagulants are required. If pancreatic tail resection is performed, postoperative blood glucose control is poor, and insulin needs to be added. Postoperative pancreatic fistula needs long-term drainage tube. Long-term fasting, abdominal infection, and abdominal bleeding may occur. If partial colectomy is performed during surgery, there may be intestinal fistula, anastomotic stenosis, and anastomotic bleeding. Secondary surgery or interventional treatment may be performed.

Intestinal preparation is required before surgery. If a doctor in our department is needed to assist during the operation, contact by phone.

5.1.6.2 Department of Anesthesiology

It is recommended to continue to optimize preoperative preparation. There was an increase in cTnI in September of 2019, and it is recommended to re-check it again. For anesthesia, it is according to the routine preparation of pheochromocytoma. The establishment of arteriovenous passage and the preparation of vascular active drugs are needed. During operation, the monitoring of changes in vital signs during surgery, the maintenance of myocardial oxygen supply and oxygen consumption balance and the guarantee of important organ perfusion are necessary. Fully explain the risk of perioperative cardiovascular and cerebrovascular accidents and major bleeding. Pay attention to the fluctuations of blood glucose, maintain water-electrolyte balance, adequately prepare blood transfusion, and recommend returning to the ICU after surgery.

5.1.6.3 Endocrinology

Take diabetic diet. Control the daily staple food within 300 g. Avoid sweet and liquid food. Please consult the nutrition department to guide the diet. Increase the daily water intake >2 L and the total daily intake >4 L, and monitor the intake and output and weight changes. If the condition allows, take proper physical activities in ground. Be careful to avoid strenuous exercise, emotional agitation, fatigue, and other triggers.

The patient's supine blood pressure is still high. The difference in recumbent blood pressure is still large. The recumbent heart rate is still fast. The monitoring HCT level is higher than before. It is recommended to increase phenol benzylamine to 10 mg one time/8 h. In the meantime, enhancing nutrition and actively increasing the amount are recommended. Closely monitor the recumbent blood pressure and heart rate (at least two times a day), and regularly re-check HCT. The Department of Anesthesiology and ICU are consulted preoperatively to assess surgical risks and closely monitor vital signs during the perioperative period. According to the patient's current blood glucose, treatment with Gwart 0.5 g three times/day and acarbose 50 mg three times/day can be maintained. Monitor blood glucose. The goals of blood glucose control are FBG 4-7 mmol/L and PBG 6-10 mmol/L. If the blood glucose is not up to standard level after a meal, the amount of acarbose can be increased with the meal to 100 mg. If drinking water is prohibited during the perioperative period, oral hypoglycemic drugs are discontinued 24 h before surgery. Intravenous fluids are given with glucose in the liquid: insulin = 2–3 g: 1 U. Blood glucose in the circulation is controlled within 7–11 mmol/L.

If headache, palpitations, sweating, and increased blood pressure occur, re-check 24-h urinary catecholamine on the day of attack and control day to assist in definitive diagnosis. Avoid the use of drugs such as gastric reassurance, morphine, and Betalek. Avoid squeezing the neck mass, and be wary of pheochromocytoma crisis.

5.1.6.4 Department of Critical Medicine

Fully explain the surgical risks and related perioperative complications. Closely monitor blood pressure and hemodynamic stability. Ensure the stability of perioperative blood pressure. Ensure the perfusion of important organs such as the heart, brain, and kidneys. Maintain the stability of electrolytes and internal environment.

5.1.6.5 Urology

The patient was a 51-year-old woman who had paroxysmal palpitations and an increased blood pressure 15 years ago. The symptoms were more obvious when excited with emotional agitations. Ten years ago, due to syncope at the time of the attack, she underwent a laparotomy in the outer hospital, but the operation was stopped because of the fluctuation of intraoperative blood pressure and heart rate. Two months ago, the patient felt that the symptoms were worsened and came to our hospital. In the outpatient consultation, blood examination, urinary catecholamines, and their metabolites were more than ten times higher than normal, mainly with increased epinephrine. MIBG and somatostatin receptor imaging were positive. Abdominal enhanced CT showed a large mass shadow of uneven soft tissue in the left splenic-renal space and adrenal region. The lesion was about 11.2 cm × 12.8 cm × 11.3 cm. The diagnosis of left adrenal pheochromocytoma was basically clear. The patient has taken phenolic benzylamine 10 mg q12h in preparation since March and today changed to 10 mg q8h and intends to undergo surgery in the near future.

- Prof. Zhang Yushi: Based on the patient's symptoms, signs, and relevant accessory examinations, the diagnosis of pheochromocytoma is basically clear. Due to the large size of the tumor, its close relationship to peripheral organs such as the spleen, pancreas, etc., its close relationship to the blood vessels such as the splenic artery, and the more serious adhesions of the abdominal organs because of an laparotomy 10 years ago, the open surgery can be performed through the original laparotomy incision. The surgeon should pay

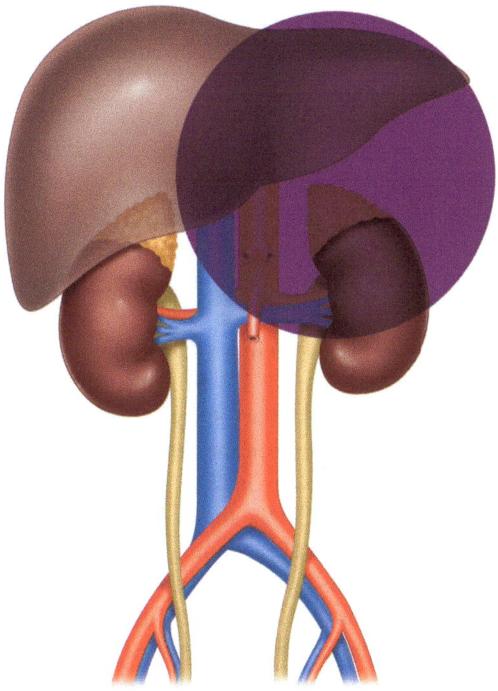

Fig. 5.4 Schematic diagram of the location of the mass

attention to meticulous dissection and be vigilant against the large amount of tumor rupture and bleeding and fully prepared before surgery.

– Professor Yan Weigang: Pay attention to fully explaining the risk of the disease to the patient before surgery, obtain informed consent, and sign an informed consent form. The open method of surgery may be more practical. The surgical procedure should be determined according to the specific situation. Careful attention should be paid to close hemostasis. Before the operation, it is necessary to demand the consultation of endocrinology, anesthesiology, intensive care medicine, general surgery, and other related departments, medical department filing, and lawyer-notarized signature of conversation. The patient will return to the ICU after surgery.

5.1.7 Surgical Approach

Laparotomy plus left adrenal pheochromocytoma resection under general anesthesia (Fig. 5.4)

5.1.8 Postoperative Pathology

Lesions are consistent with pheochromocytoma, with bleeding and necrosis.

5.2 Case 5.2

Patient: Female, 43 years old

5.2.1 Complaints

Episodic headache with heavy sweating for more than 10 years. The aggravation has been noticed with hypertension for 9 months.

5.2.2 History of Present Illness

First hospitalization (August 17, 2018, to August 22, 2018)

More than 10 years ago, the patient had, with no obvious cause of trigger, episodic head pain, accompanied by heavy sweating. She had visited the local hospital many times for more than 10 years. Blood pressure was measured. The electrocardiogram was checked. No obvious abnormalities were found, and no further diagnosis and treatment were taken. During the past 2 years, the headache has worsened progressively, accompanied by palpitation, nausea, and occasional vomiting of stomach contents. On May 24, 2018, she had, with no obvious cause of trigger, a sudden severe head pain, accompanied by dizziness, nausea, and vomiting of stomach contents. She was treated in the emergency department of Anzhen Hospital. The ECG showed V1-V3 ST-T changes; echocardiography showed abnormalities of segmental ventricular wall movement, left ventricular enlargement, and left ventricular dysfunction loss; NT-proBNP, 2980.00 ng/L; and cTnI, 0.71 ng/mL. After considering the diagnosis of acute myocardial infarction of non-ST-segment elevation and heart failure, she was treated with aspirin 0.1G qd + polivi 75 mg once a day × 10 days. The patient's dizziness and nausea symptoms were improved, and the myocardial enzymes returned to normal. Echocardiography showed abnormalities of segmental ventricular wall movement; multiple occupancy of the left ventricular, which was related to mural thrombosis; and left ventricular enlargement. Adjust the combination of aspirin and povidone antiplatelet to warfarin anticoagulant therapy. The fluctuations of blood pressure are controlled between 110 and 120/70 and 80 mmHg during the treatment period. On June 26, 2018, the patient had, with no obvious trigger, a severe headache, accompanied by dizziness, sweating, nausea, and vomiting of stomach contents. She visited Ningjin County People's Hospital. The abdominal enhanced CT showed a retroperitoneal circular mass, about 62 mm in size×67 mm, with the density of soft tissue. After the enhancement scan, the tumor was unevenly strengthened, and the central area of low density was not significantly strengthened. Urinary ultrasound found no obvious occupancy in both kidney and adrenal areas. Echocardiography showed abnormalities of segmental myocardial movement, enlargement of left ventricle, and slight widening of the ascending aorta. On July 2, 2018, the patient had, with no obvious trigger, sudden convulsions, accompanied by loss of consciousness. The convulsions lasted for more than 10 s and could be relieved on their own. However, the unconsciousness persisted. Epilepsy prevention, sedation, nutritional support, and other treatments were adopted. Convulsions were recurrent three times, and fluctuations of blood pressure were obvious during the period. Systolic blood pressure fluctuations were between 90 and 220 mmHg, and the diastolic blood pressure was unknown. She was transferred to Qilu Hospital of Shandong University for a further treatment. Her abdominal ultrasound showed cystic solid nodules near the gallbladder at the renal blood vessels under the posterior liver. Echocardiograph showed the thickening of the ventricular septum and abnormal filling of the left ventricle. CT of abdominal enhancement in the outer courtyard showed a retroperitoneal cystic solid mass. Pheochromocytoma may be probable, excluding the possible origin of duodenum. With the additional treatment of nimodipine 30 mg three times/day + cardura 1 mg one time/day, blood pressure can be maintained at 130–150/70–90 mmHg. The patient was further diagnosed and treated in our hospital on July 19, 2018. The urine catecholamine was checked: 24hNE 113.71 μg, 24hE 6.19 μg, and 24hDA 234.07 μg. Somatostatin receptor imaging, (−); ^{131} I-MIBG, abnormal in right upper abdomen, conforming to pheochromocytoma, with internal necrosis; CTU, a circular low-density shadow with predominantly mixed density in front of right kidney and beside para-abdominal aortic. The scan CT value was about 19–40 HU, with maximum cross-sectional size of about 6.7 cm × 7.0 cm. Enhanced scanning of cortical medullary stage showed the significant strengthening in the solid part of mass. These indicators were in line with paraganglioma. Blood supply to the tumor was provided by from the branch of abdominal aorta branch, closely related to the branch of superior mesenteric artery. Our outpatient clinic doctors considered that the patient's diagnosis of retroperitoneal tumor is clear. Paraganglioma is probable. In order to a further treatment into our ward, the patient was admitted to complete routine examinations and to monitor the blood pressure in the recumbent position. On August 19, 2018, she began to take oral phenol benzylamine 10 mg two times/day. No obvious orthostatic hypotension was found during hospitalization. She was allowed to be discharged on August 22, 2018.

Second hospitalization (November 2, 2018, to November 9, 2018)

The patient took oral administration of phenolic benzylamine 10 mg bid before surgery, 10 mg bid in the first week of discharge, and later changed to 10 mg tid. Supine blood pressure was 120–140/8–100 mmHg with a heart rate of 64–80 beats/min. Standing blood pressure was 87–110/65–70 mmHg with a heart rate of 85–125 beats/min. In the past 2 months, there had been no increase in blood pressure, palpitations, and hyperhidrosis. She got a weight gain of about 8 kg. After the admission to the hospital, on the afternoon of November 6, 2018, sudden palpitations and dizziness occurred. The heart rate was 120 times/min. Endocrinology consultation was asked. It was thought that the patient's current heart rate and blood pressure were still unstable. Continuation of medical treatment was needed. On November 8, 2018, drug preparation of oral benzylamine 20 mg twice/day was started, and she was discharged from the hospital on November 9, 2018.

Third hospitalization (December 11, 2018, to December 18, 2018)

After the last discharge, the patient continued to take oral phenolic benzylamine 20 mg/day. The blood pressure was stable. The supine blood pressure was 110–140/70–90 mmHg with a the heart rate of 60–80 beats/min, and the standing blood pressure was 100–120/60–90 mmHg with a heart rate of 90–120 beats/min. In January, there was no more discomfort such as headache and sweating. There was a pronounced nasal congestion, accompanied by dry mouth, mild palpitations, dizziness, nausea, drowsiness, and other discomforts. The self-reported weight gain was about 3 kg. After the admission, blood routine suggested leukopenia and anemia. After an endocrinology consultation, it is considered that the patient's current fluctuations of recumbent blood pressure were obvious. Surgery was not recommended, and the dosage of phenol benzylamine was adjusted to 15 mg qd8 + 15 mg qd16 + 10 mg qd22. She was discharged on December 18, 2018.

Present hospitalization record (February 28, 2019, to present)

After the patient was discharged from the hospital, oral phenol benzylamine 15 mg qd8+ 15 mg qd16+ 10 mg qd22 was prepared before surgery. Oral leucogen was taken to increase leukocytes, and ferrous sulfate supplementation was taken for iron deficiency. The supine blood pressure and heart rate were regularly monitored. Blood pressure and heart rate were stable. Supine blood pressure was 110–130/70–80 mmHg with the heart rate of 60–80 beats/min, and the standing blood pressure was 110–120/60–70 mmHg with a heart rate of 80–90 beats/min. She complained of intermittent episodes of dizziness, accompanied by mild palpitation. No episodic headache, nausea, vomiting, and other discomfort are found. In the local hospital, fluguiglizine hydrochloride capsules 5 mg qd and metoprolol 12.5 mg Q12h (later reduced to 6.25 mg qd) were taken to treat the symptoms. Dizziness and palpitation symptoms can be alleviated. Since the onset of disease, the patient's spirit has been acceptable, eating and sleeping normally, with regular passing of stool and urination. Self-reported weight gain is 5Kg for a period of nearly 2 months. Patient is now admitted to the ward for further treatment.

5.2.3 Past, Personal, Marital, Childbearing, and Familial History

Patient had hypertension and coronary heart disease as mentioned above. Warfarin has been discontinued for 3 months. Patient had been anemic for more than 20 years and now takes oral iron supplementation. Recent hemoglobin is normal; excessive menstrual volume caused by uterine fibroids; resection of right breast lipoma resection 8 years ago; dissection of large saphenous vein for the left lower extremity 5 years ago; nothing special about personal and family history

5.2.4 Accessory Examination

Physical examination: no bulge or percussion in both renal areas, no tenderness along both sides of the ureter, and no filling in the bladder area. The anus and external genitalia were not examined.

On August 17, 2018, 131I-MIBG showed abnormal lesion in the right upper abdomen. Pheochromocytoma is considered. Internal necrosis is seen. No lesions with clear hyperexpression of somatostatin receptor are seen in the remaining areas.

On July 27, 2018, somatostatin receptor imaging showed no significant abnormalities.

On August 3, 2018, CTU (Fig. 5.5) results were the following: In combination with clinical results, a retroperitoneal mass corresponds with paraganglioma. The junction of left adrenal gland is thickened. Local parenchyma in the bilateral kidney is slightly thinner with patches of decreased strengthening. Please combine clinical results to exclude ischemic changes. Uterine cavity is widened with effusion. Please combine the results of ultrasound to consider a cystic hypodense in the left adnexal area. A little of effusion is seen in the pelvic floor. Hepatic mul-

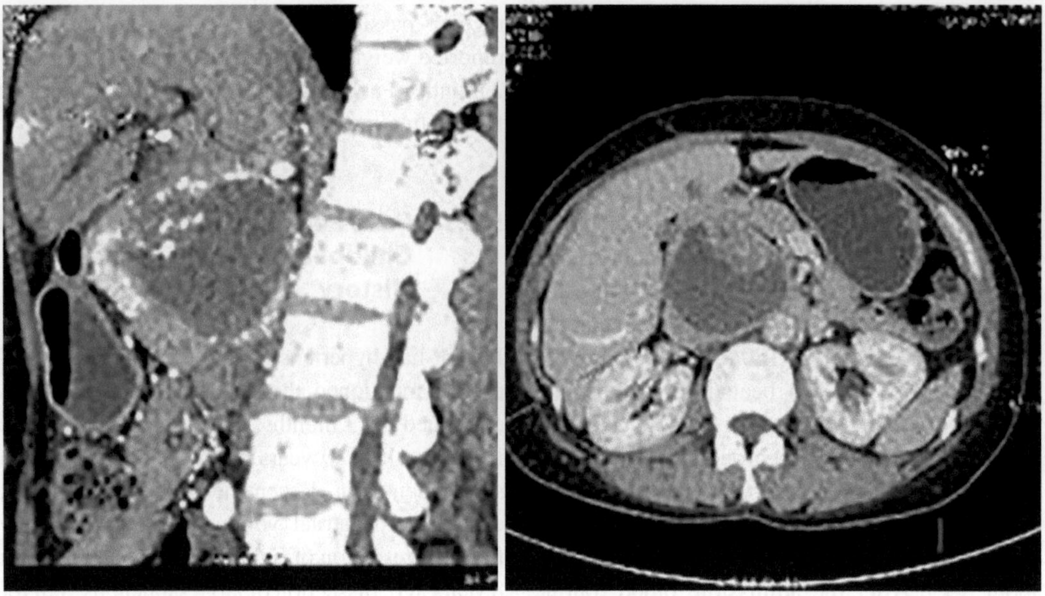

Fig. 5.5 Adrenal scan + enhanced CT

tiple hemangiomas are found with small cysts in the left lobe of the liver. Slightly thicker gallbladder wall with strengthening is seen. Cholestasis may be possible. Slight bone hyperplasia in lumbar spine is found.

In front of the right kidney and beside abdominal para-aortic, a round and mainly low-density shadow is seen with the mixed density. The flat scan CT value is about 19–40 HU, and the maximum cross-sectional size is about 6.7 cm × 7.0 cm. After enhancement, the tumor is significantly strengthened. The blood supply to the tumor comes from the branch of the abdominal aorta, which is closely related to the branch of the superior mesenteric artery.

5.2.5 Current Diagnoses

Right retroperitoneal paraganglioma
Hypertension
Past heart attack
Multiple hemangiomas of the liver
Cyst of the left lobe of the liver
Uterine fibroids
Past maceration of the great saphenous vein of the left lower extremity
Past right breast lipoma resection

5.2.6 MDT Discussion

5.2.6.1 Endocrinology

Appropriately increase the amount of high-sodium diet. Maintain the daily intake of more than 4 L. Monitor the 24 h intake and output (divided into day and night urine volume), weight, and stool. Continue to monitor the blood pressure and heart rate in the recumbent position. Monitor HCT.

The patient has been treated with phenolic benzylamine for 6 months. The current anemia has been corrected. There is no episodic increase in blood pressure. There is a slight orthostatic hypotension. Combined with the current situation of blood pressure control, it is recommended that after a further expansion (if the re-check of HCT decreases), optional surgical treatment can be selected. Avoid squeezing the abdomen and vigorous exercise, maintain electrolyte and blood glucose stability, and pay attention to the perioperative period to be vigilant against the onset of chromium crisis.

5.2.6.2 Department of Anesthesiology

Patients with paraganglioma. Previous history of myocardial infarction. Complete ECG, UCG, and heart. Tumors are closely related to large blood vessels; adequate blood preparation is necessary. Account for the risk of cardiovascular accidents in the perioperative period. Anesthesia procedure is according to pheochromocytoma preparation: the establishment of arteriovenous veins, preparation of vascular active drugs, and intraoperative strengthening of monitoring. Postoperative return to the ICU.

5.2.6.3 ICU

Fully account for the risks and complications associated with the perioperative period, maintain the stability of blood pressure during the perioperative period, and return to the ICU after surgery.

5.2.7 Surgical Approach

Transperitonealoscopic resection of right retroperitoneal paraganglioma under general anesthesia (Fig. 5.6)

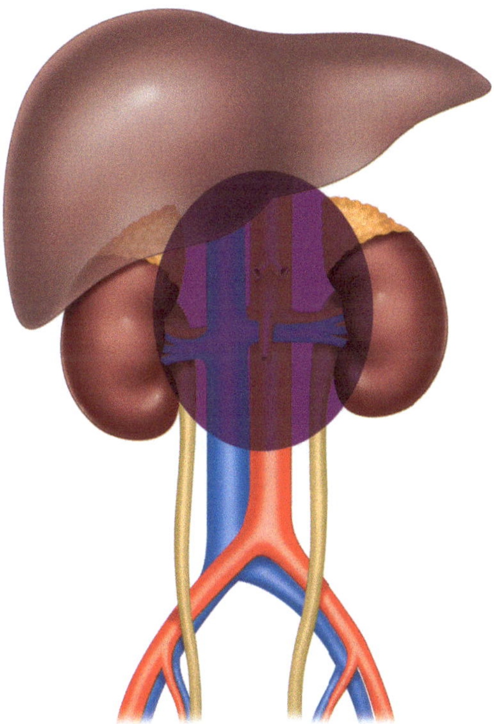

Fig. 5.6 Schematic diagram of the location of the mass

5.2.8 Postoperative Pathology

(Retroperitoneal mass) is consistent with paraganglioma.

Immunohistochemical results: Melan-A(−), AE1/AE3(−), CgA(+), Ki-67(index2%), S-100(Supports cells+), α-inhibin(−)

5.3 Case 5.3

Patient: Male, 55 years old

5.3.1 Complaints

Episodic hypertension for more than 1 year

5.3.2 History of Present Illness

In March 2020, the patient felt that the symptoms reappeared, the nature was the same, and the blood pressure was self-measured at the time of the attack, 220–230/120–130 mmHg, relieved when standing in a different position. He visited the local hospital again. Right paraganglioma was considered (no report) when the CT was checked. He reported that there was no endocrine-related test. It was recommended to take surgery in the higher hospital, and he took orally phenol benzylamine 10 mg q12h. Around May 2020, he went to the outpatient clinic, the right paraganglioma was considered, and oral phenol benzylamine was continued. Surgery was postponed due to insufficient blood preparation. During this period, the patient did not have obvious episodic manifestations.

In November 2020, he visited the outpatient clinic of our hospital and was checked: NMN 10.76 nmol/L↑, MN 3.39 nmol/L↑. Twenty-four-hour urinary catecholamines was repeated on December 01, 2020, with the following results: DA 341.68 μg/24 h↑, NE 37.03 μg/24 h, and E 4.58 μg/24 h. Reexamination of the abdominal pelvis on enhanced CT suggested that there is an oval hybrid density mass of 3.3 × 6.9 × 8.4 cm with a mild-moderate intensification in the right posterior diaphragm space. Somatostatin receptor imaging suggests abnormal lesions and possible paragangliomas. Adjust phenol benzylamine 10 mg q8h. Patient self-reports no significant manifestations of episodic hypertension and orthostatic hypotension. The possibility of right retroperitoneal paraganglioma is currently considered.

5.3.3 Past, Personal, Marital, Childbearing, and Familial History

Nothing special

5.3.4 Accessory Examination

Somatostatin receptor imaging prompt (Fig. 5.7): on the right side of the abdominal aorta, in equivalent to the T10–L1 vertebral level, behind the inferior vena cava, there is a solid mass, about 7.3 × 3.6 × 9.4 cm in size, with an increased radioactivity and lightly higher intensity than the liver. Right retroperitoneal mass may correspond to paraganglioma.

Tips for abdominal pelvic enhanced CT, three-dimensional reconstruction (Figs. 5.8 and 5.9) **and 3D visual reconstruction** (Fig. 5.10): In about posterior T10–L1 level, in front of the right mediastinal spine (right diaphragmatic foot posterior space), there is a class of oval hybrid density shadow with a smooth border, about 3.3 × 6.9 × 8.4 cm in size, about 33 Hu in the solid part of the flat scan, mild-moderate intensification after enhancement, and arterial and portal phase CT values of about 54Hu–77Hu. Low-strengthening area is seen in the center, and the right lower lung lesion adjacent is patchy shadow. The abdominal aorta is tortuous, and no obvious abnormalities are seen in the abdominal aorta, major branches, and portal vein system. In the posterior mediastinum (right diaphragmatic foot posterior space), there is a soft tissue mass. It may be of nerve source. Malignancy cannot be excluded.

In equivalent to the T10–L1 vertebral level on the right side of the abdominal aorta and behind the inferior vena cava, there is a mass with the size about 7.3 × 3.6 × 9.4 cm. The radiation uptake is increased, and the intensity is slightly higher than that of the liver.

In about posterior T10–L1 level, in front of right mediastinal spine (right diaphragm retrosteplomen space), there is a class of oval hybrid density shadow with a smooth border, about 3.3 × 6.9 × 8.4 cm in size, about 33 Hu in the solid part of the flat scan, mild-moderate intensification after enhancement, and arterial and portal phase CT values of about 54Hu–77Hu. Low-strengthening area is seen at the center.

5.3.5 Current Diagnoses

Right retroperitoneal paraganglioma

Hypertension (grade 3, very high risk)

5.3.6 MDT Discussion

5.3.6.1 Department of Anesthesiology

It is recommended to check the echocardiogram results to see if there is a significant abnormality. Follow-up in our department is recommended. It is recommended to demand the endocrinologist to assist in evaluating the patient's preoperative and adequate blood preparation, monitor intraoperative strength, and account for risks of perioperative cardiovascular and cerebrovascular events, heart failure, arrhythmia, hemorrhagic shock, delayed extubation, etc. It is also recommended that patient be returned to the ICU for further treatment after surgery.

5.3.6.2 Endocrinology

Ensure the amount of input, monitor the blood pressure and heart rate in the recumbent position, and avoid inducing episodic hypertension. The patient's preoperative preparation is basically sufficient. During the perioperative period, monitor blood pressure, heart rate, and intake and out-

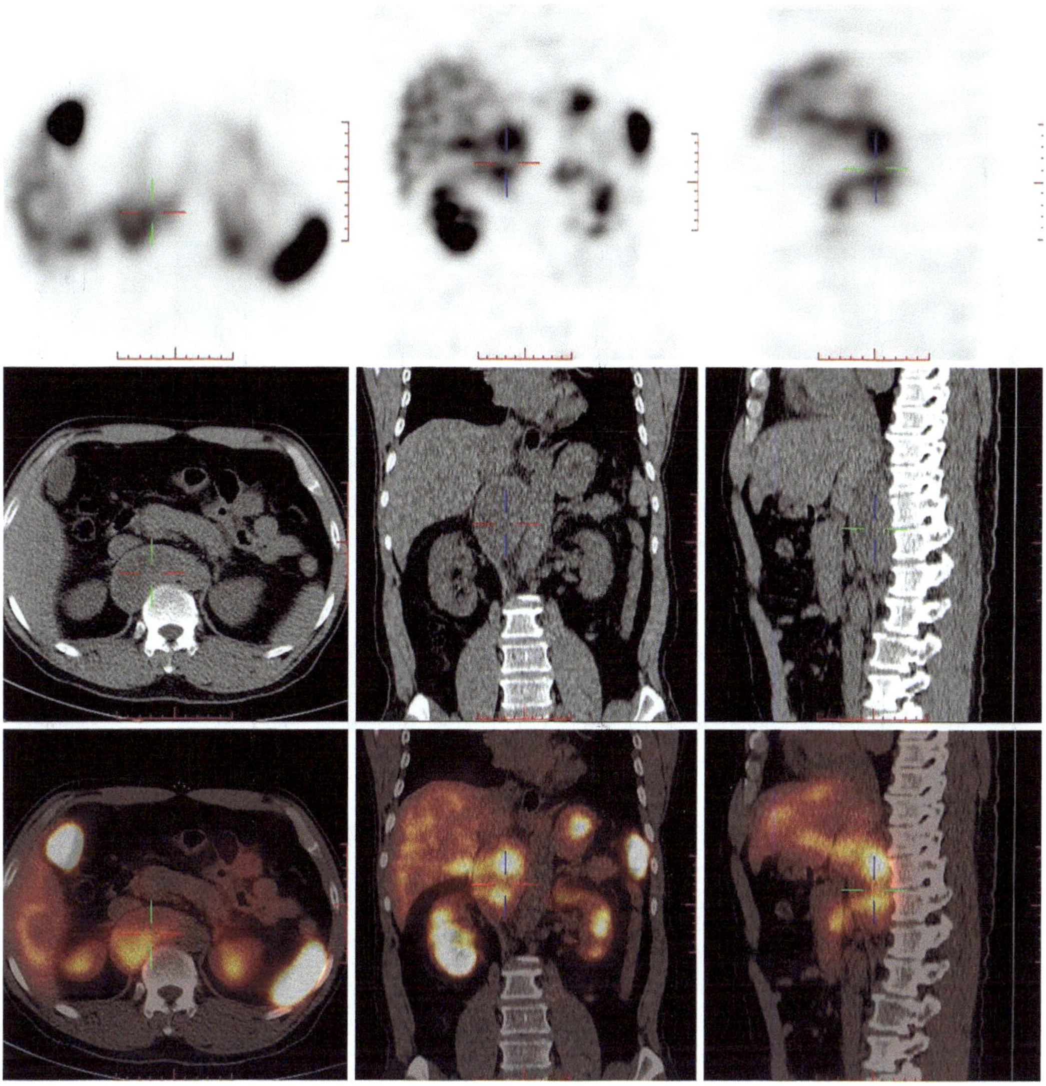

Fig. 5.7 Somatostatin receptor imaging

put. Complete the relevant screening and consultation with relevant departments. Patient is at extremely high risk during surgery, so explain it to the patient.

5.3.6.3 Orthopedics

The film shows that there is a soft tissue space between the mass and the vertebral body. The tumor is considered to be retroperitoneal. In combination with clinic results, paraganglioma is considered.

5.3.6.4 Hepatic Surgery

There is still a gap between the lesion and the liver. It is more likely to consider the retroperitoneal origin. The paraganglioma may be largely probable in combination with the medical history. The perioperative risk is fully explained.

5.3.6.5 Thoracic Surgery

The patient is diagnosed with a clear retroperitoneal mass, adjacent to the chest cavity. Depending on the patient's imaging tests and

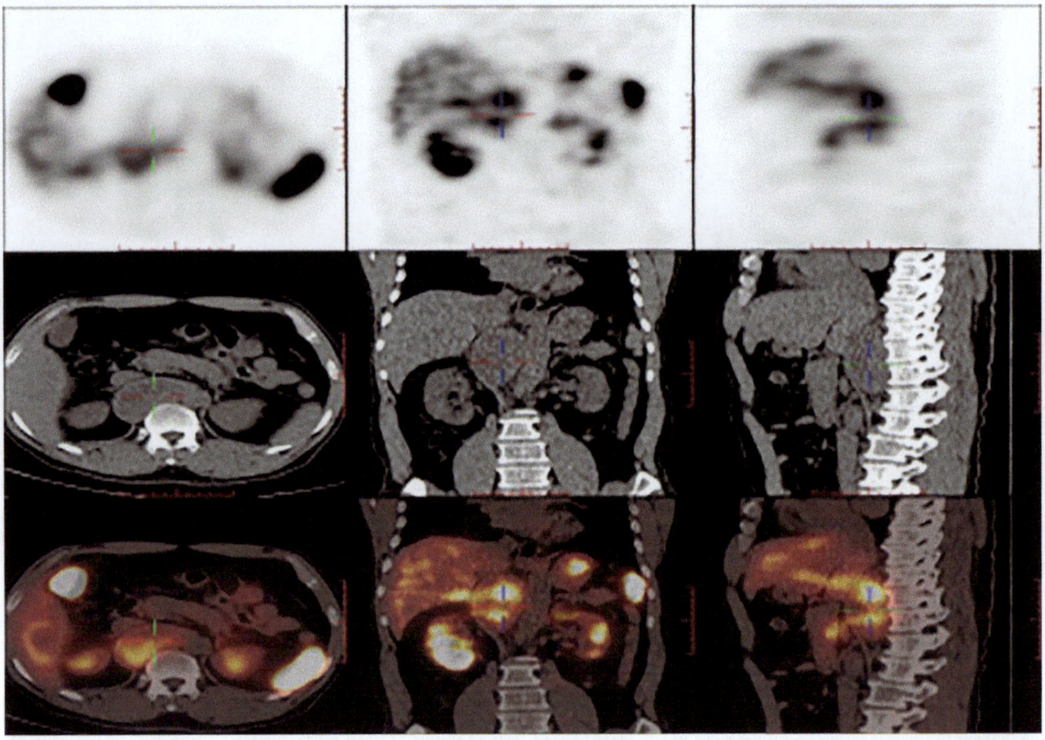

Fig. 5.8 Adrenal scan + enhanced CT

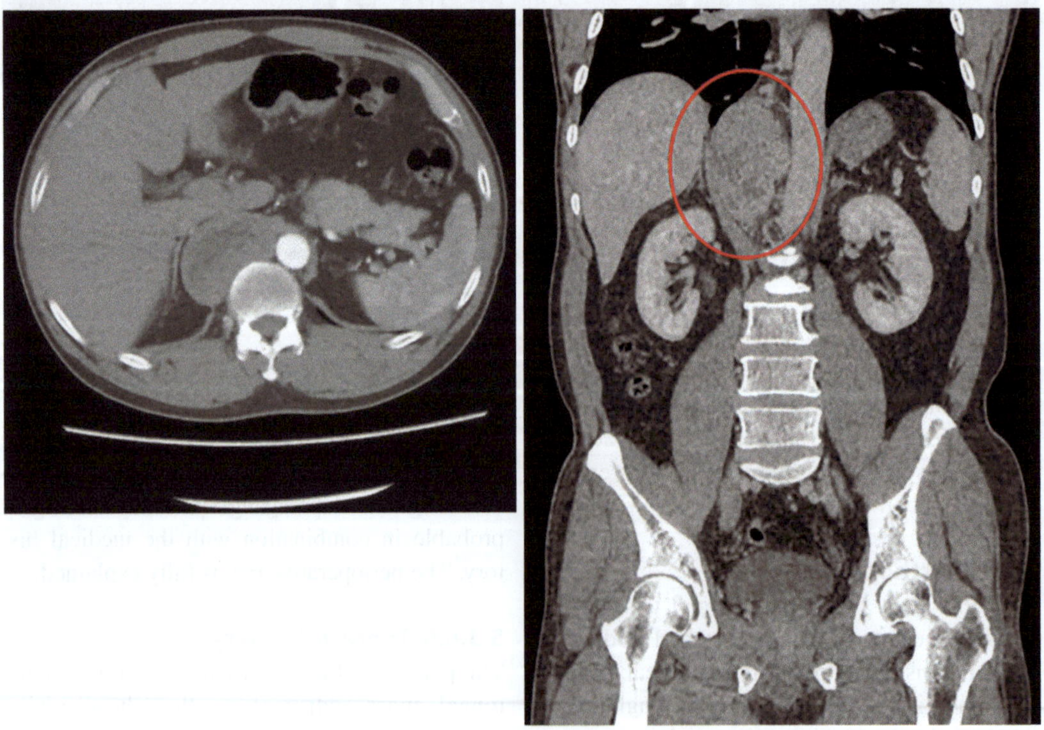

Fig. 5.9 Three-dimensional reconstruction

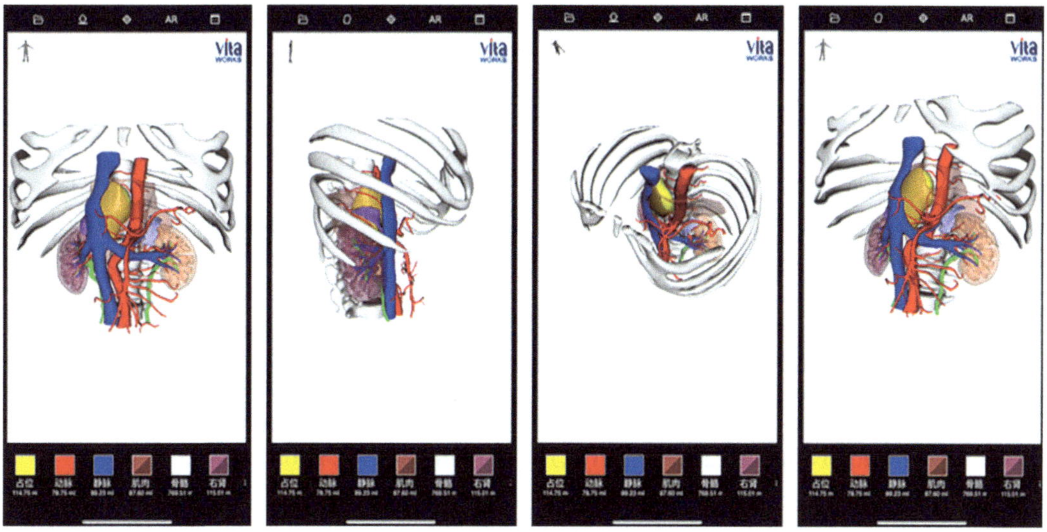

Fig. 5.10 3D visual reconstruction (mass labeled with the brownish yellow)

condition and after a full discussion with the urologic professor of surgery, a thoracic-combined laparoscopy is planned to perform for the exploration and resection of right paraganglioma (possible right nephrectomy) on Monday. The operation is extremely risky, and the patient and his family will be fully explained with the condition and surgical risks before surgery.

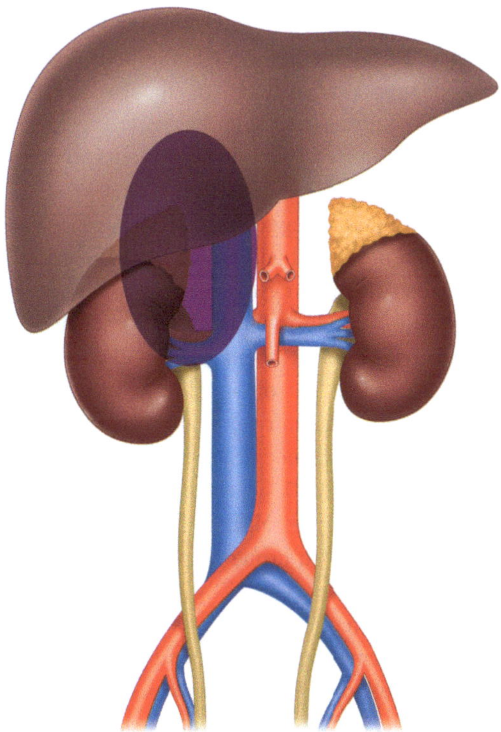

Fig. 5.11 Schematic diagram of the location of the mass

5.3.7 Surgical Approach

Thoracic laparoscopic assisted resection of right retroperitoneal paraganglioma under general anesthesia (Fig. 5.11)

5.3.8 Postoperative Pathology

(Paraganglioma) Complex paraganglioma (paraganglioma, ganglion cell neurofibroma, and a small number of ganglioneuroblastoma components may be seen).

Immunohistochemical results: Melan-A(−), AE1/AE3(−), CgA(+), Ki-67(index 1%), S-100(+), α-inhibin(−), Syn(+), SDHB(+), NeuN(−), SOX10(−), NSE(+), NF(−)

Remarks: this case has undergone a discussion with difficult pathology in the department (KH11223).

5.4 Case 5.4

Patient: Male, 43 years old

5.4.1 Complaints

Dizziness and blood pressure increased for 9 months; left adrenal tumor found for 8 months

5.4.2 History of Present Illness

First Hospitalization (July 22, 2020, to July 27, 2020)

Patients first experienced an episodic dizziness in April 2020, accompanied by an increased blood pressure, up to 240/130 mmHg. Dizziness could be relieved after a few minutes of rest, and when at rest, blood pressure returned to normal. In May 2020, due to lower abdominal discomfort, patient was checked at the local clinic. Abdominal ultrasound suggested a left retroperitoneal mass, about 11 cm in size×8 cm (no report was seen).

Abdominal CT suggests the shadow of a round mass seen in the left adrenal region. The density is uneven. Multiple cystic necrosis areas can be seen inside. The lesion's boundary is clear. The size is about 11 cm × 8 cm. The solid part of the enhanced scan is obviously and unevenly strengthened. The left adrenal gland is poorly revealed. Pheochromocytoma is considered.

On June 10, 2020, he visited our hospital for endocrine screening: NMN 12.12 nmol/L, MN 12.93 nmol/L; 24-h urinary catecholamines: NE 43.38 μg/24 h, E 48.67 μg/24 h, and DA 266.29 μg/24 h

No abnormalities were found in 24-h urine cortisol, dehydroepiandrosterone sulfate (DS), plasma ACTH (8 AM), and aldosterone (standup). 131I-MIBG suggests a large circular area of radiative concentration seen in the left upper abdomen. A hypogenic region is seen inside. Pheochromocytoma is considered with the possibility of internal necrosis.

Somatostatin receptor imaging suggests the hyperexpression focus of somatostatin receptor in the left upper quadrant. The possibility of neuroendocrine tumor with partially organic necrosis is considered.

Thoracoabdominal pelvic flat scan: a mass shadow of soft tissue density can be seen in the left adrenal region, about 11.4 × 8.5 cm. Multiple cystic low-density shadows and dot-like high-density shadows are seen internally with clear boundaries. After the admission, the patient was given phenol benzylamine for preoperative preparation with the dose of 10 mg Q8h. The patient was discharged after taking the drug.

Second Hospitalization (August 31, 2020, to September 17, 2020)

The patient was in good condition after taking the drug. After taking the drug, he complained of nasal congestion, occasional palpitations, and heart rate in 75–100 times/min. Swelling in the upper abdomen, left lower abdomen, and posterior waist was found, which could be relieved. He did not complain of fever, nausea, vomiting, dizziness, headache, and other discomforts. Now blood pressure could be controlled with the standing blood pressure of about 120/80 mmHg. There was no irregular presentation of lying blood pressure and no postural hypotension. Surgical treatment was proposed in our department. After admission, the relevant examinations were completed. Blood pressure was controlled. Due to the shortage of blood supply, the patient was temporarily discharged from the hospital for an elective surgery. The patient was instructed to continue oral phenol benzylamine (10 mg once/8 h); monitor the blood pressure and heart rate in the recumbent position daily (at least once in the morning and afternoon); be vigilant against palpitations, dizziness, cold limbs, and other discomforts or significant fluctuations in blood pressure; promptly visit the emergency department; and adjust the dose of the drug if necessary. During drug preparation, move slowly up and down, drink water appropriately (mainly light salt water), and pay attention to weight changes. An elective surgical treatment would be proposed.

(This Hospitalization, January 6, 2021)

The patient has been in good condition after taking the drug since the last discharge. He does not complain of special discomfort. HR was 75–100bmp. He does not complain of fever, malignancy, vomiting, dizziness, headache, and other discomforts. Blood pressure can be controlled with a vertical blood pressure of about 130/90 mmHg and a lying blood pressure of about 120/80 mmHg. There is no recent manifestation of orthostatic hypotension. This time, he is ready for a surgical treatment in our department. Since the onset of the disease, the patient has been mentally active, slept well, had a good appetite, had normal stool and urination, and gained 4 kg of weight since the last discharge.

5.4.3 Past, Personal, Marital, Childbearing, and Familial History

Hyperuricemia for more than 9 months with an oral febuxostat treatment.

No special for personal history, family history.

5.4.4 Accessory Examination

Abdominal pelvic enhanced CT and three-dimensional reconstruction (Figs. 5.12 and 5.13): The shadow of a round mass can be seen in the left adrenal region. The density is uneven. Multiple cystic necrosis areas can be seen inside. The lesion's boundary is clear. The size is about 11.4 cm × 8.5 cm × 8.6 cm. The solid part of the enhanced scan is obviously and unevenly strengthened. The left adrenal gland is poorly revealed. Pheochromocytoma is considered.

The shadow of a round mass can be seen in the left adrenal region. The density is uneven. Multiple cystic necrosis areas can be seen inside. The lesion's boundary is clear. The size is about 11 cm × 8 cm. The solid part of the enhanced scan is obviously and unevenly strengthened. The left adrenal gland is poorly revealed. Pheochromocytoma is considered.

5.4.5 Current Diagnoses

Left giant pheochromocytoma

Hypertension (grade 3 extremely high risk)

Hyperuricemia

5.4.6 MDT Discussion

5.4.6.1 Endocrinology

Monitor the 24-h intake and output. Ensure that the daily intake is greater than 3–4 L. Monitor the weight, HCT, and blood pressure in the recumbent position. It is considered that the surgical preparation is sufficient. Surgical treatment can be selected. Complete the screening to exclude the possibility of MEN.

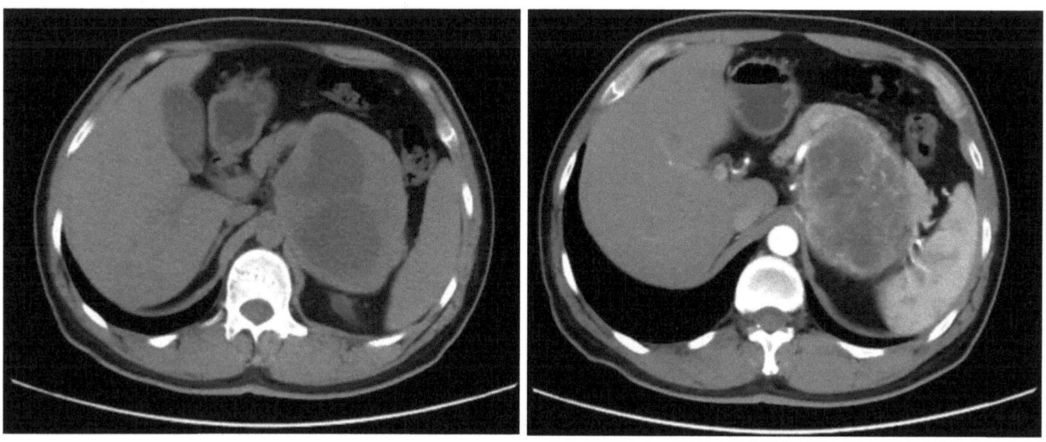

Fig. 5.12 Abdominal pelvic enhancement CT

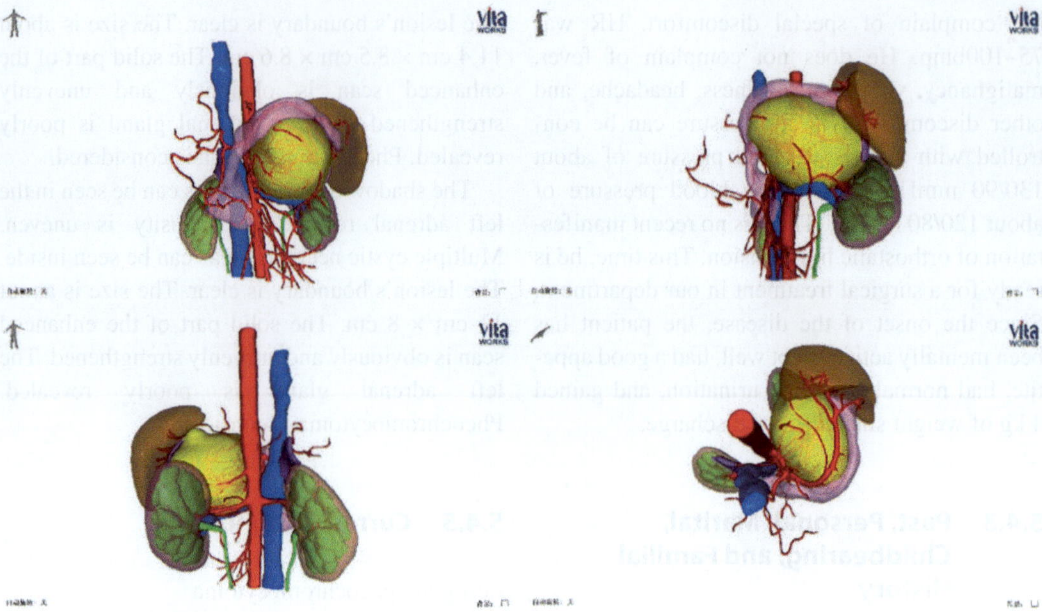

Fig. 5.13 3D visual reconstruction image

5.4.6.2 Department of Anesthesiology

ASA Class I and an elective surgery. The patient is prepared according to chromaffin anesthesia. The risk of anesthesia is high. The risk of hemodynamic fluctuations and cardiovascular and cerebrovascular events is explained to the patient. Postoperative return to the ICU.

5.4.6.3 ICU

Fully account for surgical risks and associated perioperative complications. Closely monitor blood pressure and hemodynamic stability.

Ensure the stability of blood pressure during the perioperative period and the perfusion of organs such as the heart, brain, and kidneys. Monitor and maintain the stability of the internal environment.

5.4.7 Surgical Approach

"Laparoscopic resection of left retroperitoneal paraganglioma" is performed under general anesthesia (Fig. 5.14).

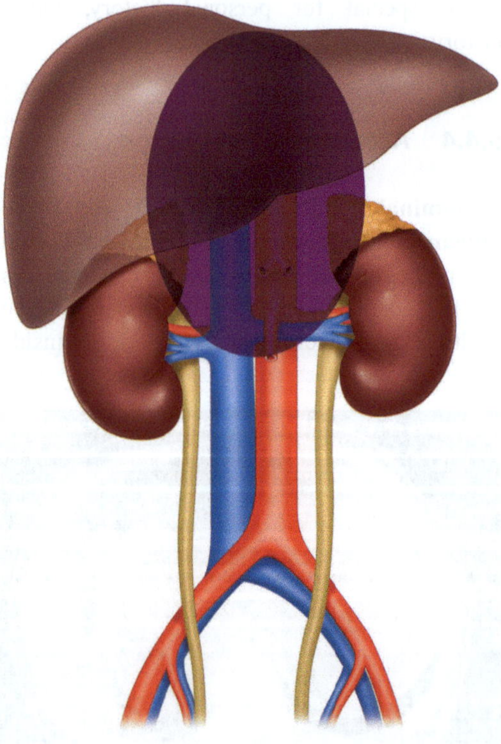

Fig. 5.14 Schematic diagram of the location of the mass

5.4.8 Postoperative Pathology

Lesions are consistent with paragangliomas.

Immunohistochemical results: CgA(+), Ki-67(index 3%), S-100(+), α-inhibin(−), Syn(+), SDHB(+), NeuN(−), SOX10(−), NSE(+), NF(−)

5.5 Case 5.5

Patient: Female, 43 years old

5.5.1 Complaints

An increase in blood pressure was found 10 years ago. A tumor in the abdomen was found 3 years ago.

5.5.2 History of Present Illness

In 2009, the patient suddenly became blindfolded, with sweating, palpitation, and transient loss of consciousness (duration unknown), when she stood up. She was relieved after rest. Blood pressure was monitored at 150/100 mmHg. Antihypertensive therapy of nifedipine 30 mg qd was given. Then blood pressure was monitored at approximately 110/70 mmHg.

In 2012, the blood pressure was about 150/100 mmHg, and she took telmisartan 40 mg qd on her own. The headaches disappeared after consciously taking the drug. The blood pressure was not measured regularly.

In 2016, CT was performed to find a "right abdominal mass" (no original film and report seen), and no further diagnosis and treatment were carried out. After annual reexamination of abdominal CT, she said that the mass increased year by year.

In April 2019, abdominal enhanced CT in another hospital shows that a circular mixed density shadow of 41 × 39 mm can be seen between the liver and stomach with clear boundaries. Inferior vena cava and portal vein are compressed. Significant strengthening of the parenchymal part is found after enhancement, but the low density in the mass is not strengthened. The possibility of "neurogenic tumors" is considered (no original film seen). No diagnosis and treatment are taken.

In November 2019, local hospital completed an enhanced MRI, which shows a "hepatic hilar and posterior peritoneal mass, diameter 45mm size, uneven strengthening, divided, enlarged when compared with the precedent scan." For a further diagnosis and treatment, she was admitted to our department on December 13, 2019.

5.5.3 Past, Personal, Marital, Childbearing, and Familial History

Mild anemia; thyroid nodules; past caesarean section. Her brother was diagnosed with hypertension in his 30 s. In November 2019, he took an abdominal CT examination, which found an "abdominal mass" (specification unknown).

5.5.4 Accessory Examination

Abdominal enhanced CT + three-dimensional reconstruction (Fig. 5.15): A round and slightly less dense mass can be seen in the hepatic hilar area. The boundary is clear, extending downward to the peritoneum. The pancreatic neck and the hepatic caudal lobes are pressurized. The size is about 39 mm × 43 mm × 44 mm. After the enhancement scan, it is unevenly and significantly strengthened. A patch of low-density shadow is visible in the lesion, and the enhancement is not significantly strengthened. The lesion is close to the pancreatic head, inferior vena cava, and portal vein trunk. The lumen of inferior vena cava is compressed and deformed. No significant abnormalities are seen in the abdominal arteries. Hepatic hilar region is rich in blood supply with multiple cysts/necrosis, which can be consistent with paraganglioma manifestations. Lesions are close to the pancreatic head, inferior vena cava, and portal vein trunk. Compression and deforma-

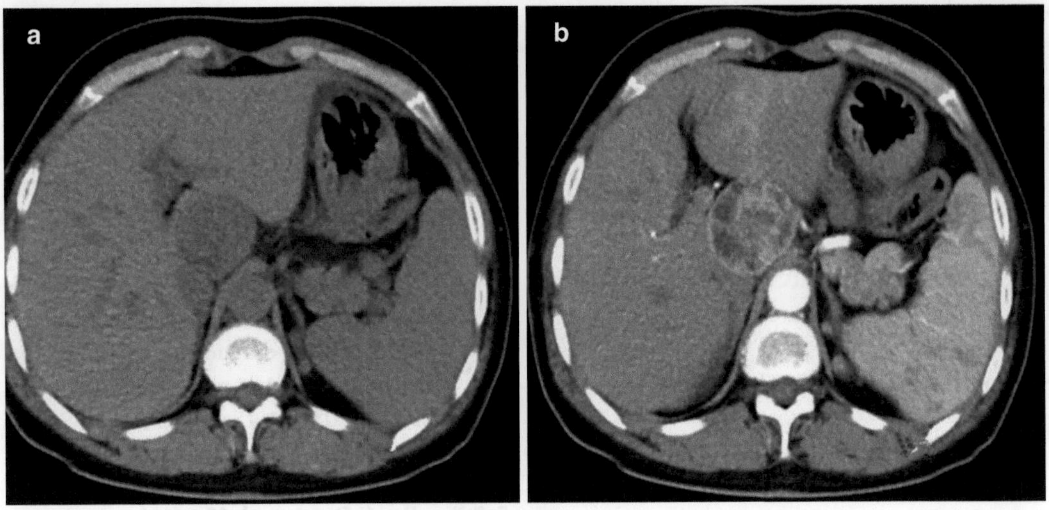

Fig. 5.15 (**a**, **b**) Abdominal pelvic flat sweep + enhanced CT

tion of lumen of the inferior vena cava are seen. There is an obvious strengthening of the left lobe of the liver in the arterial stage. Transient abnormal perfusion may occur. There are multiple small lymph nodes at the root of the mesenteric membrane and retroperitoneum.

Somatostatin receptor imaging: diffuse thyroid lesions may occur.

A round and slightly less dense mass can be seen in the hepatic hilar area. The boundary is clear, extending downward to the peritoneum. Pancreatic neck and hepatic caudal lobes are pressurized. The size is about 39 mm × 43 mm × 44 mm. After the enhancement scan, it is unevenly and significantly strengthened. The patchy of low-density shadow is visible in the lesion, and the enhancement is not significantly strengthened. The lesion is close to the pancreatic head, inferior vena cava, and portal vein trunk. The lumen of inferior vena cava is compressed and deformed.

5.5.5 Current Diagnoses

Right retroperitoneal paraganglioma
Mild anemia
Right lobe nodules of the thyroid gland
Past caesarean section

5.5.6 MDT Discussion

5.5.6.1 Endocrinology

Daily monitoring of blood pressure and heart rate in the recumbent position is recommended to evaluate the drug regimen.

5.5.6.2 Department of Anesthesiology

It is recommended to complete the myocardial enzyme profile before surgery. Fully explain to patients and their families the perioperative hemodynamic fluctuations to the patient and her family and the possibility of the risk of myocardial infarction, cerebral infarction, cerebral hemorrhage, etc. during the perioperative period. It is recommended to return to the ICU after surgery. It is recommended to prepare a cell saver during operation.

5.5.6.3 Endocrinology

Continue to monitor the intake of 24 h with a high sodium diet. Ensure that the daily intake is greater than 4. Continue to take phenol benzamine therapy. Monitor blood pressure and heart rate in the lying position. The patient's current standing HR is significantly faster than in the lying position, which suggests an insufficient expansion. Avoid squeezing the abdomen and drastic postural changes. Avoid using morphine.

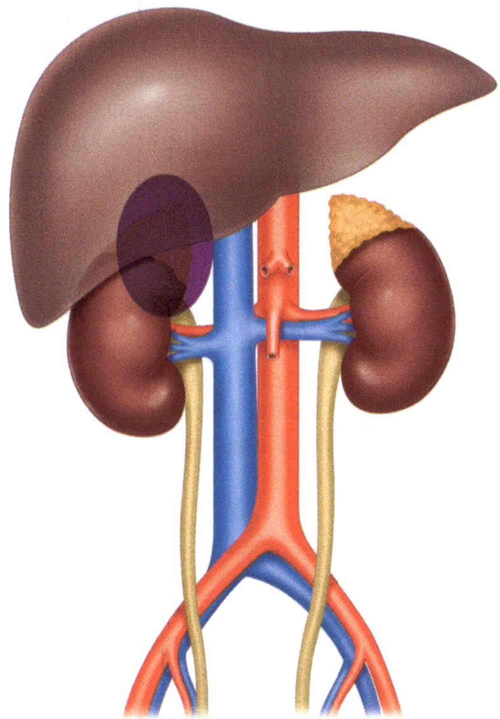

Fig. 5.16 Schematic diagram of the location of the mass

5.5.6.4 Liver Surgery
The patient's tumor is located in the hepatic hilar area, closely related to the peripheral blood vessels. The risk of surgery is high, and it is recommended to explain to the patient and the family. If the patient will be operated on, we are willing to assist during surgery.

5.5.7 Surgical Approach

"Laparoscopic exploration, retroperitoneal mass resection (posterior to the hilar)" under general anesthesia (Fig. 5.16)

5.5.8 Postoperative Pathology

Retroperitoneal mass in combination with immunohistochemistry, consistent with paraganglioma.

Lymph nodes appear with chronic inflammation (block 13 0/1).

Immunohistochemical results: Melan-A(−), AE1/AE3(−), CgA(+), Ki-67(index 1%), S-100(+), α-inhibin(−).

5.6 Case 5.6

Patient: Male, 54 years old

5.6.1 Complaints

Hypertension was found 5 years ago, aggravated with paroxysmal dizziness and palpitations 5 months ago.

5.6.2 History of Present Illness

In 2014, an increase in blood pressure of 200/110 mmHg was found. HR was unknown. A treatment of telmisartan 40 mg qd was taken. Post-monitoring found a BP of 130/80 mmHg with a HR of 70–80 bpm. Paroxysmal dizziness, palpitations, and heavy sweating occurred during change of position in July 2019, and a BP reading of 170–180/100–110 mmHg with a HR of 90–100 bpm was found. The symptoms lasted for several minutes and disappeared spontaneously. A BP reading of 140/90 mmHg and HR of 70–80 bpm were noticed between episodes. In August 2019, the endocrinology clinic of our hospital checked the patient and found the following results: NMN 6.80↑nmol/L, MN1.57↑nmol/L; 24 h urinary catecholamines found NE 518.55↑μg/24 h, E 48.61↑μg/24 h, and DA 396.59↑μg/24 h. He was instructed to take a high-sodium diet and drink plenty of water. Phenol benzylamine 5 mg q12h (October 18–November 9) was changed to 10 mg Q12h (November 10–November 21), 10 mg Q8h (November 22–November 28), 15 mg Q8h (November 29–December 14), and 20/15/20 mg Q8h (December 14 to present). I/O was about 4000–5000 mL/3000–4000 mL, nocturia two to three times, and nocturia volume of about 2000–2400 mL. He gained weight from 52 to 57 kg in the last 2 months. He defecated one stool per day.

5.6.3 Past, Personal, Marital, Childbearing, and Familial History

History of diabetes

5.6.4 Accessory Examination

Somatostatin receptor imaging: somatostatin receptor expression in soft tissues in the right adrenal region is slightly increased, not excluding pheochromocytoma. Adrenal medullary MIBG: no significant abnormalities were seen.

On September 10, 2019, adrenal thin sweep + enhanced MRI showed right adrenal mass-like abnormal shadow with a significant strengthening (39 mm × 27 mm) and necrosis of the internal plaque. Pheochromocytoma is considered. Compression stenosis of the inferior vena cava around the lesion. Malformation of bilateral subrenal polar fusion.

December 16, 2019 parietal pelvic enhanced CT + CTA (Figs. 5.17 and 5.18) showed mass-like complex density in right adrenal region (about 35 mm × 19 mm). Please combine with clinical information to consider a diagnosis. Lesion receives blood supply from a small branch of the proximal right renal artery. There is a small pararenal artery on the ventral side of lesion. The inferior vena cava and the root of left renal vein are pressed forward, and the right renal artery is compressed backward.

No obvious abnormalities were found in blood routine, liver and kidney function, and blood coagulation; 8 blood transfusions (−). HbA1c was 5.9%.

Echocardiography: LVEF 68%; mild bicuspid valve insufficiency; decreased left ventricular compliance. Myocardial enzyme (−), NT-proBNP 12 pg/mL. CT chest: micronodules of the right lung, shadow of the lower lobe of the left lung. Lung function: no significant abnormalities were seen.

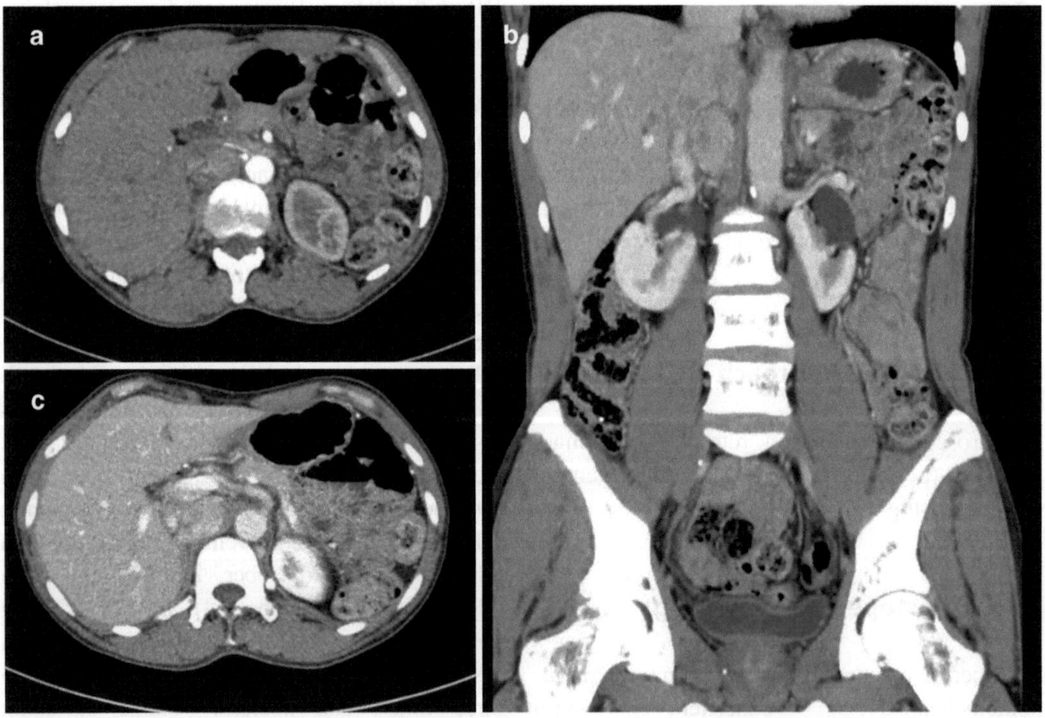

Fig. 5.17 (a–c) Abdominal pelvic enhanced CT

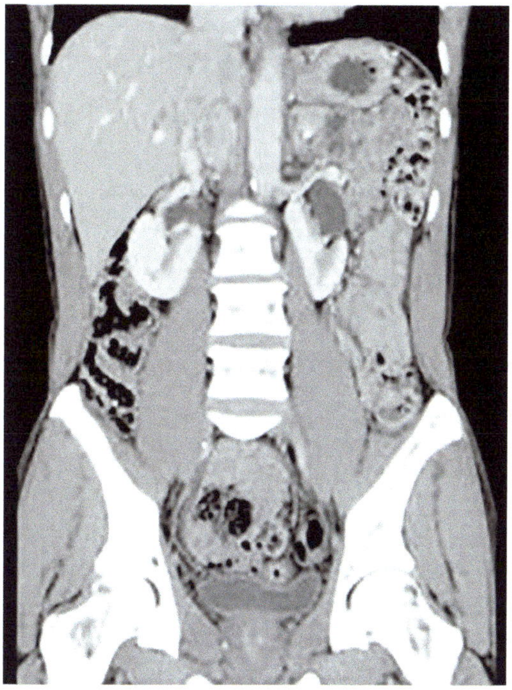

Fig. 5.18 CTA

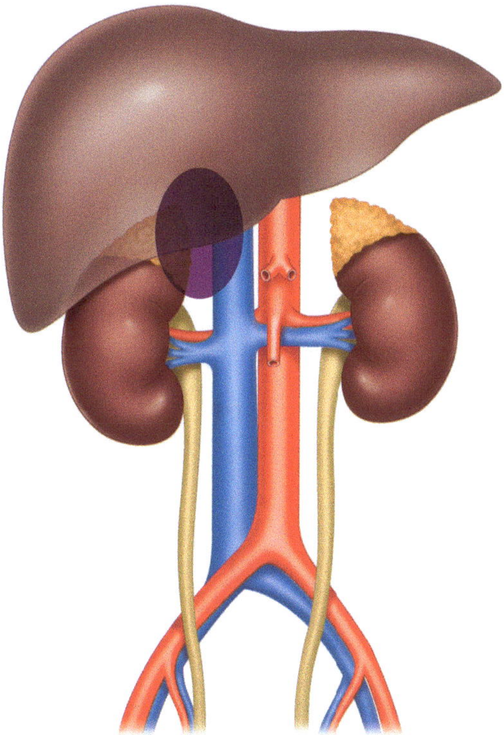

Fig. 5.19 Schematic diagram of the location of the mass

5.6.5 Current Diagnoses

Right adrenal pheochromocytoma

Type 2 diabetes

Thyroid nodules

Horseshoe kidneys

The right adrenal region has a mixed-density lumpy of about 35 mm × 19 mm in size.

The lesion receives blood supply from a small branch of the proximal right renal artery. There is a small pararenal artery on the ventral side of lesion. The inferior vena cava and the root of left renal vein are pressed forward, and the right renal artery is compressed backward.

5.6.6 MDT Discussion

5.6.6.1 Urology

Current diagnoses consider the likelihood of paragangliomas. The patient has surgical indications. However, the surgery is at very high risk, which was repeatedly explained to the patient. The patient is actively prepared with drugs and monitored for blood pressure and heart rate.

5.6.6.2 Department of Critical Medicine

Fully explain the surgical risks and related perioperative complications to the patient. Closely monitor blood pressure and hemodynamic stability. Ensure the stability of perioperative blood pressure. Ensure the perfusion of cardio-cerebral, kidney, and other important organs. Monitor and maintain changes in electrolytes and internal environment. Return to the ICU after surgery.

5.6.7 Surgical Approach

"Laparoscopic exploration and resection of right retroperitoneal paraganglioma" under general anesthesia (Fig. 5.19)

5.6.8 Postoperative Pathology

Paragangliomas. Tumor invades peripheral nerve tissue.

6 Multidisciplinary Treatment of Paragangliomas in the Vascular Area of the Epigastric Region

Quan Zong Mao, Shi Jun Wang, Jin Wen, Hua Fan, and Xiao Qiang Xue

6.1 Case 6.1

Patient: Male, 73 years old

6.1.1 Complaints

Examination has revealed retroperitoneal mass for more than 10 months.

6.1.2 History of Present Illness

Ten months ago, a retroperitoneal mass was found through physical examination and enhanced CT at the local hospital. Mass has poor borders and unevenly strengthened. No treatment was pursued. So, he was admitted to our hospital.

Quan Zong Mao and Shi Jun Wang contributed equally to this work.

Q. Z. Mao · S. J. Wang · J. Wen (✉) · H. Fan · X. Q. Xue
Department of Urology, Peking Union Medical College Hospital, Beijing, China

6.1.3 Past, Personal, Marital and Childbearing, Family History

Coronary heart disease for 4 years, asymptomatic, long-term anti-platelet trzeament, lipid adjustment treatment

6.1.4 Accessory Examination

Abdominal pelvic enhanced CT (Fig. 6.1): A cystic solid mass on the medial side of the left renal hilar, about 3.5 cm in size, with poorly defined boundaries and uneven reinforcement

Endocrine examination: 24 h urinary catecholamines: NE 118.07 μg/24 h, E 5.56 μg/24 h, DA 505.62 μg/24 h. Blood NMN 1.72 nmol/L

Somatostatin receptor imaging: somatostatin receptors in the positional capsule solid nodules are highly expressive, and a neuroendocrine tumor is more likely to be considered.

131I-MIBG: a cystic solid mass on the medial side of the left hilar, about 3.5 cm in size, with increased radio-absorption. A cystic solid nodule is seen at the right anterior and duodenal level, about 2.5 cm in diameter, with no radio-absorption.

J. Wen (ed.), *Surgical Management of Pheochromocytoma and Retroperitoneal Paraganglioma*,
https://doi.org/10.1007/978-981-99-8421-3_6

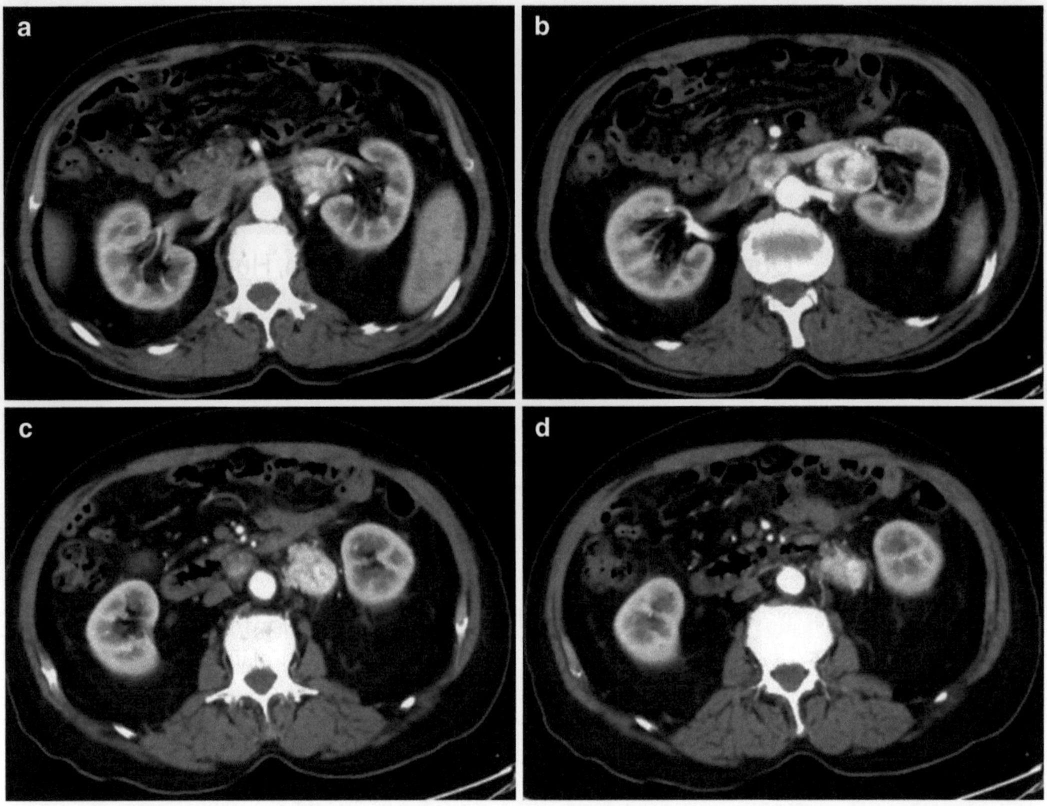

Fig. 6.1 Enhanced CT. (**a–d**) A solid mass is found in the medial side of the left renal hilum, about 3.5 cm in size, with a poorly defined border and uneven reinforcement

6.1.5 Current Diagnoses

Retroperitoneal paraganglioma

Coronary heart disease

6.1.6 MDT Discussion

6.1.6.1 Endocrinology

Treatment with phenylbenzylamine 10 mg bid and doxazosin mesylate 4 mg qd can be continued. Ensure the intake >3 L/day. Continue to monitor the blood pressure and heart rate in the recumbent position and repeat HCT weekly.

6.1.6.2 Department of Anesthesiology

Stop the drug on the day of surgery, prepare cell saver, and fully explain the risks.

6.1.6.3 ICU

Prepare the bed for patient after the surgery.

6.1.7 Surgical Approach

Laparoscopic resection of retroperitoneal mass is performed with general anesthesia (Fig. 6.2).

6.1.8 Postoperative Pathology

(Retroperitoneal mass and left kidney) is consistent with paraganglioma.

Fibrous proliferation, microplasia, adhesions, and infiltration of inflammatory cells are found in part of the renal membrane.

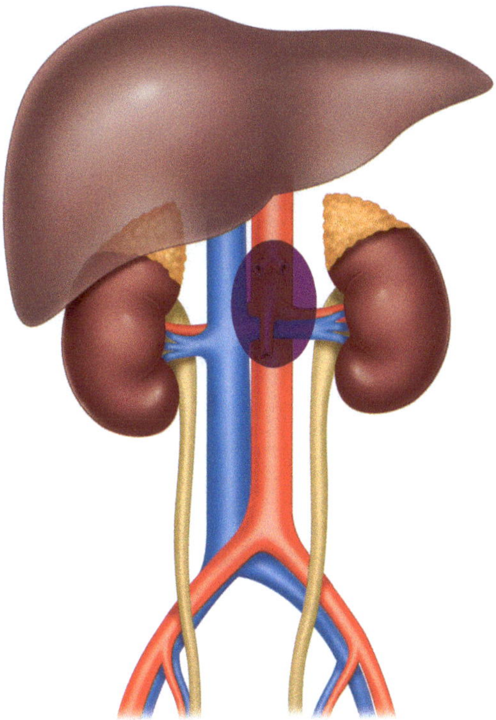

Fig. 6.2 Schematic diagram of the location of the mass

No abnormality in the renal parenchyma, ureteral segmentation, and vascular disconnection. No special finding for ureteric and blood ends. Immunohistochemical results: Melan-A(−), AE1/AE3(−), CgA(+), Ki-67(index 6%), S-100(+), α-inhibin(+), CD10(−), PAX-8(−), Vimentin(+), RCC(−), Syn(+).

6.2 Case 6.2

Patient: Female, 37 years old

6.2.1 Complaints

Sweating for more than 2 years; episodic dizziness, headache, and an increase in blood pressure for 1 year; discovery of retroperitoneal tumor 3 months ago

6.2.2 History of Present Illness

Sweating for more than 2 years; episodic dizziness, headache, and an increase in blood pressure for 1 year; discovery of retroperitoneal tumor 3 months ago; high blood pressure for 2 years

6.2.3 Past, Personal, Marital and Childbearing, Family History

Diabetes mellitus; past caesarean section

6.2.4 Accessory Examination

Abdominal pelvic enhanced CT (Fig. 6.3a, b): A solid mass of the right medial hilar, about 3.2 cm in size, with poorly defined boundaries and uneven reinforcement

Endocrine examination: 3-Methoxy norepinephrine (NMN) 5.95 nmol/L, 3-methoxyephrine (MN) 0.10 nmol/L; 24 h urinary catecholamine NE 548.83 μg/24 h; E 6.18 μg/24 h; DA 262.82 μg/24 h.

6.2.5 Diagnosis

Right retroperitoneal paraganglioma
Secondary hypertension
Type 2 diabetes
Past caesarean section

6.2.6 MDT Discussion

6.2.6.1 Basic Surgery

Explain the conditions to the patient, and there is a possibility of joint organ resection during surgery. Intraoperative assistance can be provided.

6.2.6.2 Endocrinology

Continue to monitor 24-h intake, actively increase inputs, and continue to assess the readiness.

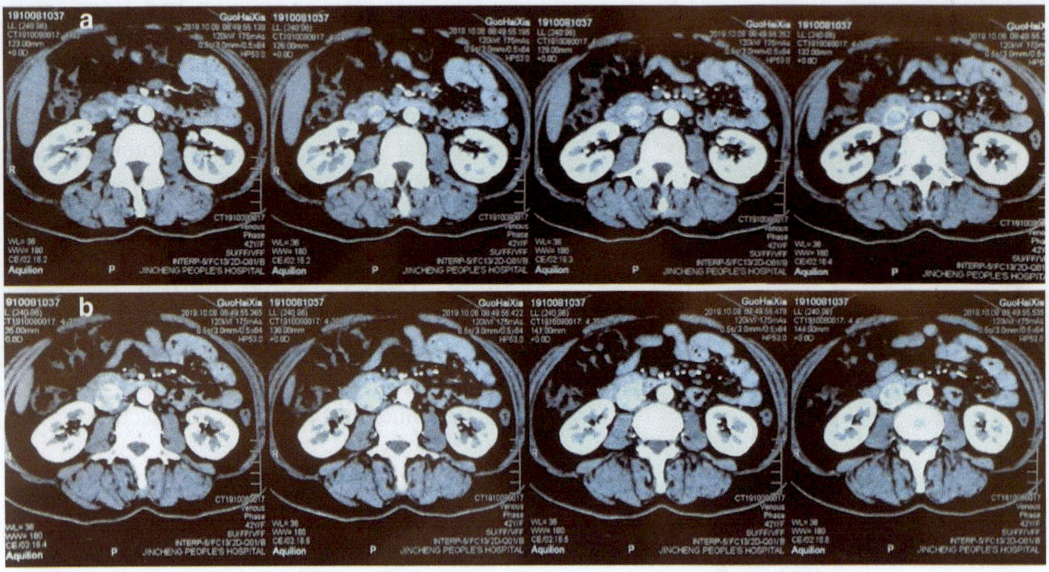

Fig. 6.3 Enhanced CT. (**a**, **b**) A solid mass is found in the medial side of the right renal hilum, about 3.2 cm in size, with an under-clear border and uneven reinforcement

Complete blood calcium and free calcium, parathyroid hormone, CEA, and other MEN.

6.2.6.3 Department of Anesthesiology

Patient is at high risk of anesthesia and is recommended to return to the ICU after surgery.

6.2.6.4 ICU

Maintain perioperative intake and output and electrolyte balance. Return to the ICU for a further treatment after surgery.

6.2.7 Surgical Approach

Laparoscopic resection of right-sided retroperitoneal paraganglioma under general anesthesia (Fig. 6.4)

6.2.8 Postoperative Pathology

(Right retroperitoneal mass) is consistent with paraganglioma.

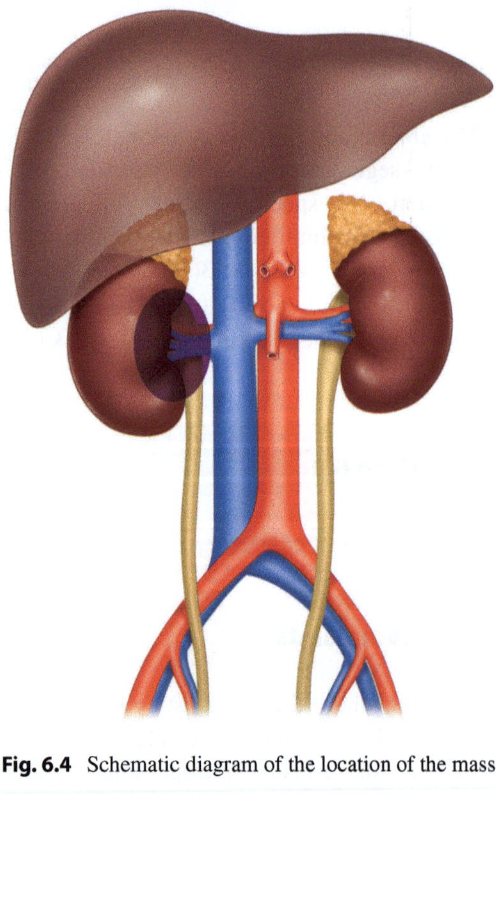

Fig. 6.4 Schematic diagram of the location of the mass

Immunohistochemical results: Melan-A(−), AE1/AE3(−), CgA(+), Ki-67(index 2%), S-100(+), α-inhibin(−), SDHB(+)

6.3 Case 6.3

Patient: Female, 65 years old

6.3.1 Complaints

Episodic sweating and nausea for 3 months and a right adrenal mass found 3 months ago

6.3.2 History of Present Illness

In October 2020, the patient had, with no obvious trigger, episodic sweating and nausea with hyposphedic discomfort. There was no occurrence of vomiting, chest pain, palpitations, dizziness, headache, or blackout or impaired consciousness. The symptoms could be relieved by themselves after about 5 min. No blood pressure and blood sugar were measured. Abdominal pelvic MRI shows a mass of about 4.5 cm in diameter in the right adrenal region, with a slightly longer T1/T2 signal and a circular and longer T2 signal seen in the lesion. The lesion is significantly strengthened. The boundary between the adjacent kidney, liver, duodenum, and the mass is not clear. The possibility of neoplastic lesions in the right adrenal region and cortical adenocarcinoma is considered.

In November 2020, the patient visited Platon General Hospital. Endocrine examination: Cortisol axis: 8 am Blood F 421.79 nmol/L (198.7~797.5), 4 pm Blood F 207.04 nmol/L (85.3~459.6), 8 am ACTH 6.06 pmol/L(<10.12), 4 pm ACTH 5.44 pmol/L; examination of RAAS: Renin (17.7uIU/mL) and aldosterone (6.7 ng/dL) are normal. Sex hormone: testosterone 0.51 nmol/L (0~1.58). The rest are normal.

Methoxytyramine (3-MT) 138.0 pmol/L (<180.0), Methoxyephrine (MN) 292.0 pmol/L (80.0~510.0, Methoxydrenephrine (NMN) 22073.3 pmol/L (120.0~1180.0).

On November 10, 2020, the patient visited our outpatient clinic. Abdominal pelvic enhanced CT shows a 5.2 cm × 4.8 cm slightly lower density mass shadow with obvious uneven strengthening in right adrenal region, and the right lobe of the liver and the inferior vena cava are not clearly visualized. Pheochromocytoma may be highly possible.

6.3.3 Past, Personal, Marital and Childbearing, Family History

Past total hysterectomy; nothing special for the rest

6.3.4 Accessory Examination

Abdominal pelvic enhancement CT suggests (Fig. 6.5) a slightly less dense mass shadow of 5.2 cm × 4.8 cm in the right adrenal, with significant uneven strengthening. The delimitation with the right lobe of the liver and the inferior vena cava is not clear.

Echocardiography: ejection fraction of 71%, degeneration of the aortic valve, mild aortic valve insufficiency, and decreased left ventricular diastolic function (grade I)

131I-MIBG: abnormally elevated uptake is seen in the right adrenal region.

There is a slightly less dense mass shadow of 5.2 cm × 4.8 cm in the right adrenal, with significant uneven strengthening. The boundary with the right lobe of the liver and the inferior vena cava is not clear.

6.3.5 Current Diagnoses

Right adrenal pheochromocytoma

Multiple cysts of the liver

Double kidney cyst

Past total hysterectomy

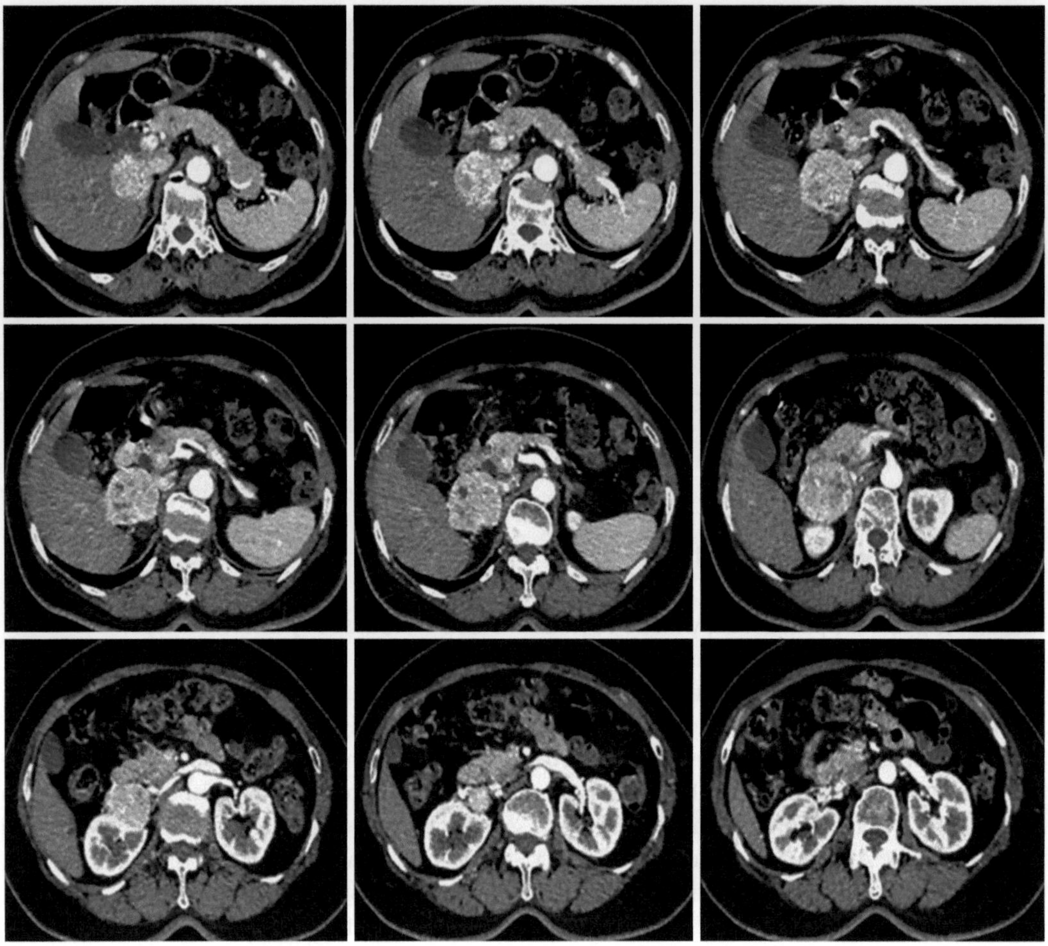

Fig. 6.5 Abdominal pelvic enhanced CT

6.3.6 MDT Discussion

6.3.6.1 Endocrinology

Ensure daily intake and continue to monitor supine blood pressure, heart rate, and weight. Avoid increased abdominal pressure, gastric reassurance, morpholine, and other drugs. Patient currently has no episodic symptoms. Blood pressure can be controlled, with no severe orthostatic hypotension. It is recommended to strengthen the intake. If necessary, adjust phenylbenzylamine to 10 mg q8h. Complete MEN-related screening. Please consult ICU and the Department of Anesthesiology. Explain the risk of surgery to the patient.

6.3.6.2 Department of Anesthesiology

Pheochromocytoma is not excluded. Anesthesia is prepared according to the pheochromocytoma routine. Preoperative blood transfusion is fully prepared. The risk is explained. Postoperative return to the ICU is recommended.

6.3.6.3 Urology

The patient's diagnosis of right adrenal pheochromocytoma is basically clear. The drug preparation is basically sufficient. Upcoming surgery is planned. Open surgery may be thought, if necessary, according to the intraoperative situation.

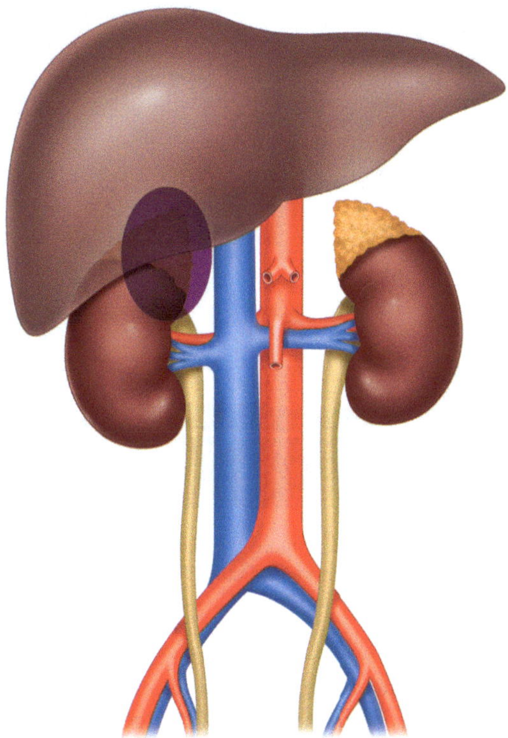

Fig. 6.6 Schematic diagram of the location of the mass

6.3.6.4 ICU

Patient is at high perioperative risk and understands the risk of surgery. If she needs to return to the ICU after surgery, contact us for bed preparation.

6.3.7 Surgical Approach

"Laparoscopic resection of right paralateral paraganglioma" under general anesthesia (Fig. 6.6)

6.3.8 Postoperative Pathology

(Right paratyle) lesions are consistent with paragangliomas.

6.4 Case 6.4

Patient: Male, 38 years old

6.4.1 Complaints

Paroxysmal increased blood pressure was found about 10 days ago.

6.4.2 History of Present Illness

Ten days ago, after fatigue during night sleep, a sudden pulsatile headache lasted more than 10 min, accompanied by palpitations and sweating, and not accompanied by nausea, jet vomiting, chest tightness, and other discomfort. Pain affected sleep. After the attack, symptoms were relieved. The symptoms recurred, with no more severe headache, mostly manifested as palpitations and sweating. Self-measured blood pressure was up to 180/110 mmHg. More often, the symptoms could be relieved on their own. During the course of the disease, no obvious change in body weight was found. No purple streaks on the skin, no full moon face, buffalo back, periodic muscle weakness, and other manifestations were seen. In order to seek further examinations, the patient went to Heilongjiang Provincial Hospital on July 7, 2020, to check the adrenal enhanced CT. CT shows that an oval soft-tissue density shadow was seen behind the right peritoneum. The size was about 34.2 × 23.3 mm with the CT value of 43HU. The right adrenal gland and inferior vena cava were not clearly demarcated. The soft tissue density behind the peritoneum was unevenly strengthened after the enhancement scan. No obvious abnormalities were found in renin, aldosterone, 24-h urinary catecholamines, serum cortisol, and blood ACTH.

6.4.3 Past, Personal, Marital and Childbearing, Family History

Nothing special

6.4.4 Accessory Examination

2020-07-22 Abdominal pelvic enhanced CT (Fig. 6.7): A nodular shadow of soft-tissue den-

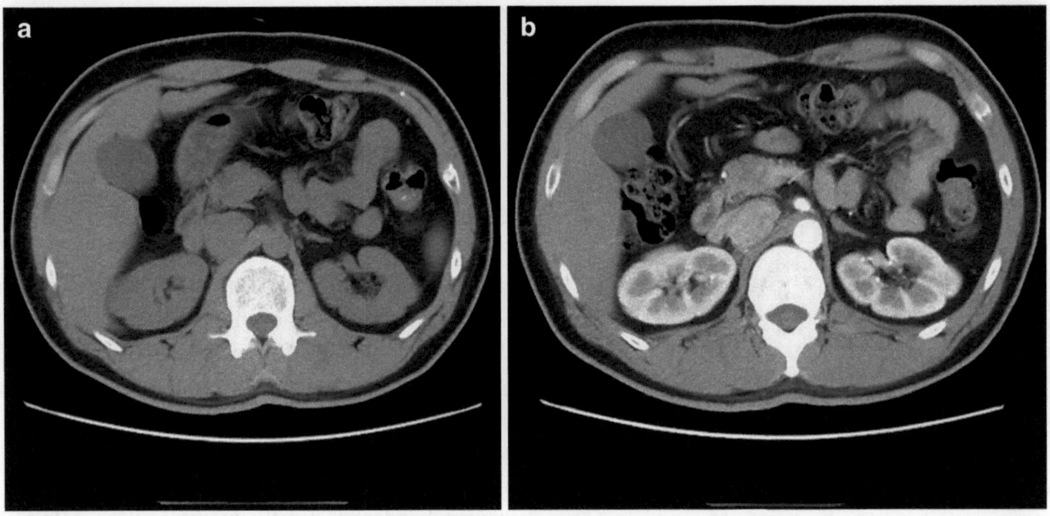

Fig. 6.7 Abdominal pelvic enhancement CT. (**a**, **b**) A nodular shadow of soft-tissue density is seen in the right retroperitoneum and beside the inferior vena cava. Enhancement shows more uniform and significant strength. The size is about 2.4 cm × 3.5 cm. The boundary is clear

sity is seen in the right retroperitoneum and beside inferior vena cava. The enhancement shows more uniform and significant strength. The size is about 2.4 cm × 3.5 cm. The boundary is clear.

Endocrine examination: 24 h urinary catecholamines: Norepinephrine 80.36 μg/24 h (16.69–40.65 μg/24 h), epinephrine 76.54 μg/24 h (1.74–6.42 μg/24 h), dopamine 405.17 μg/24 h (120.93–330.59 μg/24 h)

6.4.5 Current Diagnosis

Paraganglioma of the right kidney

6.4.6 MDT Discussion

6.4.6.1 Endocrinology

Monitor the body weight and 24 h intake and output, and measure blood pressure and heart rate in the vertical position two to three times a day. Prescribe a diabetic diet, and control the daily staple food to about 400 g. Avoid sweets and liquid food, and regularly check the spectrum of blood glucose. If the condition allows, increase appropriately physical activity. Check HCT every week, pay attention to cardiovascular symptoms and stool conditions, and avoid defecation effort. Dumic and other auxiliary laxatives can be taken. Avoid emotional agitation, fatigue, infection, severe postural changes, and compression of the abdomen. Avoid the use of morphine, gastric reassurance, and other drugs.

In terms of blood pressure, phenolic benzylamine can be increased. A difference in blood pressure in lying position is obvious. Standing heart rate is fast. After the increase of drug, the amount of intake should be increased. Daily water intake can be increased to nearly 4 L. In terms of hypoglycemia, diet and exercise control are the mainstays. If the blood glucose is still high after the meal, acarbose 50 mg (taken with the first meal) can be added before the meal. The targets of blood glucose are FBG 4–7 mmol/L and PBG 6–10 mmol/L. Demand consultations from the Department of Anesthesiology and ICU to assess perioperative risk.

6.4.6.2 Department of Anesthesiology

Middle-aged men, ASA grade III, limited-term surgery. Paraganglioma is more likely. Patient is considered to undergo surgery after taking phenylbenzylamine for 14 days. Closely monitor the blood pressure in the recumbent position. The surgeon has communicated with the patient about the sharp fluctuations in hemodynamics before and after tumor resection, which result in myocardial injury, myocardial ischemia, cerebral ischemia, AKI, cerebral hemorrhage, malignant arrhythmia, cardiac arrest, and risk of circulatory failure. The tumor and inferior vena cava are not clearly demarcated. The risk of intraoperative bleeding is high. Adequate preparation for blood transfusion is necessary. Cell saver can be prepared. Postoperative return to ICU.

6.4.6.3 Vascular Surgery

Considering that the right retroperitoneal mass is closely related to the inferior vena cava, there is a risk of vascular damage during surgery, and the risk of major bleeding. It is recommended to fully explain to the patient before surgery. Our department can provide assistance during surgery.

6.4.6.4 ICU

The diagnosis of paraganglioma is clear. The risk of perioperative hypertensive crisis is explained. The risk of stress cardiomyopathy and arrhythmia is explained. The postoperative return to the ICU is explained.

6.4.7 Surgical Approach

"Robot-assisted laparoscopic resection of right paraganglioma" under general anesthesia (Figs. 6.8 and 6.9).

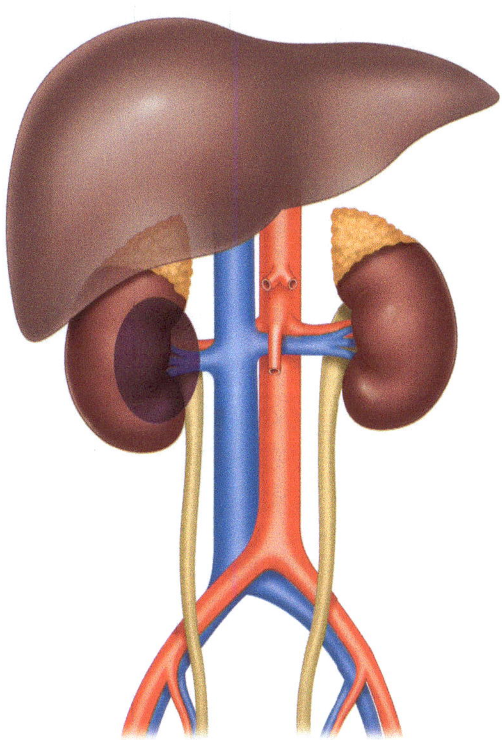

Fig. 6.8 Schematic diagram of the location of the mass

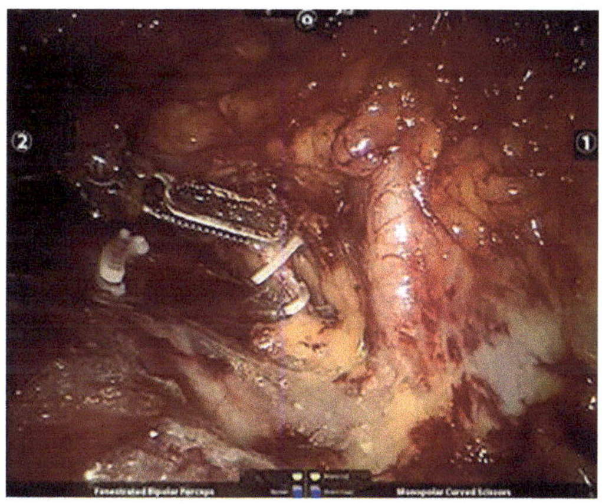

Fig. 6.9 Intraoperative condition of robot-assisted laparoscopic surgery

6.4.8 Postoperative Pathology

Lesions (retroperitoneal masses) are consistent with paragangliomas.

Immunohistochemical results: Melan-A(−), AE1/AE3(−), CgA(+), Ki-67(index 1%), S-100(+), α-inhibin(−), CD34(vascular +).

6.5 Case 6.5

Patient: Female, 56 years old

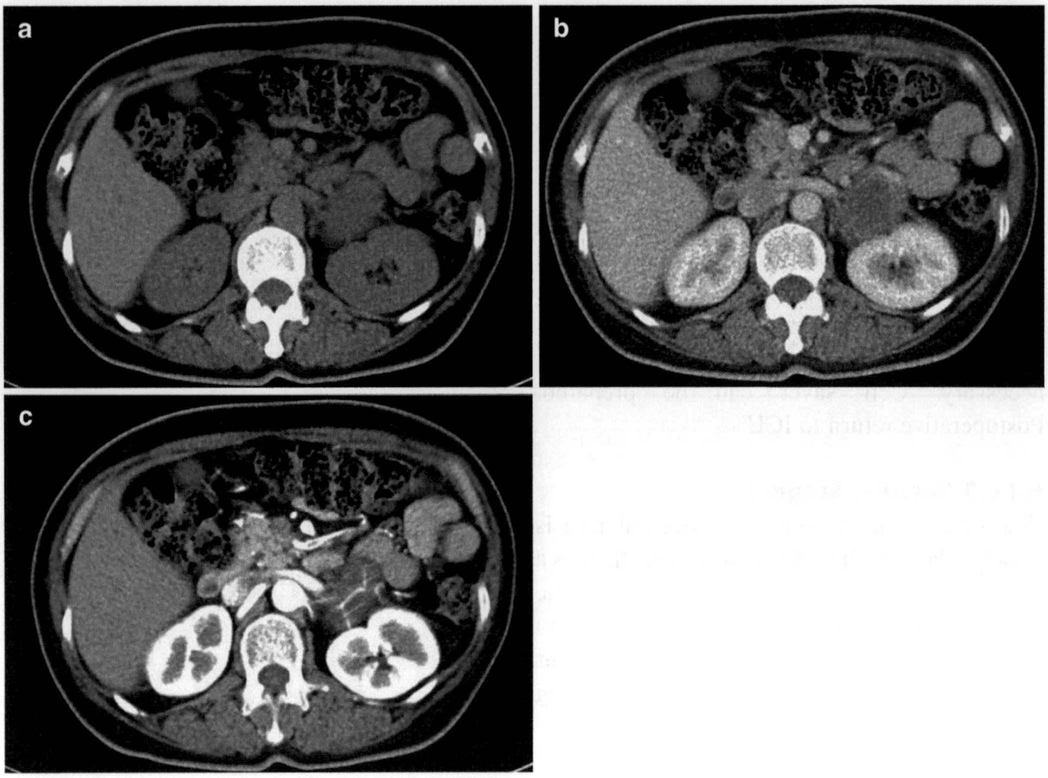

Fig. 6.10 Adrenal enhancement CT. (**a–c**) A circular cystic solid mass in the left adrenal region is found. Enhanced scanning shows that the solid component is strengthened significantly, while the low-density area is not strengthened. The size of lesion is about 5.7 cm × 4.8 cm × 4.6 cm

6.5.1 Complaints

Paroxysmal palpitations, easy sweating, and a mass in left adrenal gland have been found for half a year.

6.5.2 History of Present Illness

The patient developed paroxysmal palpitations and easy sweating half a year ago. She did not measure blood pressure at the onset of symptoms and reported no history of hypertension. She went to the local hospital for physical examination and had the double kidney B ultrasound. Left adrenal mass was found. She came to our hospital for treatment. Adrenal enhanced CT + three-dimensional reconstruction + CTA (Fig. 6.10a–c) suggest a circular cystic solid mass in the left adrenal region. The enhanced scanning shows that the solid component is strengthened significantly, while low-density area is not strengthened. The size of the lesion is about 5.7 cm × 4.8 cm × 4.6 cm. Urinary catecholamine examination at 24 h found NE 433.73 μg/24 h (10.7 times), E 238.55 μg/24 h (37.2 times), and DA 477.11 μg/24 h (1.4 times). Somatostatin receptor imaging was not significantly abnormal. Because of the possibility of pheochromocytoma, phenol benzamine 10 mg Q8H was given orally, and the patient stopped the drug after taking one box due to dry mouth and obvious nasal congestion. Two months ago, she came to our hospital for outpatient follow-up, and 24-h urinary catecholamines was checked and found NE 43.02 μg/24 h (1.06 times), E 64.54 μg/24 h (10.1 times), and DA 189.31 μg/24 h.

It is recommended to continue the preparation of phenylbenzylamine drugs. Currently, she has warm fingertips. The supine blood pressure is 127/83 mmHg with a heart rate of 80 bpm. The standing blood pressure is 151/90 mmHg with a heart rate of 87 bpm. Ther is no dry mouth and no nasal congestion. Patient began oral phenoxybenzamine 10 mg qd × 2 day → 10 mg q12h × 4 day → 10 mg q8h × 2 day on December 31. At present, the symptoms of dry mouth and nasal congestion are obvious. The supine blood pressure is 121/80 mmHg with a heart rate of 84 bpm, and the standing blood pressure is 114/76 mmHg with a heart rate of 103 bpm. There was no significant increase in body weight. HCT is changed from 40% to 38.8%.

6.5.3 Past, Personal, Marital and Childbearing, Family History

Blood glucose has increased for 3 years. Fasting blood glucose is 11–13 mmol/L. Postprandial blood glucose is 15–18 mmol/L. Takes oral acarbose two tablets tid per day.

6.5.4 Accessory Examination

There are no significant abnormalities in somatostatin receptor imaging.

Endocrine examination: 24-h urinary catecholamine tests suggest NE 43.02 μg/24 h and E 64.54 μg/24 h.

6.5.5 Current Diagnoses

Left paratyle paraganglioma

Diabetes

Past bilateral breast fibroadenoma resection

6.5.6 MDT Discussion

6.5.6.1 Department of Anesthesiology

Middle-aged and elderly women, ASA grade III, elective surgery. Pheochromocytoma is likely. Secreting epinephrine is the mainstay. Preoperative preparation is acceptable. Instruct patient to continue to take drugs before surgery and drink water to increase the capacity. The possibility of severe fluctuations in perioperative hemodynamics, as well as myocardial infarction, heart failure, malignant arrhythmias, cardiac arrest, cerebral infarction, cerebral hemorrhage, and other risks need to be explained to the patient. Intraoperative preparation of artery-vein passage and vasoactive drugs. Diabetes control is poor, and perioperative stress may further lead to hyperglycemia, which increases the risk of acute cardiovascular and cerebrovascular events. Endocrinology is asked to assist in assessing perioperative glycemic management, if necessary.

6.5.6.2 Department of Severe Medicine

Complete the screening of new crown antibodies before surgery. Fully explain the surgical risks and related perioperative complications, monitor blood pressure and hemodynamic stability, ensure the stability of perioperative blood pressure and perfusion of important organs such as cardio-cerebral kidneys, and monitor changes in electrolytes and internal environment during the perioperative period.

6.5.7 Surgical Approach

"Laparoscopic resection of left parastyle paraganglioma" is performed under general anesthesia (Fig. 6.11)

6.5.8 Postoperative Pathology

Paraganglioma (left side of the renal pedicle)

Immunohistochemical results: Melan-A(−), AE1/AE3(−), CgA(+), Ki-67(index 5%), S-100(+), α-inhibin(−).

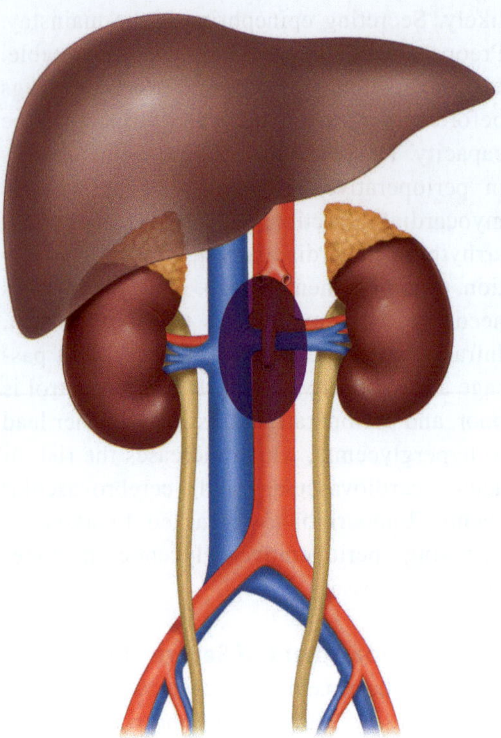

Fig. 6.11 Schematic diagram of the location of the mass

6.6 Case 6.6

Patient: Male, 38 years old

6.6.1 Complaints

An increase in blood pressure was found 6 months ago, and a retroperitoneal mass was found 2 months ago.

6.6.2 History of Present Illness

In October 2018, physical examination of the patient found an increase in blood pressure. BP was 160/90 mmHg. He did not take it seriously. In January 2019, after a poor night's rest, he had persistent dizziness, palpitations, and other discomfort. The symptoms were relieved after rest. He denied occurrence of sweating, denied abdominal pain, nausea, vomiting, etc. He visited the outer hospital and took the abdominal CT, which found a retroperitoneal mass (no report seen). He was then admitted to our clinic on February 2019. His routine blood test result shows HCT 47.1%, and 24 h urinary catecholamine results are as follows: NE 320.33 μg/24 h↑, E 5.68 μg/24 h, and DA 361.67 μg/24 h↑. Plasma catecholamines and metabolites show NMN 4.19 nmol/L↑, MN 0.11 nmol/L; (standing) PRA2 0.32 ng/mL/h↓, ALD2 16.15 ng/mL, AT-II2 44.04 pg/mL. Residual blood ACTH, blood F, DHEAS, etc. were negative. Scan of the adrenal glands shows that the left adrenal junction is slightly full. A shallow lobular soft tissue mass (31.9 × 33.6 mm) is seen in the lower edge of the left renal vein on the right margin of the retroperitoneal abdominal aorta. The enhancement scan is (Figs. 6.12 and 6.13) obviously less uniformly strengthened, and the flaky low-strengthening area is seen, Paraganglioma cell tumor is not excluded. The adrenal medullary MIBG imaging and somatostatin receptor imaging are all (+). Consideration of paraganglioma in outpatient department, he started taking phenylbenzylamine 10 mg Bid drug on March 5, 2019. After taking the drugs, BP in sitting position was 125–140/70–80 mmHg, and BP in standing position was 105–125/60–75 mmHg. However, changes in orthostatic heart rate were obvious (recumbent → position): 60–80 bpm → 120–130 bpm. During this period, there was fatigue and tiredness. Betalek 25 mg tablets taken bid were added to control the heart rate. The change in orthostatic heart rate was significantly better. On March 22, phenoxybenzamine was increased to 10 mg Q8H. Currently, BP in seated position is 105–125/60–80 mmHg with a HR of 60–75 bpm, while standing BP is 100–130/60–100 mmHg with a HR of 75–100 bpm. He has warm extremity ends. He is now admitted in our department for further treatment.

During the course of the disease, sleeping pattern and diet have been normal. Bowel movement is normal, and there is no significant weight gain after taking the phenylbenzylamine drug for preparation.

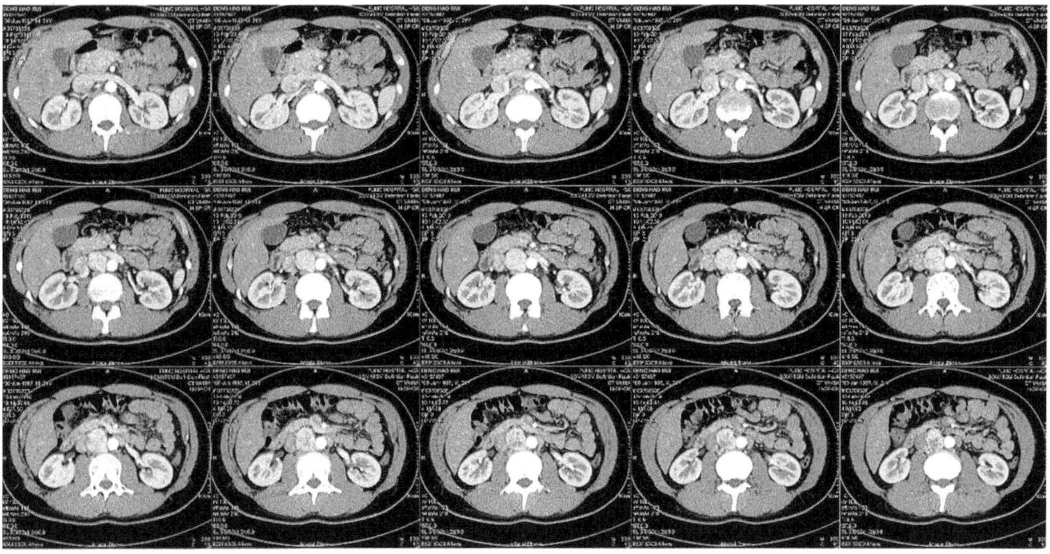

Fig. 6.12 Adrenal enhancement CT

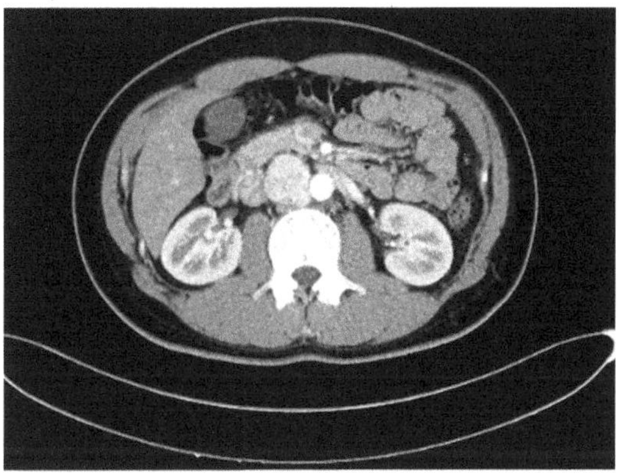

Fig. 6.13 Enhanced CT

On March 27, 2019, somatostatin receptor imaging: expression of somatostatin receptors in lesions of the right middle abdomen. In combination with adrenal medullary imaging on February 27, 2019, paraganglioma is more likely.

Superficial lobed soft-tissue mass (31.9 mm × 33.6 mm) at the lower edge of the left renal vein and at the right margin of the retroperitoneal ventral aorta

After enhancement, soft-tissue mass in the retroperitoneum is significantly less uniformly strengthened, and flaky areas of low strengthening are seen internally

6.6.3 Past, Personal, Marital and Childbearing, Family History

Nothing special

6.6.4 Accessory Examination

On March 1, 2019, 131I-MIBG: An abnormal mass is seen in the right middle abdomen. The possibility of pheochromocytoma is considered. Local tomography for localization was recommended.

6.6.5 Current Diagnoses

Right Paraganglioma (adjacent to the left renal pedicle)

Hypertension (grade 2, moderate-risk group)

6.6.6 MDT Discussion

6.6.6.1 ICU

Fully explain the risks and complications associated with the perioperative period, monitor and maintain the stability of blood pressure and hemodynamic blood during the perioperative period, avoid the fluctuations of blood pressure, and return the patient to the ICU after surgery.

6.6.6.2 Department of Anesthesiology

(1) ASA grade III, limited-time surgery; (2) The patient has a paraganglioma, who is recommended to improve the three cardiac parameters before surgery to further evaluate cardiac function. He is also adviced to quit smoking and strengthen respiratory exercise. (3) Patient anesthesia is according to pheochromocytoma routine preparation: the establishment of arteriovenous veins, preparation of vascular active drugs, intraoperative strengthening, monitoring of changes in vital signs, maintenance of myocardial oxygen supply and oxygen consumption balance, and ensuring the perfusion of important organs are important. (4) Fully explain to the patient the risk of perioperative cardiovascular and cerebrovascular accidents and major bleeding. Pay attention to fluctuations of blood glucose, maintain water-electrolyte balance, and fully prepare blood supply. (5) Recommend return to ICU after surgery.

6.6.7 Surgical Approach

"Laparoscopic resection of right retroperitoneal paraganglioma" under general anesthesia (Fig. 6.14)

6.6.8 Postoperative Pathology

Lesion is consistent with paraganglioma and chronic inflammation of lymph node (0/5).

Immunohistochemical results: S-100(+), CgA(+), Melan-A(−), α-inhibin(−), AE1/AE3(−), Ki-67(index 2%).

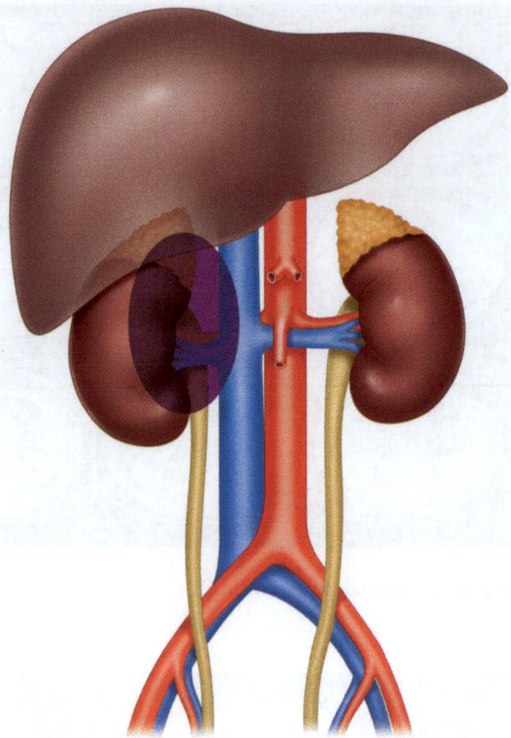

Fig. 6.14 Schematic diagram of the location of the mass

6.7 Case 6.7

Patient: Female, 26 years of age

6.7.1 Complaints

Physical examination revealed a mass in left abdomen more than 2 months ago.

6.7.2 History of Present Illness

In August 2018, the patient's physical examination of ultrasound revealed that the left abdomen was occupied by a mass (specification unknown).

The patient reported no paroxysmal palpitations, hypertension, headache, sweating, waist pain, low back pain, bloating, and abdominal pain. For further diagnosis and treatment, the patient came to our hospital and checked through CTU, which shows a high strengthening mass below the pancreatic body and tail and below the anterior left kidney. The size is about 10 cm × 8 cm × 9.7 cm. Its internal density is uneven, the edges are still clear, and the flat scan CT value is about 33HU. The cortical phase of enhanced scanning is uneven and significantly strengthened. Further check of the somatostatin receptor imaging shows a hyperexpression lesion of somatostatin receptor hyperexpression lesion below the left kidney, middle and lower level (left retroperitoneal part). 131I-MIBG shows a large area of radioactive concentration in the left mid-abdomen, which suggests an ectopic pheochromocytoma. On September 3, 2018, 24-h urine catecholamine results show NE 19.20 μg/24 h, DA 169.40 μg/24 h, and E 1.92 μg/24 h. On September 29, 2018, 24-h urine catecholamine results show NE 23.97 μg/24 h, E 2.28 μg/24 h, and DA 141.29 μg/24 h. According to instructions by outpatient department, she took phenylbenzylamine preparation. From September 17, 2018, to October 17, 2018, she took an oral phenylbenzylamine 5 mg tid. From October 17, 2018 to present, she took an oral phenylbenzylamine 10 mg tid. Self-monitoring of supine blood pressure reads 100–140/60–80 mmHg with a heart rate of 65–75 beats/min. Standing blood pressure is 100–130/60–70 mmHg with a heart rate of 70–90 beats/min. Patient has warm extremities.

6.7.3 Past, Personal, Marital and Childbearing, Family History

Nothing special

6.7.4 Accessory Examination

131I-MIBG Abnormal lesion in left mid-abdominal abnormality is considered as an ectopic pheochromocytoma. No significant abnormalities are seen in the remaining areas.

Somatostatin receptor imaging: a hyperexpression lesion of somatostatin receptor at the left lower middle and lower level (equivalent to the retroperitoneal site of the left peritoneum). In combination with adrenal medullary imaging, pheochromocytoma is considered.

CTU (Figs. 6.15 and 6.16):

An irregular mass shadow is seen below the pancreatic body and tail of the left abdomen and in front of lower left kidney. The size is about 10 cm × 8 cm × 9.7 cm. Its internal density is uneven, the edges are still clear, and the scan CT value is about 33 HU. The cortical phase of enhanced scanning is unevenly and significantly strengthened. The parenchymal phase is slightly reduced. There are multiple flakes without obvious strengthening in the lesion. The posterior lesion is close to the left kidney. The local boundary is slightly unclear. The abdominal segment of the left ureter is close to the lesion, and the lumen is slightly changed with pressure

The upper edge of the lesion is locally adjacent to the tail of the pancreas, and the demarcation is still clear. The blood supply of the lesion seems to come from the branch of sub-mesenteric artery and from fine branches of the abdominal aorta. The inferior mesenteric vein undergoes upward and outward compression changes, and the lesion appears to show drainage from the inferior mesenteric vein branch.

6.7.5 Current Diagnoses

Left retroperitoneal giant paraganglioma

6.7.6 MDT Discussion

6.7.6.1 ICU

Patient is fully accounted for the surgical risks. It is recommended to return to the ICU after surgery.

6.7.6.2 Endocrinology

The patient's diagnosis of left paraganglioma is relatively clear. The current drug preparation is

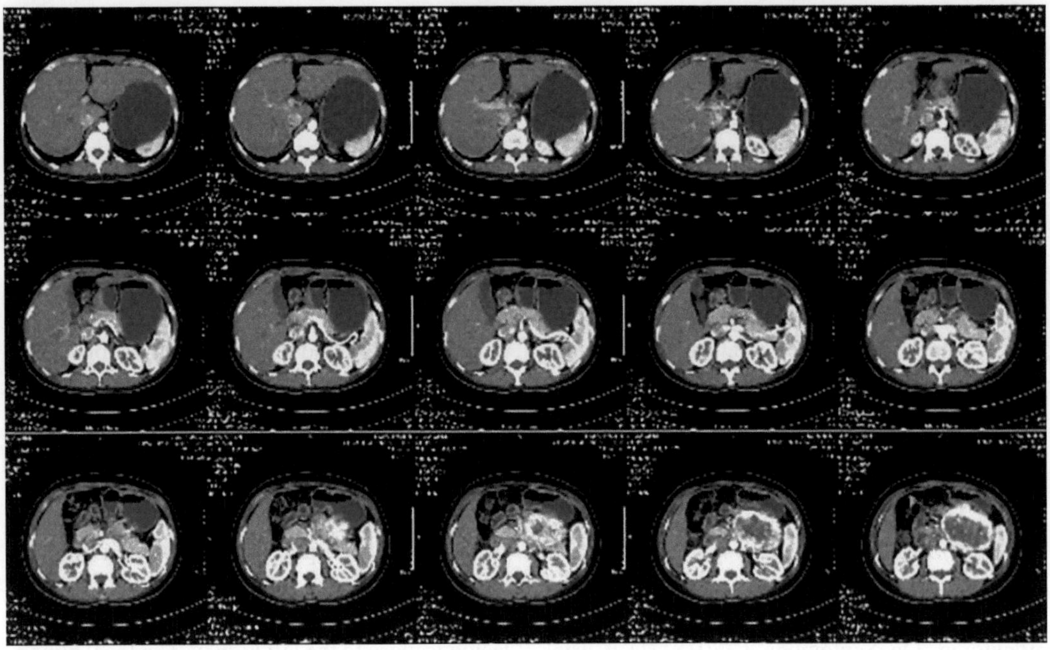

Fig. 6.15 Adrenal enhancement CT

relatively adequate. The recumbent position BP, HR, weight, and HCT are monitored. MEN is screened.

6.7.6.3 Department of Anesthesiology

Surgery is risky, and cardiopulmonary function is fully assessed.

6.7.6.4 Basic Surgery

Our department is willing to assist on the stage of operation and explain the possibility of local pancreatic resection, pancreatic tail resection, and splenectomy.

6.7.6.5 Vascular Surgery

Our department is willing to actively assist on the stage of operation and fully explain to the patient the risk of intraoperative damage to large blood vessels and even the possibility of blood vessel reconstruction.

6.7.6.6 Ophthalmology

No contraindications to anesthesia

6.7.7 Surgical Approach

"Laparoscopic assisted resection of the left paraganglioma" under general anesthesia (Fig. 6.17).

6.7.8 Postoperative Pathology

(Left paraganglioma) Paraganglioma with partial bleeding, edema, degeneration, and active local growth

Immunohistochemical results: Melan-A(−), AE1/AE3(−), CgA(+), Syn(+), Ki-67 (index approx. 5%), S-100 (partial+), α-inhibin (partial+)

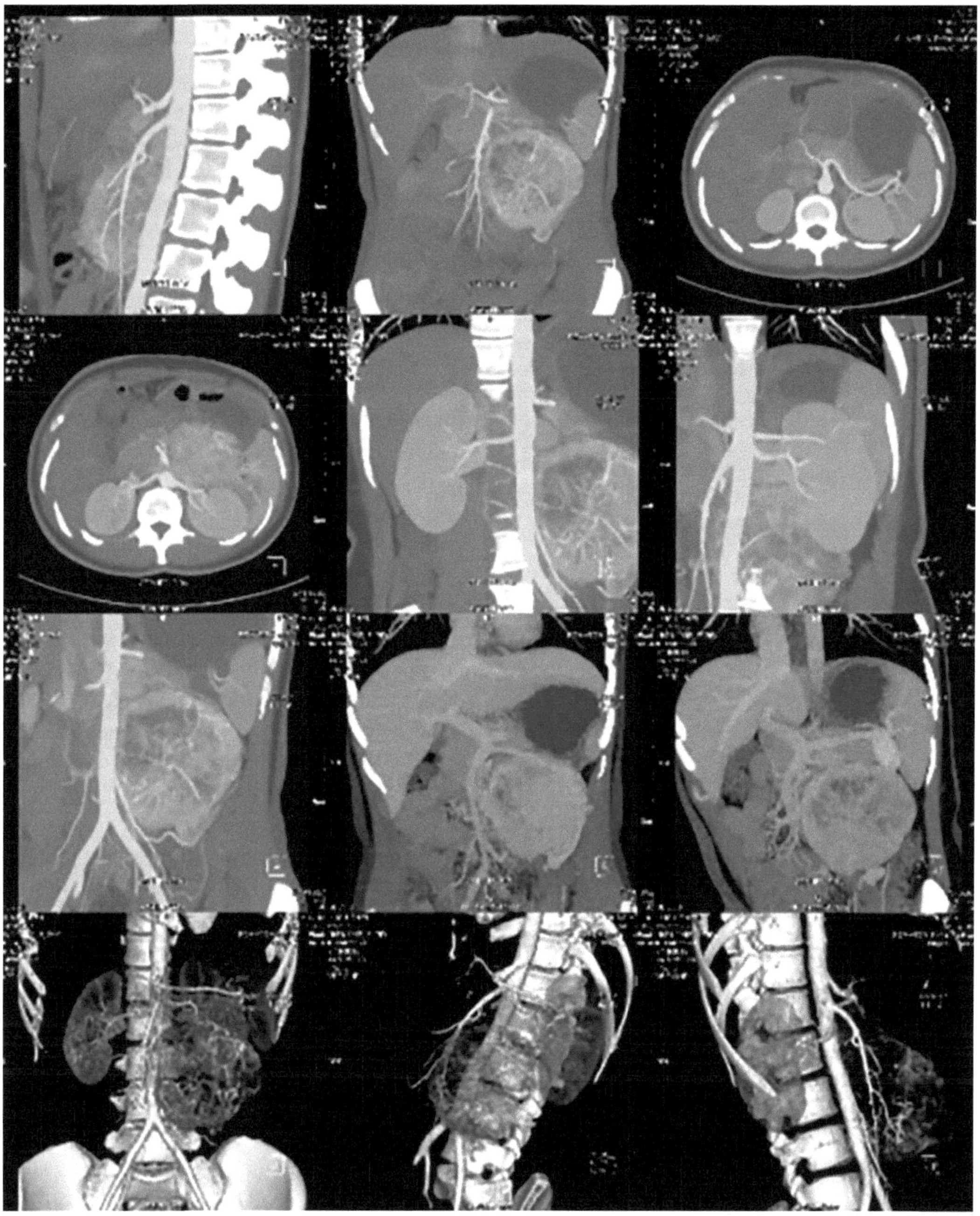

Fig. 6.16 Abdominal enhancement CTA

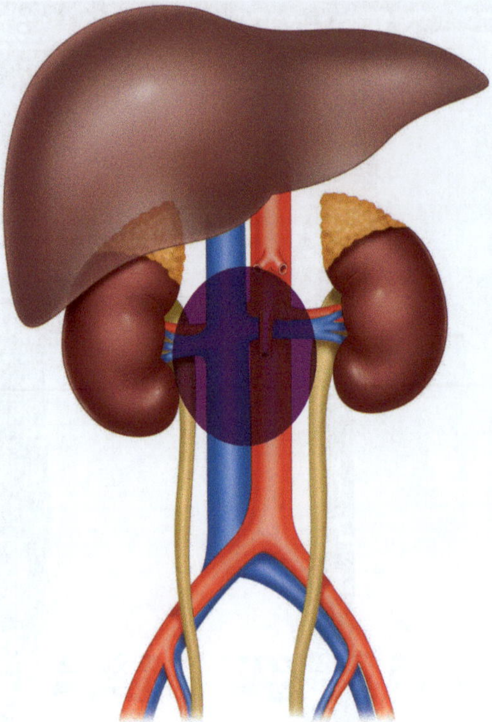

Fig. 6.17 Schematic diagram of the location of the mass

6.8 Case 6.8

Patient: Female, 32 years old

6.8.1 Complaints

Intermittent headache for 3 years, hypertension found 3 months ago

6.8.2 History of Present Illness

In 2015, the patient had intermittent headache without obvious precipitating causes. Patient felt paroxysmal dull pain in the occipital region without nausea, vomiting, and blurred vision. It was spontaneously relieved after a few minutes of each attack. Blood pressure was not measured and further diagnosis and treatment were not sought. In April 2018, the patient had headache again without obvious precipitating causes. The location and nature were the same, accompanied by heavy sweating, lasting about 9 h without spontaneous relief. Blood pressure was checked by local hospital staff with a 230/120 mmHg reading. She was treated with drugs such as losartan and nifedipine. Blood pressure was reduced to normal, and headache symptoms were relieved.

The patient visited our outpatient clinic in May 2018 and 24-h urinary catecholamine was checked and found NE 126.00 μg/24 h↑, E 4.55 μg/24 h, and DA 259.37 μg/24 h. Somatostatin receptor imaging shows a lesion of a slight increase in radiation uptake in the right jaw position and a circular foci of increased radiation uptake in the left middle quadrant. MIBG systemic imaging shows an area of radiogenic uptake elevation in the left mid-upper quadrant. There are no abnormal radiation concentrations or attenuated areas in the bilateral adrenal glands and other parts of the body. In combination with somatostatin receptor tomography, it is consistent with the possibility of retroperitoneal abdominal para-aortic paraganglia. Chest-abdominal pelvic enhanced CT shows a round soft tissue nodule at the lower edge of the left renal artery of the abdominal aorta, with uniform internal density, smooth edges, and about 25 × 26 mm in size. The arterial stage of enhanced examination shows that it is significantly strengthened. The decrease is seen at the portal phase and the delayed phase. The boundary with the surrounding tissues is clear. The relationship with the left renal vein is closer. No significantly enlarged lymph nodes are seen retroperitoneally. Left retroperitoneal mass may be consistent with paraganglioma presentation. Head and neck CTA shows a nodule of soft tissue density above the bifurcation of right common carotid artery, about 9 mm × 7 mm in size, significantly strengthened after enhancement scan, no strengthening area inside, blood supply by the branch of right external carotid artery. The possibility of paraganglioma is considered. Outpatient clinic considers the possibility of multiple paragangliomas. On May 24, 2018, she took phenylbenzylamine 5 mg q12h, now adjusted to 15 mg 8 am, 15 mg 12 noon, 10 mg 4 pm. After taking the drug, patient complained of nasal congestion. Blood pressure was monitored, with normal heart rate, no obvious orthostatic hypotension, headache, palpitations, and sweating. Patient had a weight gain of about 1 kg. She was admitted for surgery. Currently, extremities are hot and humid with peripheral vascular signs (−).

6.8.3 Past, Personal, Marital and Childbearing, Family History

Suspected allergy to cephalosporin antibiotic; nothing special for the rest

6.8.4 Accessory Examination

On June 1, 2018, somatostatin receptor imaging shows a lesion of a slight increase in radiation uptake in the right jaw position and a circular foci of increased radiation uptake in the left middle quadrant. The thyroid gland is faintly demonstrated. The liver, spleen, kidneys, bladder, and intestines are normally demonstrated. There is no abnormal radiation reduction or concentration areas seen in all parts of the remaining body. For high expression lesion of somatostatin receptor in left mid-upper quadrant, the possibility of neuroendocrine tumor is considered. It is recommended to further clarify by the positioning of tomography. For an expression lesion of somatostatin receptor in equivalent to the right jaw position, the nature is to be determine. It is recommended to further differentiate it by tomography.

On June 22, 2018, chest-abdominal pelvic enhanced CT shows a round soft tissue nodule at the lower edge of the left renal artery of the abdominal aorta, with uniform internal density, smooth edges, and a size of about 25 mm × 26 mm. The arterial stage of enhanced examination show that it is significantly strengthened. The decrease is seen at the portal phase and the delayed phase. The boundary with the surrounding tissues is clear. The relationship with the left renal vein is closer. No significantly enlarged lymph nodes are seen retroperitoneally. The bladder is full, and the morphology is normal. The bladder wall is smooth, and no significant thickening is seen. The prostate gland is normal in size, and no abnormal density is seen. The seminal vesicle glands are roughly symmetrical and normal in morphology and size, and no abnormal density is seen. The rectal wall is not thickened. There are no abnormally enlarged lymph nodes in the pelvic and bilateral inguinal folds. Left retroperitoneal mass may be consistent with paraganglioma presentations. Lesions are closely related to left renal veins. Fatty liver is considered.

On June 8, 2018, 131I-MIBG: Intravenous tracer 1 or 2 days of systemic imaging shows an area of radiogenic uptake elevation in the left mid-upper quadrant. There are no abnormal radiation concentrations or attenuated areas in the bilateral adrenal glands and other parts of the body. Bilateral salivary glands and the liver are normally demonstrated. Elevated foci in the left mid-upper abdomen, in combination with somatostatin receptor tomography on June 1, 2018, are consistent with the possibility of retroperitoneal para-aortic paraganglioma.

On July 12, 2018, head and neck CTA (Figs. 6.18 and 6.19) shows a nodule of soft-tissue density above the bifurcation of the right common carotid artery, about 9 mm × 7 mm in size, significantly strengthened after enhancement scan, with no strengthening area inside and blood supply by the branch of the right external carotid artery. Please combine clinical presentations to consider the possibility of paragangli-

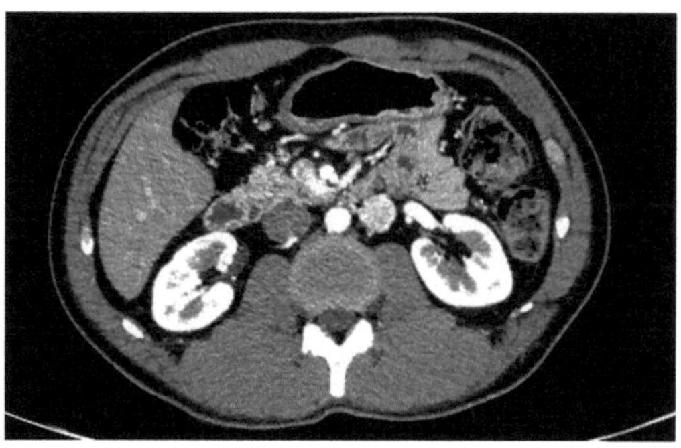

Fig. 6.18 Abdominal pelvis enhancement CT

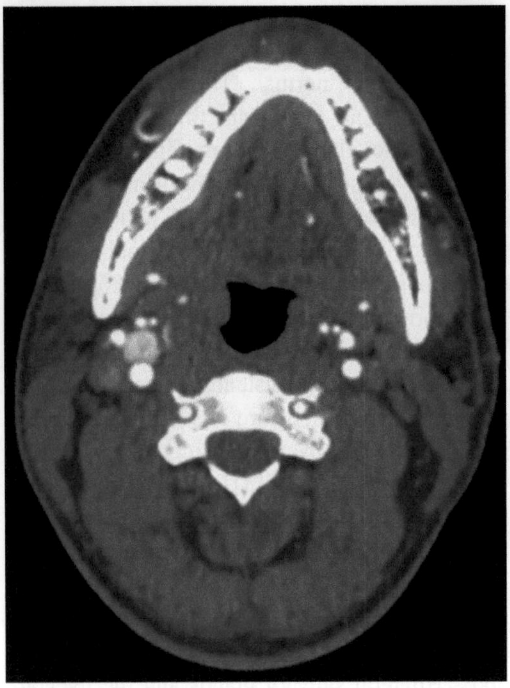

Fig. 6.19 Head and neck CTA

oma. Left mucosal thickening of sphenoid sinus and multiple small lymph nodes in bilateral neck are found.

Endocrine Examination: 24 h urinary catecholamines: NE 126.00 μg/24 h, E 4.55 μg/24 h, DA 259.37 μg/24 h;

Blood ACTH 54.9 pg/mL, blood F 19.22 μg/dL, 24hUFC 63.14 μg/24 h;

PRA2 1.91 ng/mL/h, AT-II2 79.25 pg/mL, ALD2 17.28 ng/dL.

A round soft tissue nodule is found at the lower edge of the left renal artery of the abdominal aorta, with uniform internal density, smooth edges, and a size of about 25 mm × 26 mm. The arterial stage of enhanced examination shows that it is significantly strengthened. The decrease is seen at the portal phase and the delayed phase. The boundary with the surrounding tissues is clear. The relationship with the left renal vein is closer

Head and neck CTA shows a nodule of soft-tissue density above the bifurcation of the right common carotid artery, about 9 mm × 7 mm in size, significantly strengthened after enhancement scan, with no strengthening area inside and blood supply by the branch of the right external carotid artery. The possibility of paraganglioma is considered

6.8.5 Current Diagnoses

Posterior peritoneal mass on the left side
  Paragangliomas
  Mass above the right common carotid artery
  Paraganglioma

6.8.6 MDT Discussion

6.8.6.1 Endocrinology

Combined with the history and the results of the examinations, it is more likely to consider multiple paragangliomas. Continue preoperative preparation of phenylbenzylamine, record the 24 h intake and output, instruct the patient to increase the amount of intake appropriately and eat a high-sodium diet, and monitor the blood pressure and heart rate in the recumbent position, blood HCT, and weight changes. The preoperative control of blood pressure is required in the normal range without dizziness attack and orthostatic hypotension. Adjust the dose of phenylbenzylamine according to the blood pressure and heart rate. The remaining treatment opinions are the same.

6.8.6.2 Department of Anesthesiology

Case is considered as ASA Grade III and elective surgery. Follow the advice of endocrinology consultation for the full preoperative preparation. Strengthen perioperative hemodynamic monitoring. Fully account for perioperative hypotension, myocardial infarction, heart failure, arrhythmia, stroke, major hemorrhage, and pulmonary complications such as lung infection and atelectasis. It is recommended to return to the ICU.

6.8.6.3 Otolaryngology

The neck mass may be considered largely to be paraganglioma. It is recommended to complete temporal bone enhancement CT, neck soft tissue MRI, and 24-h urinary MN/NMN. Optional resection of neck mass may be considered.

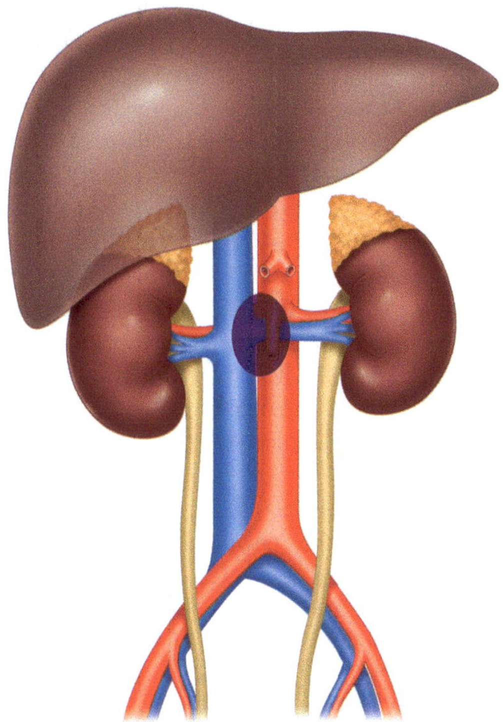

Fig. 6.20 Schematic diagram of the location of the mass

6.8.7 Surgical Approach

"Thoracic laparoscopic assisted resection of left retroperitoneal paraganglioma" under general anesthesia (Fig. 6.20)

6.8.8 Postoperative Pathology

Lesions (left paraganglioma) are consistent with paragangliomas. Peripheral lymph nodes show chronic inflammation (0/2).

Immunohistochemical results: AE1/AE3(−), CgA(+), Ki-67(index 2%), S-100(Supports cells+), Syn(+), SDHB(−)

6.9 Case 6.9

Patient: Female, 30 years old

6.9.1 Complaints

Intermittent dizziness and palpitations for more than 5 years

6.9.2 History of Present Illness

First admission (May 24, 2018, to June 22, 2018)

In June 2012, the patient started to experience intermittent dizziness, rotation of non-looking objects, blurred vision, syncope, black scorpion, etc. Blood pressure was occasionally measured at 140/90 mmHg, but she did not pay attention to the diagnosis and treatment. After that, dizziness was gradually increased, especially when the body position was changed, accompanied by headache and pain. NRS was three points with intermittent palpitations and sweating. Self-measured blood pressure was up to 200/130 mmHg with a pulse of 130 beats/min. Symptoms were relieved after rest. She went to another hospital. She was treated with Betaloc, Norvox, valsartan, and other drugs successively, and her blood pressure was basically controlled at 130–140/90–100 mmHg. In November 2014, she was admitted to Anzhen Hospital. PRA in the supine position was 5.15 ng/mL/h (0.93–6.56) and ALD 0.1 ng/mL (0.059–0.174). Renal artery ultrasound, abdominal ultrasound, and adrenal CT scan showed no abnormalities. Essential hypertension was considered. She took olmesartan 20 mg qd and Kangxin 5 mg qd. Blood pressure was controlled at 120–130/80–90 mmHg, occasionally greater than 140/90 mmHg. Dizziness and palpitations were less than before. In June 2016, the antihypertensive drug was changed to labetalol 200 mg tid because of the preparation for pregnancy. The dizziness and palpitations were more frequent than before, and the blood pressure increased again. Treatment with Baixintong 30 mg qd did not control blood pressure. In December 2016, the pregnancy was terminated under hysteroscopy due to the disappearance of umbilical blood flow at 24 weeks of pregnancy. The antihypertensive drug was adjusted to oral treatment of olmesartan 20 mg qd + Kangxin 5 mg qd. Blood pressure was not controlled well, still more than 140/90 mmHg, especially at night, with the highest at 180/120 mmHg. In March 2018, she was admitted to Anzhen Hospital again. Her blood test showed the following: NE 771–1424 pg/mL (70–550) and NMN 866–1362 pg/mL (0–140). DA, E, and MN were normal. Twenty-four hours UFC was 149.77 μg/24 h (58–403). Contrast-enhanced CT of the abdomen found a retroperitoneal space-occupying lesion with rich blood supply, about 37 × 27 × 29 mm in size. No necrosis was excluded, and no obvious enlarged lymph nodes were found in the abdominal cavity. The possibility of ectopic pheochromocytoma was considered. She was treated with amlodipine 5 mg qd, Kangxin 5 mg qd, and mazanil 1 mg qn. The blood pressure at night and in supine position was still 150–180/100 mm Hg. She felt dizzy when changing rapidly positions. Black lobster was obvious. At the same time, there were palpitations and sweating after waking up, which last for 1 min to recover. In April 2018, she visited the endocrinology clinic of our hospital, and 24-h urine CA was checked and found the following: NE 820.47, 823.01 μg/24 h, DA 241.07, 304.47 μg/24 h, and E 1.79. Somatostatin receptor tomography showed a lesion of slightly higher expression of somatostatin receptors on the left abdominal main para-arterial (L3 level). Pheochromocytoma was not excluded. CTU showed a retroperitoneal mass on the left side of the abdominal aorta, suggesting the clinical possibility of paraganglioma. Small branches of the abdominal aorta provided blood supply, and it was drained venously to the left renal vein. On April 23, phenoxybenzamine 10 mg q12h and Betaloc 25 mg q12h were added. Supine blood pressure fluctuations were monitored between 150 and 160/90 and 100 mmHg. The standing blood pressure was 120/80 mmHg. The patient went to the outpatient department of urology and was recommended to undergo surgical treatment. She was admitted to our department on May 24. Accessory examination: 24 h urine catecholamines showed NE 531.00 μg/24 h, E 9.91 μg/24 h, and DA 298.11 μg/24 h; urine volume 5900 mL; 12 h urine catecholamines (8 am–8 pm) showed 12hNE 318.69 μg/12 h, 12hE 2.66 μg/12 h, and 12hDA 130.46 μg/12 h; 12 h urine catecholamines (8 pm–8 am) showed 12hNE 267.79 μg/12 h, 12hE 5.18 μg/12 h, and 12hDA 87.29 μg/12 h. Twenty-four hours ambulatory blood pressure monitoring showed a mean blood pressure of 134/92 mmHg. Night blood pressure was significantly higher than daily blood pressure. 131I-MIBG: a lesion of increased radioactivity in the left middle abdomen. Blood F[8 AM]: 15.60 μg/dL. Twenty-four hours UFC: 62.22 μg/24 h. Urine output: 5100 mL. Thyroid function 2+ thyroid function 3: normal. 6 gonads: FSH 4.75 IU/L, E2 63.60 pg/mL, P 4.41 ng/mL, T 0.39 ng/mL, LH 2.00 IU/L, and PRL 8.49 ng/mL. PTH: 90.5 pg/mL. Free calcium: 1.13 mmol/L (Ph 7.34). Ca: 2.18 mmol/L. P: 1.25 mmol/L. 24 h UCa: 16.36 mmol/24 h. 24 h UP: 37.72 mmol/24 h, 24 h U-V: 4100 mL. ALP: 74 U/L, β-CTX: 0.901 ng/mL. T-25OHD: 18.7 ng/mL. CT less than 1.5 pg/mL. GASTRIN 37.2 pg/mL. Glucagon: 116.66 pg/mL. Parathyroid ultrasound: no obvious abnormality. Echocardiography: LVEF 55% and mild mitral insufficiency. Conventional MRI of the head +T2 × WI: scattered punctuations of abnormal signals in the bilateral frontal and parietal lobes, non-specific changes, and cyst in right maxillary sinus. Thyroid and neck lymph nodes ultrasound: no obvious abnormality. Whole-body bone imaging: the abnormal findings of the lateral sternoclavicular joint were considered highly likely to be inflammatory lesions. Renal blood flow function imaging: the blood perfusion and function of both kidneys were normal, and the drainage of the left renal pelvis was slightly less smooth. After admission, phenoxybenzamine was administered to control blood pressure. After monitoring of supine-standing blood pressure, gradual increase the dose of phenoxybenzamine was instructed. At the same time, the patient was instructed to increase intake, take appropriate high-salt diet, ensure adequate blood volume, enhance nutrition, and maintain stable weight gain. After taking phenoxybenzamine and ensuring the intake, the patient still had a rapid heart rate. Betaloc was given to control the heart rate.

The patient felt depressed and requested to be discharged from the hospital. She would return to the hospital to evaluate whether surgical treatment was feasible 2 weeks later. Her conditions and related risks were fully explained to the patient and her family. The patient still insisted on being discharged from the hospital.

Second admission (June 22, 2018–present)

After discharge, patient continued oral therapy of phenoxybenzamine at 8:00 10MG, 14:00 20MG, 20:00 15MG, and 02:00 10MG and Betaloc 25 mg bid. Blood pressure basically fluctuated between 130 and 160/70 and 100 mmHg and heart rate between 70 and 90 bpm. Occasionally, she had head swelling pain, during which blood pressure measured up to 176/119 mmHg. After taking nitrendipine 10 mg, the blood pressure could be reduced to less than 140/90 mmHg. In the early morning, the blood pressure dropped by 30–40 mmHg from a recumbent position to a vertical position, while the heart rate increased by 30–40 bpm with self-consciousness of dizziness, weakness, and palpitations. For the rest of the time, the difference of blood pressure in the recumbent position was 10–20 mmHg. She is now admitted in our ward for further diagnosis and treatment.

During the course of the disease, the patient had no obvious fatigue and discomfort, fear of heat and cold, general sweating, limb convulsions, confusion or loss of consciousness, face or lower limb puffiness, night paroxysmal dyspnea, chest pain, left shoulder or back or left upper extremity pain and other discomforts, vomiting, diarrhea, blood in the stool, numbness or coldness of hands and feet and cotton sensation of the feet, half-body sweating, full moon face, bloody appearance, streaks of purple skin, triggering lactation, enlargement of hands and feet or ugly face, limb paralysis, bone pain in the lower back and limbs, getting shorter, fractures or urinary excretion of stone, absence of visual field loss, slurred speech, limb movement disorder, absence of morning consciousness disorder, wandering erythema of the skin, absence of personality, or temper changes. Mental health and appetite are usual. She has poor sleep, manifested by difficulty in falling asleep. She defecates once a day, and the stool is dry. Intermittent oral Dumic is taken for a laxative therapy. Urination is normal. There is a weight gain of 3 kg after the last discharge.

6.9.3 Past, Personal, Marital and Childbearing, Family History

Her father suffers from hypertension (diagnosed after the age of 40, drug control is good) and cerebrovascular disease (specification unknown). Nothing special for past, personal, menstrual, marital, and childbearing history. 1.5 cm × 2.5 cm milk coffee spot is visible on the epigastric skin; no full moon face, buffalo back, and supraclavicular fat pads; and no streaks of skin purple, acne, and pigmentation. The skin is not moist. The temperature of the hands and feet is slightly lower, and there is no yellow stain on the mucous membranes of the whole body, and there are no palms or spider moles.

6.9.4 Accessory Examination

CTU (Fig. 6.21): a retroperitoneal mass on the left side of the abdominal aorta, suggesting the clinical possibility of paraganglioma. Small branches of abdominal aorta provided blood supply, and it was drained venously to the left renal vein. Physiological changes may occur in bilateral annex areas. Small pelvic effusion is seen.

Somatostatin receptor imaging: a lesion of slightly higher expression of somatostatin receptors in the mid-abdominal midline, and tomography is recommended for the further clarification.

131I-MIBG: a lesion equivalent to the radiotrophic elevation zone in the left mid-abdomen. In combination with somatostatin receptor imaging on May 2, 2018, retroperitoneal pheochromocytoma is considered.

A tumor in the left side of the retroperitoneal abdominal aorta is seen. Paraganglioma is more likely in combination with clinical considerations. The small branches of the abdominal aorta provide blood supply to the tumor and the blood is drained to the left renal vein

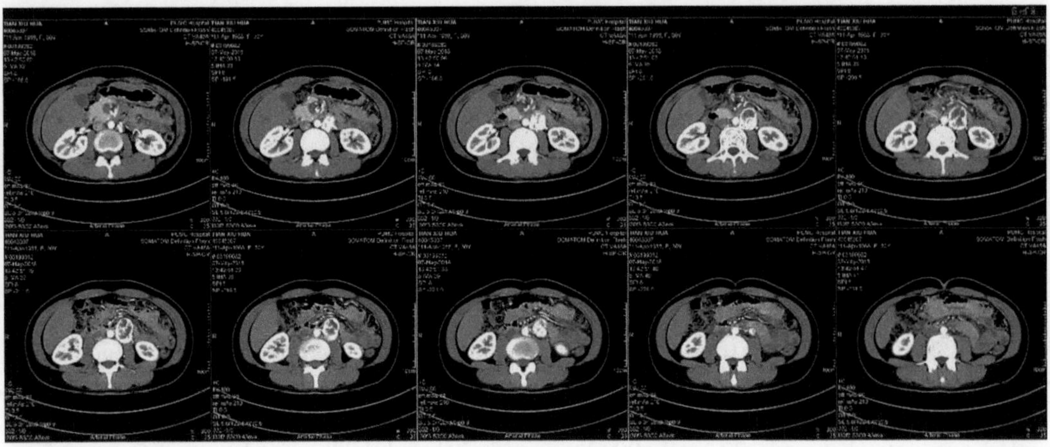

Fig. 6.21 Abdominal pelvic enhancement CT

6.9.5 Current Diagnoses

Retroperitoneal paraganglioma
Secondary hypertension
Abnormal liver function
Cyst of right maxillary sinus

6.9.6 MDT Discussion

6.9.6.1 Urology

(1) At present, the diagnosis of paraganglioma is clear, no distant metastases are seen, and there are indications for surgical management. (2) At present, blood pressure and heart rate control are not good, and it is recommended to continue drug preparation and monitor changes in blood pressure and heart rate. (3) Fully explain to the patient and his family the necessity of surgery, the risk of intraoperative left renal resection, perioperative bleeding, and cardiopulmonary risk. (4) Follow-up.

6.9.6.2 Department of Anesthesiology

(1) Patient regarded as ASA grade III, limited-time surgery. (2) Strengthen monitoring during surgery, maintain the balance of myocardial oxygen supply and consumption, and ensure the perfusion of important organs. (3) Fully explain the perioperative cardiovascular and cerebrovascular accidents and large vascular risks, and maintain water-electrolyte balance. (4) Prepare for adequate blood transfusion. (5) Return patient to ICU after surgery.

6.9.6.3 ICU

Patients with a retroperitoneal mass, not excluding paragangliomas. Explain that the perioperative fluctuations of blood circulation are large. Cardiovascular and cerebrovascular events may be possible.

6.9.7 Surgical Approach

Laparoscopic resection of left retroperitoneal paraganglioma under general anesthesia (Fig. 6.22)

6.9.8 Postoperative Pathology

Left retroperitoneal paraganglioma lesions conform to paragangliomas, with invasion of the envelope. Immunohistochemical results: Calretinin(−), CgA(+), Ki-67(index 1%), Syn(+), Vimentin(+), α-inhibin(灶+), AE1/AE3(−), CAM5.2(−)

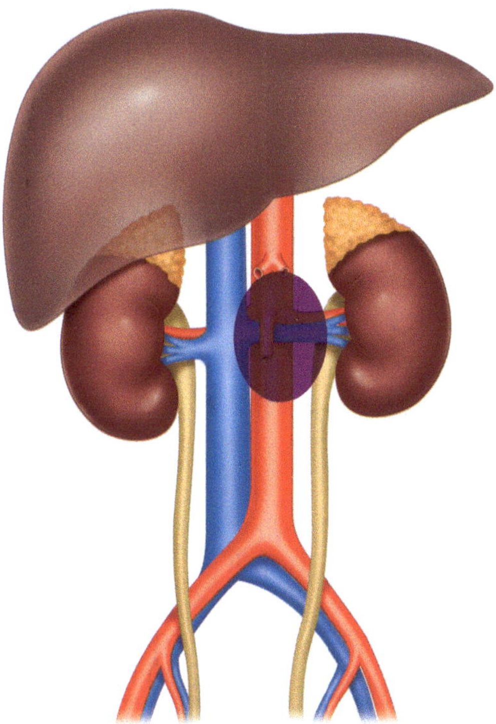

Fig. 6.22 Schematic diagram of the location of the mass

6.10 Case 6.10

Patient: Male, 45 years old

6.10.1 Complaints

Physical examination revealed a lesion in the left peritoneum more than 2 months ago.

6.10.2 History of Present Illness

In October 2018, the patient's left renal ultrasound revealed a low-echo nodule of about 4.7 cm × 3.0 cm × 3.2 cm in size next to the left side of the spine and adjacent to the left renal artery, with clear boundaries. A retroperitoneal solid mass was suggested. External renal MR flat scan + enhancement showed that a tumor of 48 mm × 47 mm × 36 mm can be seen in the left anterior area of the central horizontal spine of the left kidney. Its internal signal is not uniform. The arterial phase of strengthening is not obvious, and lesions are unevenly strengthened during the venous phase and delayed phase. Neurogenic tumor was considered. No special treatment was given by the outer hospital. Patient occasionally had mild dizziness and palpitations during the self-reported course of the disease. There were no abnormalities in the outpatient's somatostatin receptor imaging and adrenal medullary imaging in our outpatient clinic. There were no obvious abnormalities in the 24-h urine CA, UFC, F, ACTH, ALD, AT, PRA, and other related endocrine examinations. The outpatient clinic admitted him with a left retroperitoneal lesion. After the patient was admitted to the hospital, he actively completed the relevant assessment. Considering the possibility of left paraganglioma, drug preparation was recommended first, and surgery was performed within a limited period of time. Oral phenylbenzylamine 10 mg Q8H was given, and the patient's condition was stable.

After the patient was discharged from the hospital, he took phenoxybenzamine 10 mg Q8H regularly. After taking the drug, he developed dry mouth, sore throat, and nasal congestion. The following were noted: NBP 105–108/63–75 mmHg (recumbent position), 95–117/75–90 mmHg (upright position); HR 65–75 bpm (recumbent position), 90–109 bpm (upright position); and Hct 44.2 → 42.8%. He had transient occipital distention on December 12, 2018, which lasted for 2 min before it was resolved spontaneously. The patient did not complain of abdominal pain, nausea, vomiting, palpitations, sweating, pallor, wet and cold limbs, and other discomfort. Appetite and sleeping pattern are normal. He exercises normally. For surgery, he was admitted to the hospital with a left retroperitoneal occupancy. Since the onset of the disease, the patient's mental health, sleep, and appetite are normal, and he urinates normally. He complains of laborious defecation. He defecates once in 2–3 days. Oral probiotics was taken. Now, he defecates once a day. The stool is dark and soft without blood and other abnormalities. He gained 2 kg in the last month.

6.10.3 Past, Personal, Marital and Childbearing, Family History

Nothing special

6.10.4 Accessory Examination

Somatostatin receptor imaging: physiological uptake of the pancreatic head in the mid-abdomen may be seen. The rest of somatostatin receptor imaging is not significantly abnormal.

131I-MIBG (November 23, 2018): No abnormalities were seen in adrenal medullary imaging.

Abdominal pelvic enhanced CT + three-dimensional reconstruction (Fig. 6.23 and 6.24): the medial limb of the left adrenal gland is thickened, and there is no obvious abnormality in the morphology, density, and size of the right adrenal gland. There are no obvious abnormalities in the size and morphological density of the both kidneys. No significant abnormal strengthening is seen in the enhancement scan. There are scattered and slightly full lymph nodes in the posterior peritoneum. Three-dimensional reconstruction: a round and slightly less dense retroperitoneal shadow below the left anterior renal vein. The size is about 3.4 cm × 3.6 cm × 5.1 cm. The flat scan CT value is about 28 HU. The enhancement of the scan is not uniform. For the circumference of the arterial stage, the lesion is more obviously strengthened and thickened, and a tortuous small blood vessel shadow can be seen above and below the lesion. For the portal vein stage and the delayed phase, CT value of the lesion

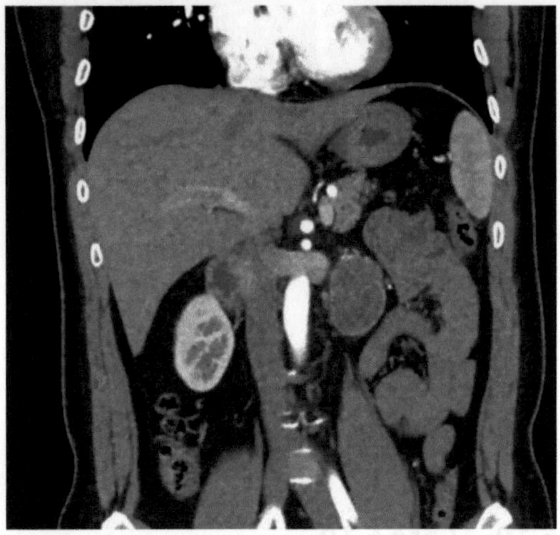

Fig. 6.24 CT 3D reconstruction

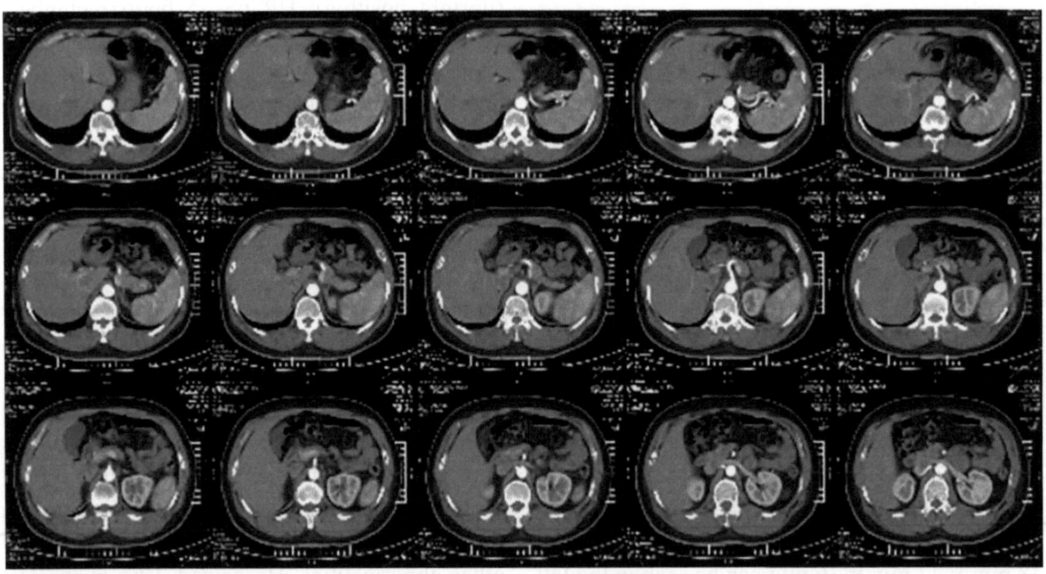

Fig. 6.23 Abdominal pelvic enhancement CT

are strengthened moderately. The lesion boundary is clear. The left renal artery and vein are slightly changed under pressure.

Endocrine examination: On October 30, 2018, 24-h urine cortisol showed urine volume 1000 mL and UFC 53.20 μg/24 h. Serum total cortisol (8 AM): F[8 AM] 9.34 μg/dL. Plasma ACTH (8 AM): ACTH 22.8 pg/mL. Twenty-four hours urinary catecholamines: NE 20.31 μg/24 h, E 2.95 μg/24 h, DA 164.79 μg/24 h, and urine output 960 mL. Aldosterone (cubic): ALD2 12.81 ng/dL. Renin activity (elevation) + angiotensin II (elevation): AT-II2 60.02 pg/mL, PRA2 1.01 ng/mL/h.

A slightly less dense and quasi-circular shadow can be seen anteriorly and below the retroperitoneal left renal vein, with a size of about 3.4 cm × 3.6 cm × 5.1 cm and a flat scan CT value of about 28 HU. The enhancement is not uniform in enhanced scanning

For the arterial stage, lesion is more obviously strengthened. A thickened and tortuous small blood vessel shadow can be seen above and below the lesion. The CT value of lesion in the portal vein stage and the delayed stage is moderately strengthened. The lesion boundary is clear, and the left renal artery and vein are slightly compressed

6.10.5 Current Diagnoses

Left retroperitoneal paraganglioma
Hyperbilirubinemia

6.10.6 MDT Discussion

6.10.6.1 Internal Medicine

Elevated bilirubin cannot exclude the possibility of a long-term elevation due to metabolic abnormalities. Monitor the results of abdominal pelvic CT. If there is no obvious abnormality in the liver system, no current special treatment is necessary. Monitor regularly liver function, and watch out for cardiac and segmental ventricular movement abnormalities. Coronary CTA is recommended to further exclude ischemic cardiomyopathy.

6.10.6.2 ICU

Fully account for the risks and complications associated with the perioperative period. Ensure the organ perfusion during the perioperative period, and return the patient to the ICU after surgery.

6.10.6.3 Department of Anesthesiology

Complete blood gas and coronary CTA. Consult to internal medicine and endocrine. Fully explain the risks of perioperative cardiovascular and cerebrovascular accidents, allergies, reflux aspiration, etc., and return the patient to the ICU after surgery.

6.10.7 Surgical Approach

"Laparoscopic resection of left retroperitoneal mass" under general anesthesia (Fig. 6.25)

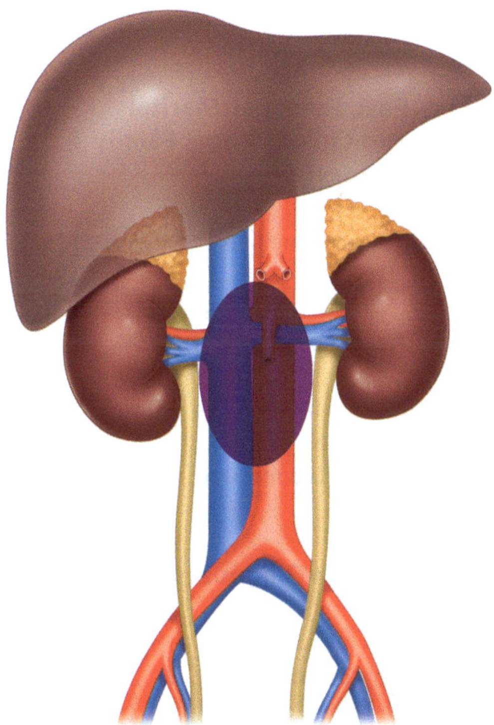

Fig. 6.25 Schematic diagram of the location of the mass

6.10.8 Postoperative Pathology

Left retroperitoneal mass is consistent with paraganglioma.

6.11 Case 6.11

Patient: Female, 42 years old

6.11.1 Complaints

Sweating for more than 2 years, episodic dizziness, headache, blood pressure increase for 1 year, and an occupying lesion found in the right peritoneum for 3 months (Fig. 6.26a–c)

6.11.2 History of Present Illness

Sweating for more than 2 years, episodic dizziness, headache, blood pressure increase for 1 year, and an occupying lesion found in the right peritoneum for 3 months. High blood pressure for 2 years

6.11.3 Past, Personal, Marital and Childbearing, Family History

History of diabetes mellitus and caesarean section

6.11.4 Accessory Examination

Endocrine examination: 24 h urine catecholamines: NE 548.83 μg/24 h, E 6.18 μg/24 h, DA 262.82 μg/24 h. The rest were normal.

6.11.5 Current Diagnoses

Retroperitoneal paraganglioma
- Secondary hypertension
- Diabetes
- Past caesarean section

6.11.6 MDT Discussion

6.11.6.1 Endocrinology

(1) Monitor the 24 h inflow and output (counting the amount of urine in the day and night), weight, and stool, continue to monitor the blood pressure and heart rate in the recumbent position, and monitor HCT. (2) There is no episodic blood pressure increase and a slight orthostatic hypotension. In combination with the current situation of blood pressure control, it is recommended that after further expansion (if the follow-up of HCT decreases), optional surgical treatment can be selected. (3) Avoid squeezing the abdomen and strenuous exercise, and maintain the balance of electrolytes. Blood glucose is stable. Perioperative attention is paid against the episodes of pheochromocytoma crisis.

6.11.6.2 Department of Anesthesiology

(1) Case is regarded as ASA grade III, limited-time surgery. (2) Patient's diagnosis is paraneuroma. Complete ECG, UCG. (3) Tumor is closely related to large blood vessels. Fully prepare blood supply, and account for the risk of perioperative cardiovascular accidents. (4) Anesthesia preparation is according to pheochromocytoma preparation: establishment of arteriovenous passage, preparation of vasoactive drugs, and intraoperative strengthening of monitoring. (5) Return patient to the ICU after surgery.

6.11.6.3 ICU

(1) Fully explain the risks and complications associated with the perioperative period. (2) Maintain blood pressure stability during the perioperative period. (3) Return the patient to the ICU after surgery.

6.11.7 Surgical Approach

Laparoscopic resection of right paraganglioma under general anesthesia (Fig. 6.27).

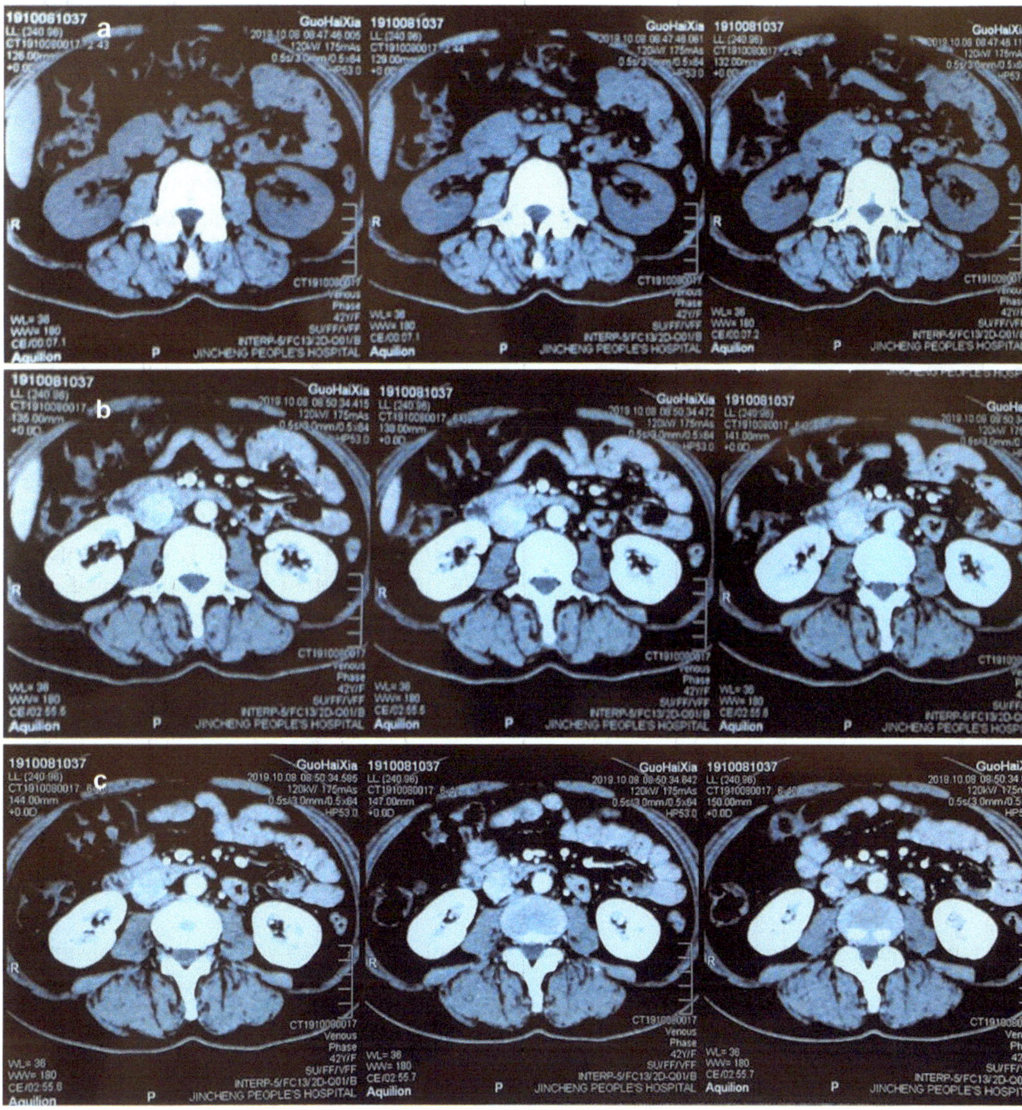

Fig. 6.26 Abdominal pelvic CT. (**a**–**c**) A retroperitoneal shadow of mass behind right renal vein, about 3.5 cm × 4.2 cm in size. During the arterial phase, lesion has a significant strengthening of the envelope, and the compressed changes are seen in the right renal artery and vein

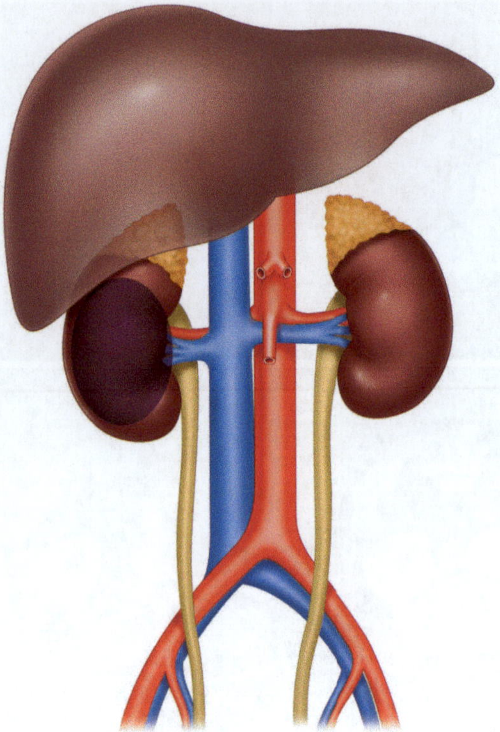

Fig. 6.27 Schematic diagram of the location of the mass

6.11.8 Postoperative Pathology

Right retroperitoneal paraganglioma

Melan-A(−), AE1/AE3(−), CgA(+), Ki-67 (2%), S-100(+), α-inhibin(−)

6.12 Case 6.12

Patient: Male, 62 years old

6.12.1 Complaints

Hypertension was found 4 years ago. Episodic sweating and a lesion at the left adrenal gland were found 3 months ago.

6.12.2 History of Present Illness

The patient was diagnosed with hypertension after physical examination 4 years ago. The maximal blood pressure could reach 220/110 mmHg with cold extremities. With antihypertensive drugs, BP could be controlled at 125/95 mmHg. In December 2016, he was admitted to our hospital because of episodic sweating, accompanied by fatigue, cold extremities, and a BP 220/110 mmHg. Antihypertensive drugs were taken once a day. Adrenal CT scan (Fig. 6.28a, b) showed left adrenal gland is occupied by a tumor of 5 cm × 2.9 cm. In December 2016, 24-h urinary CA showed NE 1177 μg/24 h (↑29 times). MIBG: (−) Renin >12 ng/mL/h↑, angiotensin II 557.27 pg/mL↑, and aldosterone 20.74 ng/dL. Renal artery ultrasound: (−). Usually, hands and feet are cold, which aggravate at the time of attack. There is no postural dizziness. He losses 10 kg, compared with 4 years ago.

6.12.3 Past, Personal, Marital and Childbearing, Family History

Alcohol abuse for 20 years, 1 lb/day; abstinence from alcohol 4 years ago; one sister has a history of retroperitoneal tumors.

6.12.4 Accessory Examination

PET-CT results: a mass of abnormally elevated metabolism in the left adrenal region, SUVmax 7.4, being considered as malignant lesion.

Somatostatin receptor imaging: highly expressive lesions of somatostatin receptors in left adrenal, and a pheochromocytoma is more likely to be considered.

131I-MIBG: Negative

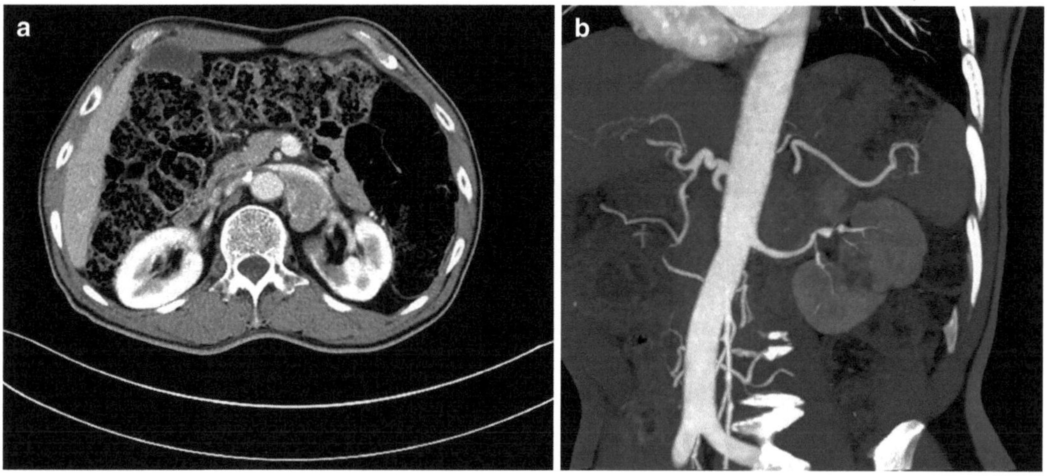

Fig. 6.28 Abdominal and pelvic CT. (**a**, **b**) A lesion beside left renal pedicle. The maximum cross-section is about 4.6 cm × 3.0 cm. The boundary is clear. After the enhanced scan, it is unevenly and significantly strengthened. Pheochromocytoma cannot be excluded. Left renal artery is compressed and altered

24-h urinary CA: NE 1177 μg/24 h (↑29 times), NE 758.57 μg/24 h (↑19 times), NE 990.00 μg/24 h (↑25 times)

6.12.5 Current Diagnoses

Left paratyle paraganglioma

Catecholamine cardiomyopathy

Arrhythmia

Diabetes

Diabetic nephropathy (urine microalbumin phase)

Multiple ischemic necrosis of the left kidney

Left renal insufficiency

Multiple aneurysms in the distal branch of the left renal artery

Multiple atherosclerosis abdominal aorta and branches of abdominal aorta.

Lumbar scoliosis.

6.12.6 MDT Discussion

6.12.6.1 Department of Anesthesiology

Ask endocrinology and internal medicine consultation to assist in preoperative optimization. Strengthen monitoring during the perioperative period, and explain the violent fluctuations in the perioperative circulation, malignant arrhythmias, risk of heart failure, and the possibility of discontinuation of surgery. After surgery, patient must return to the first ward of the ICU.

6.12.6.2 Endocrinology

Continue the current preoperative preparation of phenylbenzylamine, and monitor the blood pressure and heart rate, blood HCT, body weight, and other indicators in the recumbent position. The blood pressure is preoperatively required to be controlled in the normal range, and there should be no obvious orthostatic hypotension, asymptomatic attack, blood HCT decline, and weight gain. Adjust the dose of phenylbenzylamine and Betaloc according to the blood pressure and heart rate at the recumbent position.

6.12.6.3 Internal Medicine

Explain the risk of perioperative cardiopulmonary complications. It is recommended that the serum potassium be maintained at 4.0–5.0 mol/L.

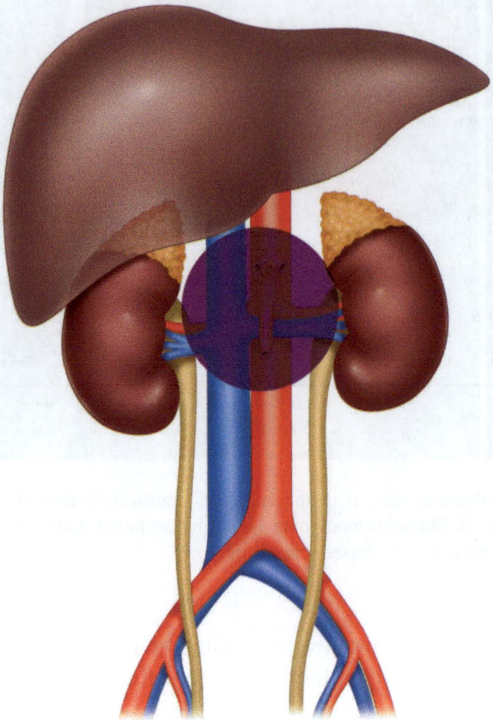

Fig. 6.29 Schematic diagram of the location of the mass

6.12.7 Surgical Approach

Laparoscopic resection of left retroperitoneal paraganglioma under general anesthesia (Fig. 6.29)

6.12.8 Pathological Results

Retroperitoneal paraganglioma

Immunohistochemical results: Melan-A(−), AE1/AE3(−), CgA(+), Ki-67(index 3%), S-100(+), α-inhibin(−)

7

Multidisciplinary Treatment of Paragangliomas in the Lower Abdominal Vascular Area

Bing Bing Shi, Zhi Jun Zhang, Jin Wen, Rui Qiang Zhang, Xue Min Gao, Meng Chao Wei, and Nan Lei

7.1 Case 7.1

Patient: Female, 55 years old

7.1.1 Complaints

Retroperitoneal mass was found more than 3 years ago.

7.1.2 History of Present Illness

In 2015, the patient was admitted to the hospital for abdominal pain, and an enlarged lymph node of about 1.5 cm × 1.6 cm × 2.3 cm in size could be seen on the right side of the abdominal aorta at the waist three level. The boundary was clear. No further diagnosis and treatment were carried out. There were no palpitations, dizziness, high blood pressure, sweating, cold extremities, and other discomfort. After regular review of abdominal CT, the mass gradually increased. In January 2018, our hospital CT showed a round nodular shadow below the level of the duodenum, abdominal aorta, and the anterior vena cava, the size of about 2.0 cm × 2.7 cm. The border is still clear. The density is still uniform. The enhancement is more obvious in the edge. The inferior vena cava is slightly compressed. The lesion is close to the abdominal aorta.

The possibility of paraganglioma is considered. Currently, the recumbent BP is 122/62 mmHg with a HR of 62 bpm, and upright BP is 116/77 mmHg with a HR of 80 bpm. Since March 29, phenol benzylamine has been taken orally, and the current dose is 10 mg q12h. Nasal congestion has been obvious in the past month. HCT decreases from 43 to 41%. There are no change in body weight, no significant change in extremity temperature, and no significant orthostatic hypotension.

7.1.3 Past, Personal, Marital and Childbearing, Family History

Nothing special

7.1.4 Accessory Examination

CT (Figs. 7.1a, b and 7.2): A circular nodular shadow below the horizontal section of the duo-

Bing Bing Shi and Zhi Jun Zhang contributed equally to this work.

B.B. Shi · Z.J. Zhang · J. Wen (✉) · R. Q. Zhang
X. M. Gao · M. C. Wei
Department of Urology, Peking Union Medical College Hospital, Beijing, China

N. Lei
China Union Medical University Press, Beijing, China

J. Wen (ed.), *Surgical Management of Pheochromocytoma and Retroperitoneal Paraganglioma*,
https://doi.org/10.1007/978-981-99-8421-3_7

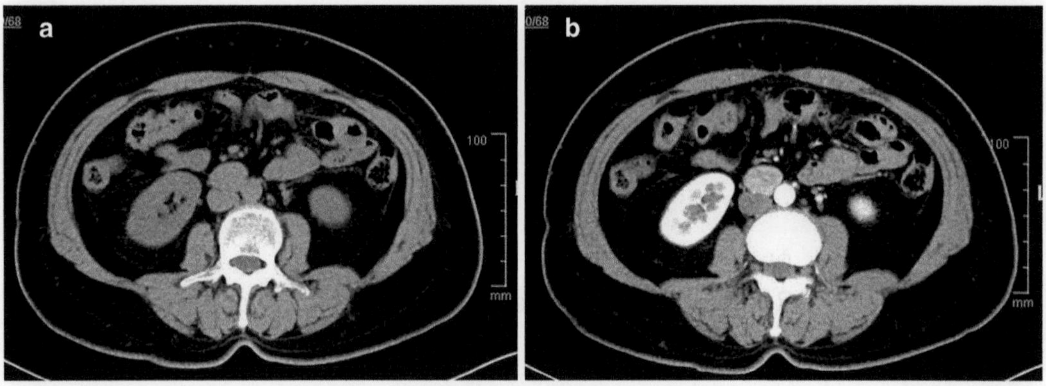

Fig. 7.1 Abdominal pelvic CT. (**a**, **b**) A circular nodular shadow was found below the horizontal section of the duodenum, abdominal aorta, and anterior inferior vena cava, about 2.0 cm in size×2.7 cm in size. The border is still clear. The density is still uniform, and the strengthening of the edge is more obvious. The inferior vena cava is slightly compressed. The lesion is close to the abdominal aorta. Paraganglioma may be considered

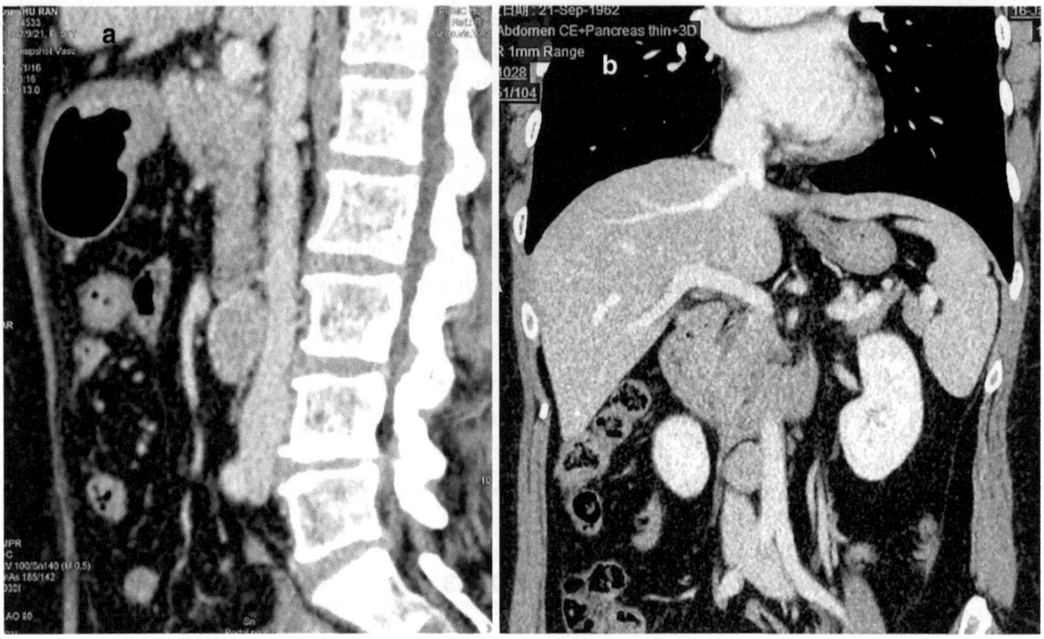

Fig. 7.2 Abdominal pelvic CT sagittal reconstruction. (**a**–**b**) The inferior vena cava is slightly compressed and the lesion is adjacent to the abdominal aorta and Inferior mesenteric artery

denum, abdominal aorta, and anterior inferior vena cava, about 2.0 cm in size×2.7 cm in size, was found. The border is still clear. The density is still uniform, and the strengthening of the edge is more obvious. The inferior vena cava is slightly compressed. The lesion is close to the abdominal aorta. Paraganglioma may be considered.

Endocrine tests:

24 h urine: NE 35.82 μg/24 h, E 3.60 μg/24 h, DA 197.05 μg/24 h. Blood methoxy norepinephrine 1.78 nmol/L↑.

131I-MIBG: a circular aera of radiation elevation was seen in the middle abdomen, which was considered a paraganglioma, and no obvious abnormalities were seen in the remaining parts.

Somatostatin receptor imaging: a hyperexpression lesion of somatostatin receptor in the middle abdomen is more likely to be considered as a paraganglioma.

Thyroid ultrasound: a very solid nodule under the right lobe of the thyroid gland

7.1.5 Current Diagnoses

Right retroperitoneal paraganglioma

The nature of thyroid nodules is to be investigated.

MEM-2?

7.1.6 MDT Discussion

7.1.6.1 Endocrinology

(1) Add the monitoring of 8–10 pm recumbent blood pressure and heart rate in the evening. Recheck HCT every week, pay attention to cardiovascular symptoms and stool conditions, and instruct patient to avoid defecation effort, emotional agitation, fatigue, infection, severe postural changes, and compression of the abdomen. Avoid the use of morphine, gastric reassurance, and other drugs. (2) Please recheck 24 h ambulatory monitoring of blood pressure, and increase the daily water intake to nearly 4 L. If the lying blood pressure is still high, nifedipine can be added. (3) Consult with the anesthesiology department and critical care to assess perioperative risk.

7.1.6.2 Department of Anesthesiology

(1) Phenol benzylamine preparation is right. Please instruct the patient to take phenol benzylamine until the morning of surgery according to the opinions of endocrinology consultation. Ensure that the daily intake is sufficient. Fully explain the intraoperative hemodynamic fluctuations leading to myocardial ischemia, heart failure, malignant arrhythmia, cerebral infarction, cerebral hemorrhage, fundus hemorrhage, and circulatory failure risk. (2) Strengthen monitoring during surgery, prepare vasoactive drugs, and maintain the balance of myocardial oxygen supply and oxygen consumption. (3) Postoperatively return to the ICU.

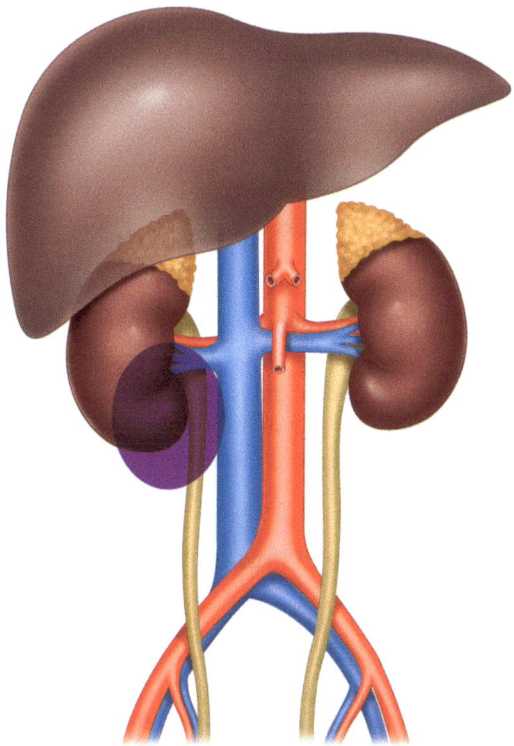

Fig. 7.3 Schematic diagram of the location of the mass

7.1.6.3 ICU

Patient is considered to have risks of paraganglioma and is intended to undergo a surgical treatment. Explain to the patient the risks of major perioperative bleeding, violent hemodynamic fluctuations, pheochromocytoma crisis, cardiovascular and cerebrovascular events, myocardial infarction, cerebral infarction, etc.

7.1.7 Surgical Approach

Trans-laparoscopic resection of right paraganglioma under general anesthesia (Fig. 7.3)

7.1.8 Postoperative Pathology

Retroperitoneal mass paraganglioma, invading the envelope. Immunohistochemical results:

CgA(+), Ki-67(index 1%), Syn(+), Vimentin(+), α-inhibin(−), S-100(−), AE1/AE3(−)

7.2 Case 7.2

Patient: Male, 37 years of age

7.2.1 Complaints

Dizziness and abdominal pain with episodic fluctuations of blood pressure for 7 days; the aggravation has been noticed for 2 days.

7.2.2 History of Present Illness

On October 13, 2018, the patient had, with no obvious precipitating factor, dizziness and abdominal pain. Abdominal pain was paroxysmal in nature. The measured blood pressure was paroxysmally elevated with a maximum of 190/100 mmHg and a minimum of 70/56 mmHg. A blood routine examination showed WBC 13.62 × 10^9, HGB 164 g/L, and a PLT of 276 × 10^9. Urine amylase: 804 U/L. Cardiac ultrasound: decreased function of left ventricular diastolic and normal left ventricular systolic function. Ultrasound of the abdomen: fatty liver (moderate). CET: lacunar lesions in bilateral basal ganglia, fourth brain ventricular dilation, and widening of the occipital pool.

The family reported that he was suspected to complain of acute pancreatitis and received infusion therapy for 3 days, cefuroxime sodium 2 g bid intravenous injection and omeprazole 40 mg qd intravenous instillation, and rehydration treatment for 3 days. The abdominal pain was relieved. Two days ago, after exerting force to defecate, the patient had abdominal pain again. The pain was worse than before. Two tablets of morphine were taken orally. He was treated in a hospital in Beijing to check the abdominal ultrasound: low echo shadow on the left side of the umbilical level was found, and the nature is to be determined. Without treatment, he was transferred to the emergency department of Beijing Friendship Hospital for paroxysmal elevation of blood pressure, up to 267/160 mmHg and as low as 67/40 mmHg.

Abdominal enhanced CT results: (1) Para-abdominal aortic lesions, nature to be determined, small blood vessel rupture? Neurogenic tumors? Other? (2) The right lobe of the liver is calcified. (3) There are more contents in the terminal ileum and colon, and there are scattered contents with higher density in the gastrointestinal tract (please combine with clinical presentations). (4) A few flocculent shadows in the bilateral groin (please combine clinical presentations).

Head CT: (1) lacunar cerebral infarction is not excluded; (2) inflammation of left sphenoid sinus. Diagnosis was made as "Cause of abdominal pain to be investigated and the nature of para-aortic lesion to be determined with a possible neuroendocrine tumor? or pheochromocytoma. Cardiac insufficiency, liver insufficiency, and renal insufficiency." After giving fasting water, anti-infective, and other symptomatic supportive treatment, abdominal pain was not relieved. He presented sweating, paroxysmal convulsions, and urinary incontinence. Today, he came to the emergency department of our hospital for medical treatment.

Blood routine: WBC 19.65 × 10^9, HGB 167 g/L, and PLT 240 × 10^9. Blood gas analysis showed PH 7.429, PCO2 28.3 mmHg PO2 55.7 mmHg, $HCO3^-$ 18.4 mmol/L, and Lac 3.7 mmol/L.

Liver and kidney function: TBIL 22.4umol/L, ALT 37 U/L, Urea 9.62 mmol/L, and Cr(E) 198umol/L.

Cardiac test: CK 293 U/L, CKMB 9.5 μg/L, cTnI 1.287 μg/L, NT-proBNP >35,000 pg/L, Myo 1865 μg/L. Patient still presents with episodic fluctuations of blood pressure, the lowest 62/50 mmHg, the highest 280/130 mmHg, with HR 120–160 times/min. So he was sent to the emergency room. Endocrinology consultation was asked. The possibility of pheochromocytoma crisis was considered. Treatment of urapidil hydrochloride by venous pumping and rapid venous expansion in the meantime was recommended. Patient was advised to avoid squeezing the abdomen and avoid taking gastric reassurance, morphine, and other drugs that can induce pheochromocytoma crisis.

At 15:56 pm, patient presented with upper and right gaze of both eyes with closed teeth, facial muscle twitches, and unconsciousness. Epilepsy was considered. He was treated with endotracheal intubation, mechanical ventilation, and analgesia and sedation. Blood pressure during the rescue room changed from 30/10 mmHg to 330/160 mmHg, with a HR of 110—170 beats/min and an excessive urine output. There were no obvious abnormalities in the head CT scan, and the thoracolumbar and abdominal pelvic CT scan showed a lesion at the vertebral level of about L2–L3 and in the left anterior position of the abdominal aorta. Pheochromocytoma was not excluded. Considering that the patient's circulation fluctuates violently and it is difficult to regulate the tranquility of blood pressure and NE medication, our department admitted him to our hospital with a diagnosis of pheochromocytoma and pheochromocytoma crisis. Since the onset of the disease, the patient has been able to eat and sleep. Constipation is obvious. There is no significant change in weight. Currently, he is in analgesic and sedative state.

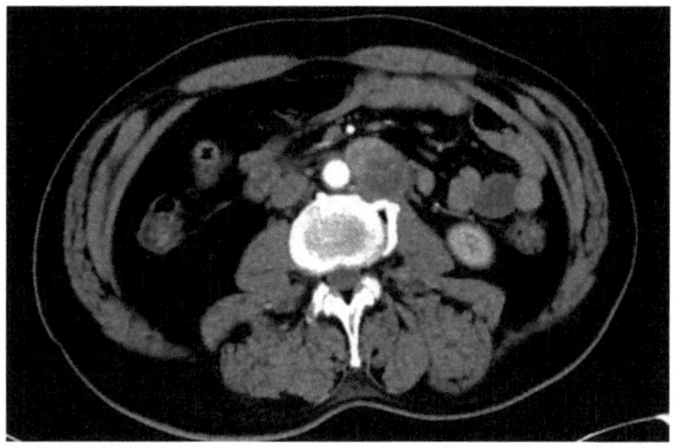

Fig. 7.4 Abdominal pelvic enhancement CT

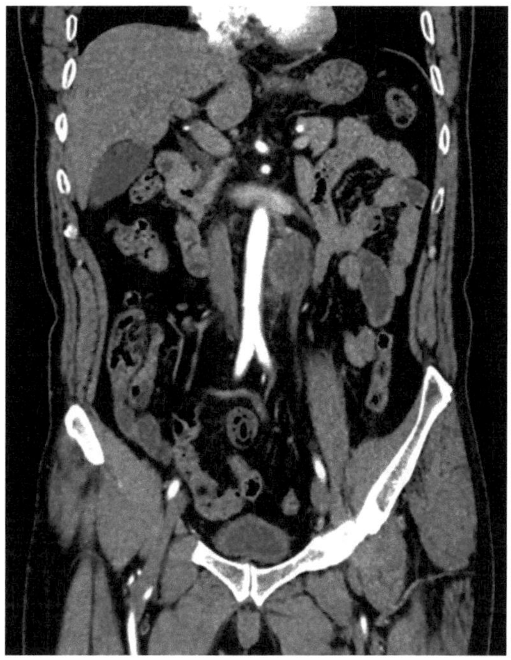

Fig. 7.5 Three-dimensional reconstruction of abdominal pelvic CT

7.2.3 Past, Personal, Marital and Childbearing, Family History

Hemorrhoids more than 10 years, 8 years after nasal polypectomy; no other special findings

7.2.4 Accessory Examination

Abdominal pelvic enhancement CT + CTA (Figs. 7.4 and 7.5): a soft tissue shadow was found in about L3 vertebral level and in front and left of abdominal aorta, about 4.3 cm in size×3.5 cm × 4.2 cm in size. Small flaky low density can be seen inside. Soft tissue components can be strengthened after enhancement, and the local boundary with the left lumbar major muscle is not clear. A few calcified and non-calcified plaques may be seen in the walls of the abdominal aorta and its branches.

131I-MIBG scintigraphy: the para-aortic mass of the abnormal elevation of radioactivity, corresponding to the mass site of the abdomen shown in diagnostic CT. There were no areas of abnormally concentrated or attenuated radiation in the area of the adrenal glands or other parts of the body. Bilateral salivary glands and liver are normally demonstrated. Mass is considered as a para-aortic pheochromocytoma.

Somatostatin receptor imaging: There are no abnormalities in somatostatin receptor imaging.

A mass shadow of soft-tissue density is seen in the left and in front of abdominal aorta at about L3 of the vertebral level, with a size of about 4.3 cm × 3.5 cm × cm 4.2 cm.

Small flaky low density can be seen inside the tumor. The soft tissue component can be strengthened after enhancement, and the local and left lumbar major muscles are not clearly demarcated.

7.2.5 Current Diagnoses

The cause of abdominal pain remains to be investigated.

Paragangliomas are more likely.
Pheochromocytoma crisis
Myocardial damage
Acute renal insufficiency
Epilepsy is not excluded.
Hemorrhoids
Past nasal polypectomy

7.2.6 MDT Discussion

7.2.6.1 Internal Medicine

(1) The patient has CAD. When conditions permit, it can be considered to add aspirin and statin therapy. Pay attention to drug side effects (he can consult cardiology outpatient evaluation after the end of surgery and stability); (2) the risk of perioperative cardiovascular events needs to be fully explained before surgery, including myocardial infarction, heart failure, arrhythmia, shock, stress heart disease, and sudden death; (3) maintain the balance of intake and output, electrolyte balance, etc. and BP stability; (4) preoperative preparation and treatment can be followed by your department and endocrinology; (5) follow-up.

7.2.6.2 Department of Anesthesiology

(1) Patient is regarded as ASA grade III. elective surgery. (2) Look for results of PFTs. Anesthesia is prepared according to the routine preparation of pheochromocytoma, strengthening monitoring of changes in vital signs during surgery and maintaining the stability of blood pressure, water, and electrolytes. (3) Fully account for perioperative myocardial infarction, arrhythmia, heart failure, severe hypotension, stroke, lung infection, atelectasis, and the risk of major bleeding; prepare for adequate blood supply. (4) Postoperative return to the ICU is recommended.

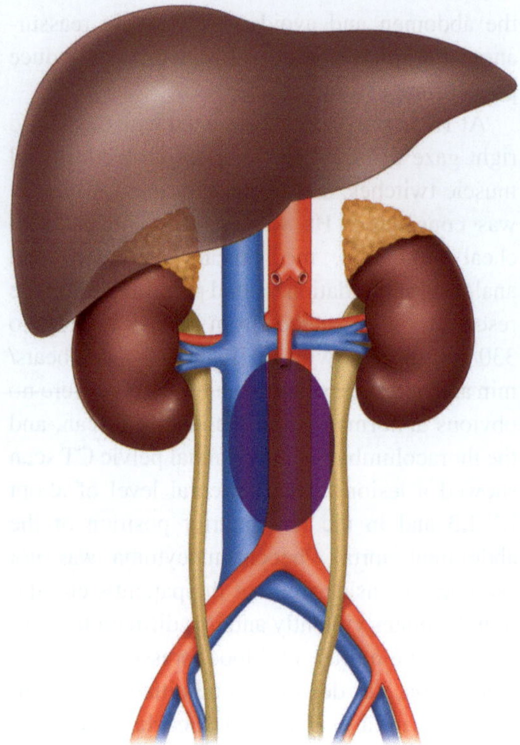

Fig. 7.6 Schematic diagram of the location of the mass

7.2.6.3 ICU

(1) Fully explain the risks and complications associated with the perioperative period. (2) Please contact the ICU to reserve a bed before surgery.

7.2.7 Surgical Approach

Laparoscopic assisted resection of left retroperitoneal paraganglioma under general anesthesia (Fig. 7.6)

7.2.8 Postoperative Pathology

Lesions are consistent with paragangliomas. Flaky necrosis is visible. Tumor invades the surrounding fibrous envelope. Nerve invasion is visible, and intravascular tumor plugs are not clear.

Immunohistochemical results: Melan-A(−), AE1/AE3(−), CgA(+), Ki-67(index 2%), S-100(+), α-inhibin(−), SDHB(+)

7.3 Case 7.3

Patient: Male, 58 years old

7.3.1 Complaints

High blood pressure was found more than 1 year, with episodic palpitation and profuse sweating for 8 months.

7.3.2 History of Present Illness

In April 2017, the patient's physical examination revealed that the blood pressure was increased, fluctuating between 130 and 140/80 and 90 mmHg. In August 2017, the patient intermittently had episodic palpitations and sweating, which occurred especially when walking. It lasted for 2–3 months/time. In September 2017, the patient was found to have a retroperitoneal mass (self-complaint 4.9 × 3.4 cm, no report seen) due to lumbar SPINE MRI. In May 2018, CT of our hospital (Fig. 7.7a–e) found a round soft tissue density shadow beside the retroperitoneal abdominal aorta (about L3–L4 vertebral level) and in front of inferior vena cava, about 3.9 × 5.0 × 4.3 cm. Flat sweep density is uneven. Multiple patches of low-density shadows are visible. Enhancement is visible, and multiple irregular patchy intensifications are seen in it. The branch of superior mesenteric vein was close to the front of the mass. The lesion is partially demarcated from the abdominal aorta and the wall of inferior vena cava. Preparation of oral phenol benzylamine has been carried out since April 19. Current doses are 20 mg (morning), 20 mg (noon), and 30 mg (evening).

On May 2 and May 6, 2018, he had sudden dizziness, blackness, and general weakness. There has been no obvious orthostatic hypotension for more than a month. He gains a weight from 62 to 66 kg. HCT has decreased from 50.9% to 46.3%.

7.3.3 Past, Personal, Marital and Childbearing, Family History

History of cervical disc herniation surgery and lumbar disc herniation surgery

There is no specification for personal history, marriage and childbirth history, and family history.

7.3.4 Accessory Examination

Endocrine-related tests:

24 h Urine CA: NE 25.4 μg/24 h, E 2.7 μg/24 h, DA 261.5 μg/24 h; 24hUFC 58.52 μg

Blood F(8 AM): 20.99 μg/dL

Blood ACTH(8 AM): 50.9 pg/mL

PRA2 0.01 ng/mL/h↓, AT-II2 59.60 pg/mL, ALD2 21.29 ng/dL

131I-MIBG imaging: retroperitoneal mass of radioactive concentration. Paraganglioma is more likely considered.

Somatostatin receptor imaging: high expression lesions of retroperitoneal somatostatin receptor. Paragangliomas are more likely considered.

7.3.5 Current Diagnoses

Submesenteric para-arterial paraganglioma

7.3.6 MDT Discussion

7.3.6.1 Gastroenterology

In combination with the medical history, hemorrhoid bleeding is likely. However, colorectal

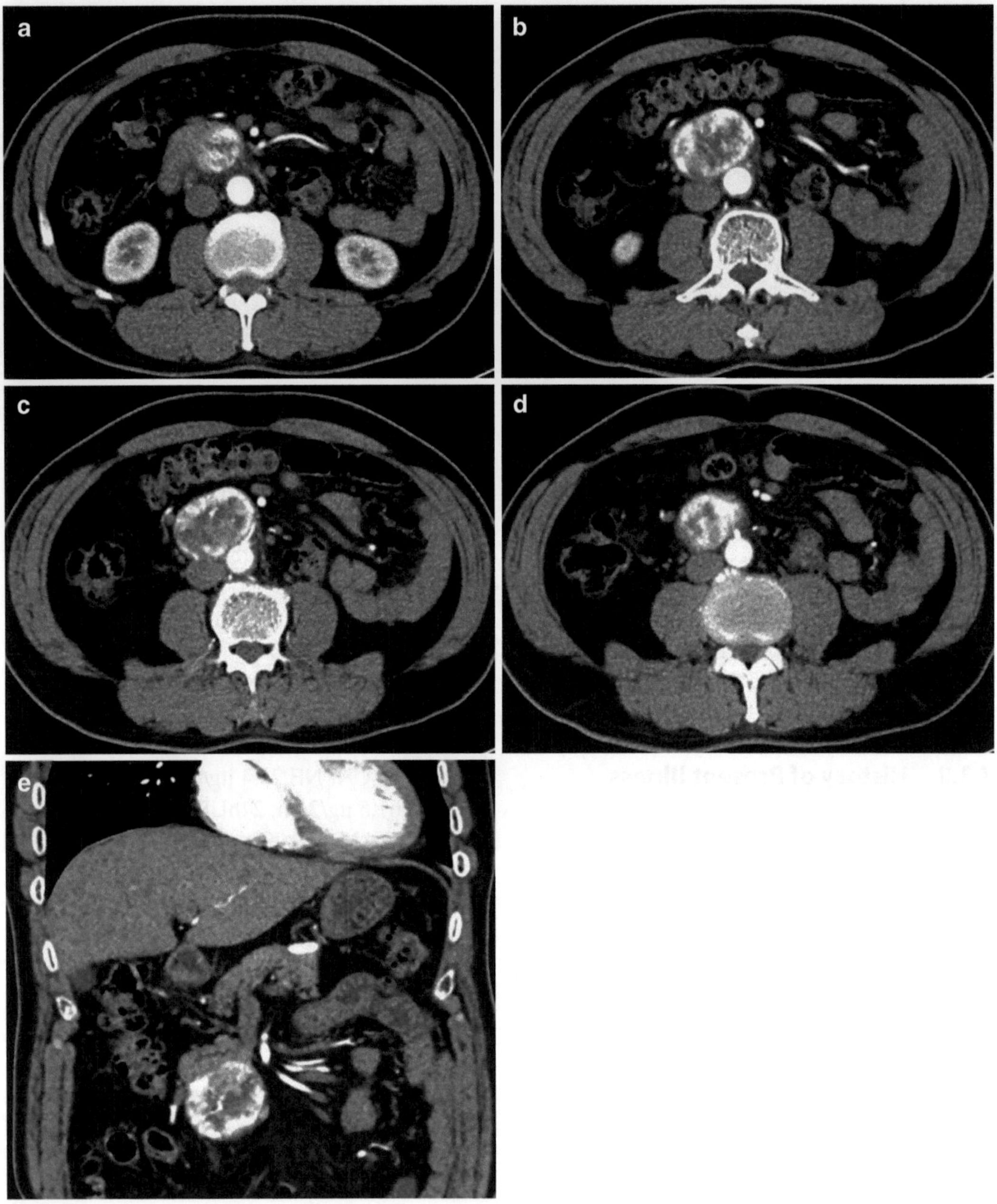

Fig. 7.7 Three-dimensional reconstruction of abdominal pelvic CT. (**a**–**e**) A round soft tissue density shadow beside retroperitoneal abdominal aorta (about L3–L4 vertebral level) and in front of inferior vena cava, about 3.9 × 5.0 × 4.3 cm. Flat sweep density is uneven. Multiple patches of low-density shadows are visible. Enhancement is visible, and multiple irregular patchy intensifications are seen in it. The branch of superior mesenteric vein was close to the front of the mass. The lesion is partially demarcated from the abdominal aorta and the wall of inferior vena cava

tumors are not yet excluded. For the time being, basic surgical consultation is asked. The external treatment of Ma Yinglong/Puzi hemorrhoids plugs can be considered. Closely observe the stool, volume, and traits, and monitor hemoglobin, blood pressure, and heart rate. If the blood in the stool is increased, it is primarily recommended to recheck the abdominal pelvic CT plus enhancement and complete the colonoscopy. If there are concerns in your department, colon CT reconstruction can be done. Follow-up in our department.

7.3.6.2 Ophthalmology

Double retinal arteriosclerosis, grade I, double senile cataract, double presbyopia

7.3.6.3 Basic Surgery

There is no obvious abnormality in the anus. Finger examination: the finger sleeve enters about 6 cm, the rectal mucosa is smooth, and the obvious mass is not touched. It is recommended to complete the CEA and CA series. Colonoscopy can be arranged. There is currently no indication for surgical intervention. Continue the follow-up.

7.3.6.4 Urology

In combination with clinical manifestations, imaging, and endocrine examination, the consideration of current retroperitoneal mass as the paraganglioma is clear. There are indications for surgical management of the retroperitoneal mass. However, the tumor is closely related to the large blood vessels and intestinal blood vessels, and the risk of surgical bleeding, intestinal vascular damage, and intestinal necrosis is high. Actively complete preoperative examinations and drug preparation, and fully explain the risks to patients and their families.

7.3.6.5 Department of Psychological Medicine

Patient currently has no clear manifestations of anxiety disorder and can continue to be observed. Patient is at high risk during disease treatment. When communicating and informing the patient of bad news, pay attention to use with SPIKE models (prepare the right environment, give preparation, understand each other's awareness and expectations, give accurate information, verify each other's understanding and feedback, appease emotions, develop a plan, and give safety nets), and reduce the patient's stress response.

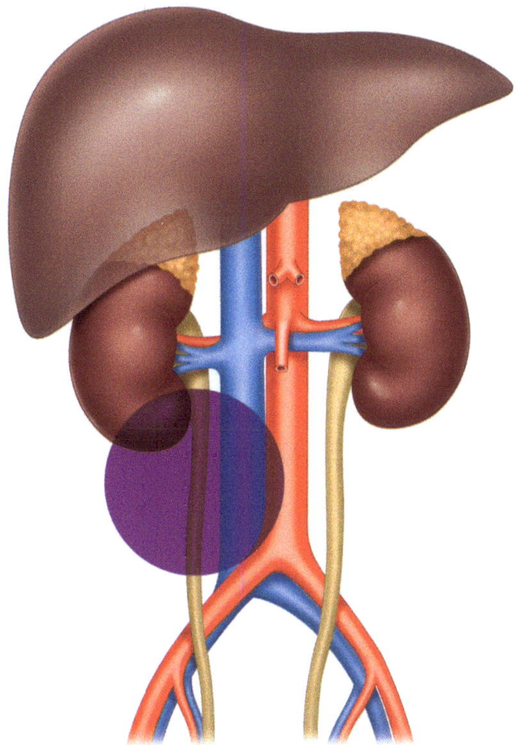

Fig. 7.8 Schematic diagram of the location of the mass

7.3.6.6 Neurology

Clinical episodes do not meet the characteristics of typical TIA or of epilepsy. If the episodic symptoms of paragangliomas in your department cannot be explained, EEG, exercise-induced test, head MRI + SWI, and TCD can be further completed during episodic attack, if necessary.

7.3.7 Surgical Approach

Laparoscopic resection of retroperitoneal mass is performed under general anesthesia (Fig. 7.8)

7.3.8 Postoperative Pathology

Retroperitoneal paraganglioma pheochromocytoma

Immunohistochemical results: Melan-A(−), AE1/AE3(−), CgA(+), Ki-67(index 1%), S-100(+), α-inhibin(+)

7.4 Case 7.4

Patient: Male, 57 years old

7.4.1 Complaints

Abdominal pain, discovery of retroperitoneal mass 6 months ago

7.4.2 History of Present Illness

On September 10, 2020, the patient suddenly had a tearing pain in the lower abdomen, accompanied by low back pain. VAS score was 8 points. He denied fever, nausea, vomiting, uncomfortable exhaust and defecation, and other symptoms. He visited the local hospital. Blood pressure was measured and found to be normal, and abdominal CT was performed, which showed a retroperitoneal lump shadow at double kidney level, about 7.4 cm × 3.5 cm in size, with an uneven density, and CT value of about 39–65HU. The inferior vena cava and abdominal aorta are not clearly demarcated. It is recommended to take a further consultation. He would see the emergency department of our hospital. Abdominal enhanced CT shows (Fig. 7.9) a mass shadow of soft-tissue density seen below posterior duodenal horizontal segments and in front of inferior vena cava and abdominal aorta. Strips of flaky shadow with slightly higher density are seen internally. Larger cross-section is of about 3.8 cm × 7.7 cm. Multiple tortuous vascular shadows (5im33–39) can be seen around the arterial stage, with possible a partial communication with the left renal vein (5im33). The lesion in arterial phase is significantly and unevenly strengthened. The strengthening in portal phase and delayed phase of is also uneven. The duodenal is pushed. 3D visualization image of reconstruction (Fig. 7.10a–d) shows that the lesion and the inferior vena cava, the leading edge of the abdominal aorta, and the inferior mesenteric artery are not clearly demarcated.

Vascular surgery consultation considers that there is no clear active bleeding on the current

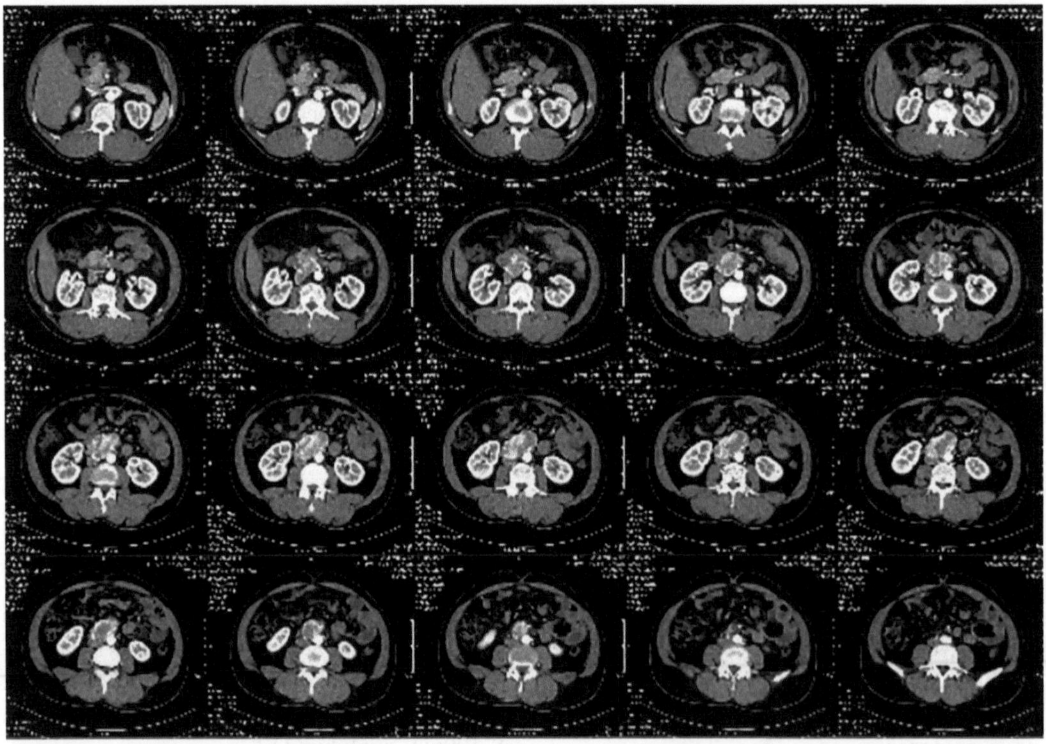

Fig. 7.9 Abdominal pelvic CT enhanced scan

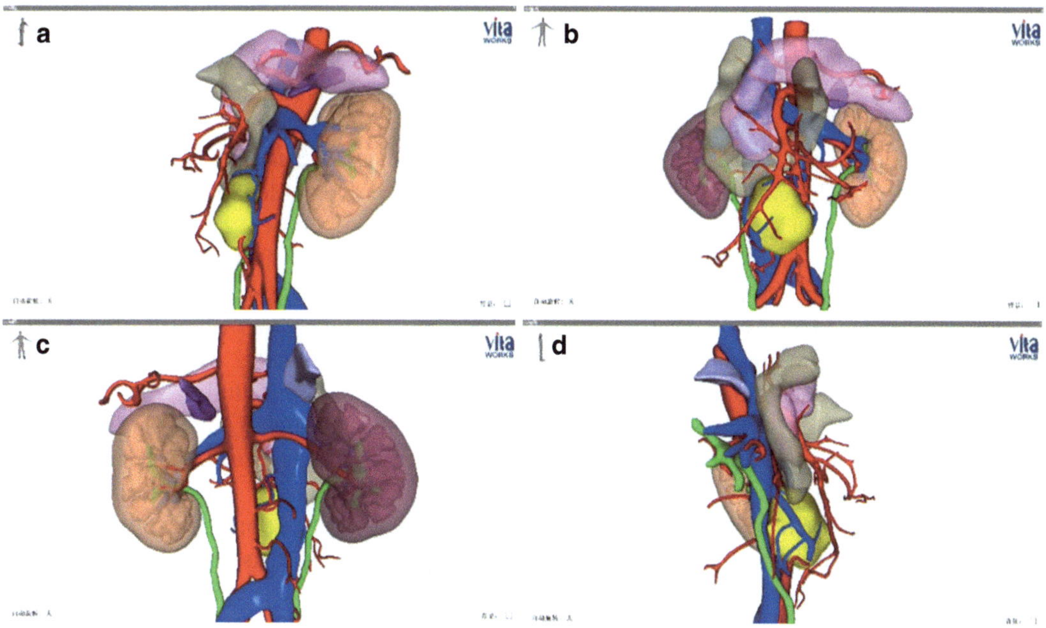

Fig. 7.10 (**a**–**d**) 3D visualization image of reconstruction (Yellow mass represents the tumor)

examination. There is no indication for an emergent intervention of vascular surgery. It is recommended to continue the primary treatment. Therefore, after symptomatic treatment such as pain relief, the abdominal pain was relieved, and the patient was recommended to go to a further specialist treatment. The patient then attended the endocrinology clinic. Endocrinology clinic considers a retroperitoneal paraganglioma. The amount of benzylbenzamide 5 mg q8h × 1 week was increased to 10 mg q12h × 2 weeks, then to 15 mg in the morning, 15 mg in the afternoon, and 10 mg in the evening. So far after taking the drug, fatigue and nasal congestion occurred. Occasional paroxysmal headaches and sweating appeared, which could be relieved after 1 min. Blood pressure fluctuated at 110–120/75–90 mmHg with a HR at 70–90 bpm in the past month.

7.4.3 Past, Personal, Marital and Childbearing, Family History

Nothing special

A mass shadow of soft-tissue density is seen below posterior duodenal horizontal segments and in front of inferior vena cava and abdominal aorta. Strips of flaky shadow with slightly higher density are seen internally. Larger cross-section is of about 3.8 cm × 7.7 cm. Multiple tortuous vascular shadows (5im33–39) can be seen around the arterial stage, with possible a partial communication with the left renal vein (5im33). The lesion in arterial phase is significantly and unevenly strengthened. The strengthening in portal phase and delayed phase of is also uneven. The duodenal is pushed. The lesion and the inferior vena cava, the leading edge of the abdominal aorta, and the inferior mesenteric artery are not clearly demarcated.

7.4.4 Current Diagnoses

Retroperitoneal paraganglioma

7.4.5 MDT Discussion

7.4.5.1 Endocrinology

(1) High-sodium and high-protein diet: ensure that the amount of intake is greater than 3000 mL, monitor the in-and-out volume and weight, mea-

sure blood pressure and heart rate at least two to three times a day, and repeat HCT once a week. Avoid drastic postural changes, laborious bowel movements, agitation, exertion, and infection. Avoid medications such as gastric reassurance and morpholine. (2) Currently, the patient is fully prepared for surgery, and it is recommended to continue the current dosage of phenol benzylamine, and it is necessary to increase the dose of phenol benzylamine to 15 mg q8h while continuing to strengthen volume management. Closely monitor inflows, recumbent blood pressure, and changes in heart rate. Adequate criteria for preoperative preparation for pheochromocytoma include normal blood pressure, no paroxysmal increase in blood pressure, palpitations, hyperhidrosis, etc. no severe orthostatic hypotension, volume recovery, and improvement in hypermetabolic syndrome. (3) Explain the risk of surgery, closely monitor the patient's vital signs and heart rhythm during the perioperative period, and be vigilant against hypertensive crisis and alternating high and low blood pressure. Preoperatively, consult with the Department of Anesthesiology and the Department of Critical Care to assist in the assessment. Full account of surgical risks. (4) It is recommended to complete PTH, free calcium, 24-h urinary calcium, blood calcium, phosphorus, ALP, 25-hydroxyvitamin D (rapid immunization), TP1NP, β-CTX, and to complete calcitonin, CEA, thyroid ultrasound, and screen for MEN.

7.4.5.2 Department of Anesthesiology

(1) Case regarded as ASA III , NYHA grade 1, limited-time surgery. (2) Patient's diagnosis is pheochromocytoma. It is recommended that anesthesia be prepared according to pheochromocytoma routine: establishment of arteriovenous passage and vasoactive drugs, strengthening the monitoring of changes in vital signs during surgery, and ensuring the perfusion of important organs. (3) The tumor is closely related to large blood vessels. Preoperative blood supply is fully prepared, and autologous blood is used when necessary, during surgery. Fully account for major bleeding and perioperative cardiovascular and cerebrovascular accidents. (4) Postoperative return to the ICU is recommended.

7.4.5.3 Vascular Surgery

(1) Patient is regarded as NYHA grade 1, limited-time surgery. (2) Patient's diagnosis is pheochromocytoma. It is recommended that anesthesia be prepared according to pheochromocytoma routine: establishment of arteriovenous passage and vasoactive drugs, strengthening the monitoring of changes in vital signs during surgery, and ensuring the perfusion of important organs. (3) The tumor is closely related to large blood vessels. Preoperative blood supply is fully prepared, and autologous blood is used when necessary during surgery. Fully account for major bleeding and perioperative cardiovascular and cerebrovascular accidents. (4) Postoperative return to the ICU is recommended.

7.4.5.4 Basic Surgery

(1) The mass is closely related to the adjacent intestinal tube, blood vessels, and pancreas, and the patient is informed of the conditions. (2) Conduct preoperative intestinal preparation, as well as full preparation for blood supply. (3) If you need our department to assist during operation, please contact in time.

7.4.6 Surgical Approach

Laparoscopic resection of retroperitoneal mass under general anesthesia (Fig. 7.11)

7.4.7 Postoperative Pathology

Retroperitoneal paraganglioma pheochromocytoma

Immunohistochemical results: Melan-A(−), AE1/AE3(−), CgA(+), Ki-67(index 1%), S-100(+), α-inhibin(+)

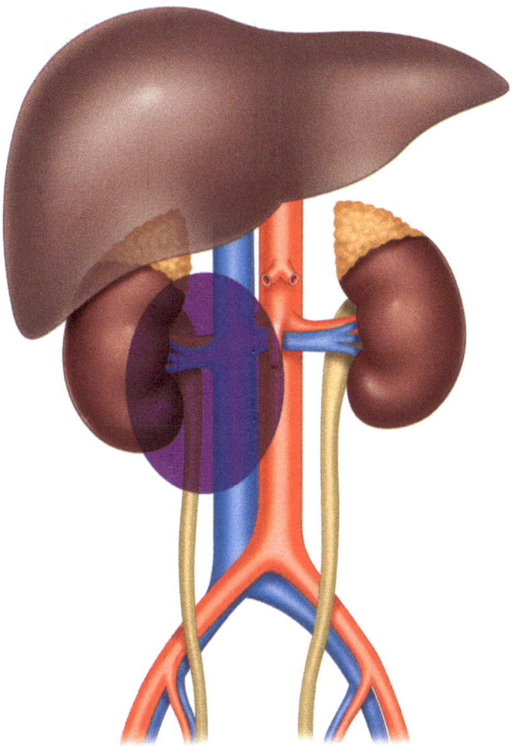

Fig. 7.11 Schematic diagram of the location of the mass

7.5 Case 7.5

Patient: Female, 29 years old

7.5.1 Complaints

Headache and palpitations for 12 years, increased blood pressure for 10 years, and the discovery of retroperitoneal tumor for half a year

7.5.2 History of Present Illness

In 2006, the patient had, without obvious incentives, occasional headaches and palpitations, without trembling hands, profuse sweating, pain in the precordial area, etc., which she did not take seriously. In 2008, the above symptoms worsened. She went to a local hospital. The measured blood pressure was at 180–190/120–130 mmHg and successively was treated with Diowen, Bebot, and Betaloc. She reported that his blood pressure could be controlled and symptoms of headache and palpitation were more eased than before. In the past 2 years, dizziness gradually appeared when squatting and standing up. Blood pressure in lying and standing position was not measured. Since the beginning of 2018, the patient's self-measured blood pressure in the afternoon has been about 150/100 mmHg. The precordial area is uncomfortable when the blood pressure rises. In the morning, the blood pressure is about 120/80 mmHg, and there is no special discomfort. She goes to another hospital and adjusts antihypertensive drugs. At the same time, she took an examination of blood catecholamines (NE 12.283 ng/mL, E < 0.005 ng/mL, DA < 0.005 ng/mL) and urine catecholamines (NMN 12195.00 μg/24 h, MN 389 μg/24 h). For a further diagnosis and treatment, she came to a hospital in Beijing to check 131I-MIBG imaging, which found a left retroperitoneal lesion, about 4.7 cm × 3.2 cm. The 131I-MIBG imaging was positive. Pheochromocytoma was considered. Later, for a further diagnosis and treatment, she visited our hospital in July 2018. The urine catecholamines were checked: 24hNE 385.71 μg/24 h. CTU: (L3 vertebral body level) retroperitoneal mass on the left side of the abdominal aorta, about 4.7 cm × 3.2 cm × 3.8 cm. The average CT value is about 31HU. The enhanced scan shows a significantly heterogeneous enhancement. Paraganglioma is considered. It is possible that the blood supply arteries come from the left renal artery, inferior mesenteric artery, and abdominal aorta, and the veins return to the inferior vena cava. Routine examinations were completed after admission, and oral phenoxybenzamine 10 mg BID drug preparation was given.

After discharge, the patient came to the endocrinology clinic of our hospital regularly, and the patient's blood pressure was adjusted with phenol benzylamine 30 mg–40 mg-20 mg tid, Lohoxi 5 mg qd, and Betaloc 25 mg tid. Blood pressure is stabilized at 120–140/80–100 mmHg with a heart rate of about 80–100 bpm. At present, patient complains of mild dizziness and nasal congestion and denies of discomfort such as palpitations, sweating, and hand tremors. For a further treatment, the outpatient clinic proposed her to be admitted to the hospital for a left retroperitoneal lesion.

7.5.3 Past, Personal, Marital and Childbearing, Family History

History of hypertension as described above. She complained of abnormal glucose tolerance. The platelet count was found to have increased since 2008, and the platelet count gradually increased after that and is currently stable at more than 500 × 109/L. In 2017, there were two episodes of numbness in the right half of the body, and the local hospital considered transient cerebral ischemia. She was treated with thrombolytic therapy twice and then did not take regular medication. There is no sequelae left. An increased proteinuria was found due to hypertensive renal damage, which was relieved after drug treatment (specification unknown). In 2009, bilateral ovary open surgery was performed because of teratoma removal. She underwent a transnasal pituitary cystectomy in 2014, after which binocular optic atrophy was found, and now binocular vision is blurred, mainly for the right eye. Nothing special for family history

7.5.4 Accessory Examination

CTU (Figs. 7.12 and 7.13): There is no significant abnormality in the morphology and density of the adrenal glands. Double kidneys show round multiple low-density foci. There is no significant strengthening after enhancement. The bladder is poorly filled. The bladder wall is smooth, and the wall is slightly thickened. Uterine morphology is acceptable, multiple patches of low-density lesions are seen in bilateral adnexal areas. The larger one is located on the right side, about 1.6 × 1.2 cm in size. The enhanced scan does not see significant abnormalities. At (L3 vertebral level) the left side of the retroperitoneal abdominal aorta, there is a soft-tissue shadow with a size of about 4.7 cm × 3.2 cm × 3.8 cm. The flat scan CT value is about 31HU. The enhanced scan shows a significantly uneven strengthening. Multiple tortuous and increased fine vascular shadows are seen around the mass. Blood supply is from the left renal artery, suborpine artery, and the small branches emitted from abdominal aorta. The vein returns to the inferior vena cava. The mass is closely related to the abdominal aorta and the left psoas major muscle. The surrounding intestinal tube is pressured and displaced. There are multiple calcifications in the abdominal aorta and its branches, and no obvious abnormalities are seen in the remaining abdominal blood vessels and renal veins.

A retroperitoneal mass on the left side of the abdominal aorta (L3 vertebral body level), about 4.7 cm × 3.2 cm × 3.8 cm. The average CT value is about 31HU. The enhanced scan shows a significantly heterogeneous enhancement. There are multiple small vascular shadows around the mass with more tortuous increases.

The tumor blood supply comes from the left renal artery, the inferior mesenteric artery, and the fine branches of the abdominal aorta, and the veins flow back to the inferior vena cava. The mass is closely related to the abdominal aorta and the left lumbar major muscle. The surrounding intestinal tubes are pressured and displaced.

7.5.5 Current Diagnoses

Left retroperitoneal paraganglioma

- Hypertension (grade 3, very high risk)
- Hypertensive renal impairment
- Double kidney cyst (Bosniak type I)
- Transient ischemic attack
- Past 2 thrombolytic treatments
- Past bilateral ovarian teratoma retraction
- Bilateral optic nerve atrophy
- Past transnasal pituitary cyst resection
- The cause of thrombocytosis is unknown

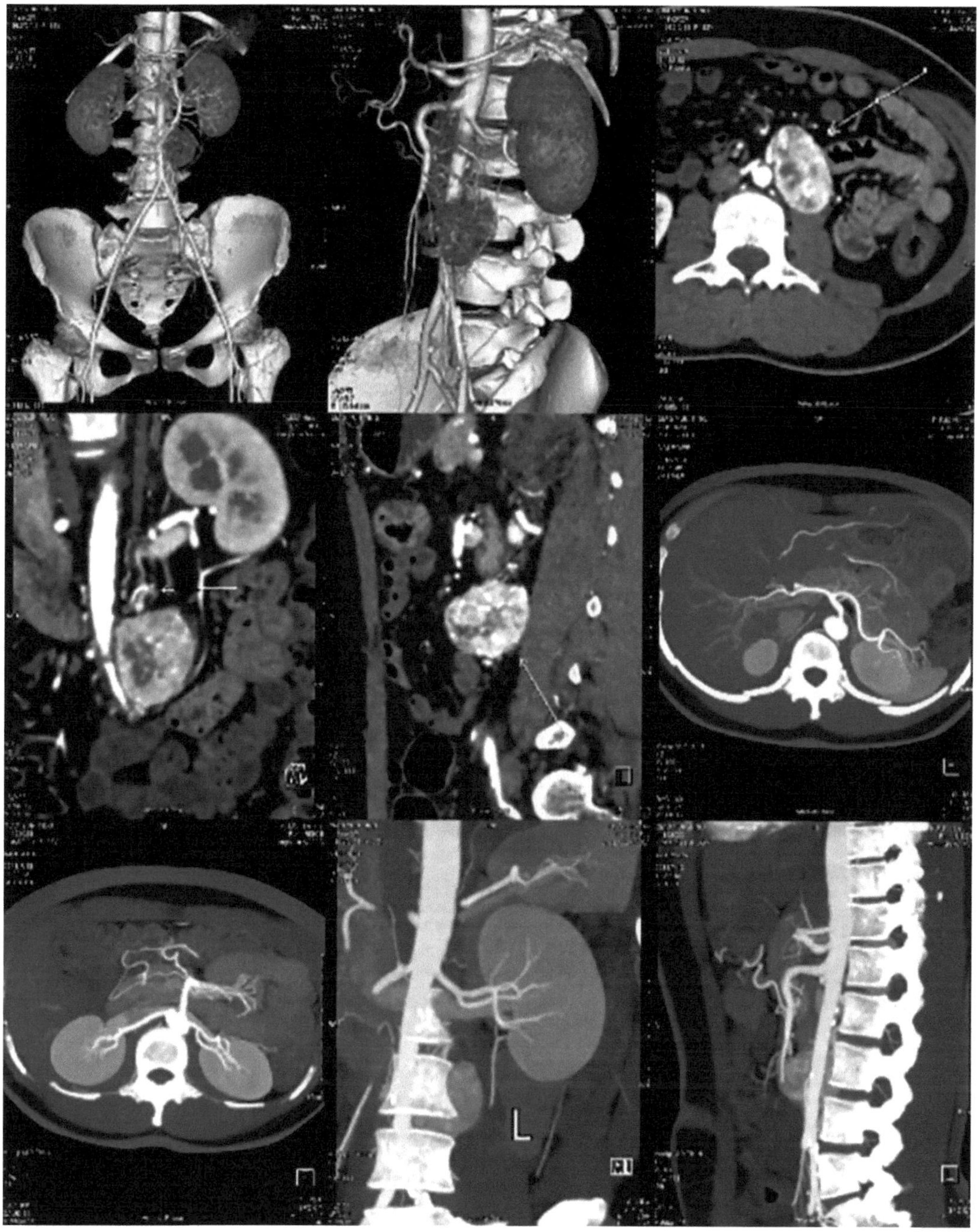

Fig. 7.12 Abdominal pelvic CT enhanced scan

7.5.6 MDT Discussion

7.5.6.1 Endocrinology

(1) Measure blood pressure and heart rate at least once a day in the recumbent position, monitor the amount of inflow and weight, and recheck HCT once a week. (2) The supine blood pressure is still high, and the amount of phenol benzylamine and codohua has been added. The change of blood pressure in the recumbent position has been observed. Daily drinking volume is 2–3 L.

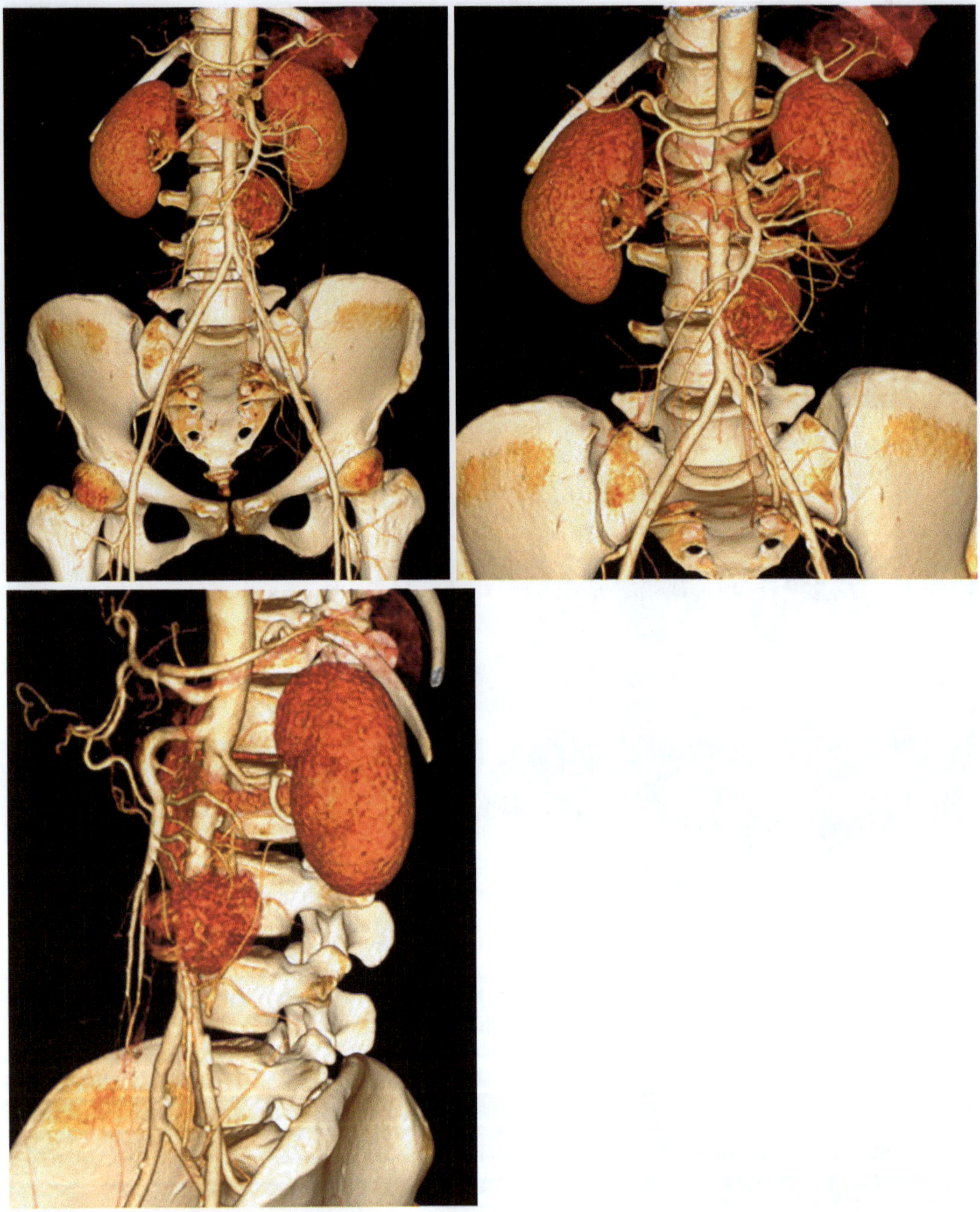

Fig. 7.13 3D reconstruction of abdominal pelvic CT

(3) The following are the full targets of preoperative preparation: no episodic symptoms, stable blood pressure, smooth stool, and decreased HCT.

7.5.6.2 Department of Anesthesiology

Agree with endocrinology, prepare according to preoperative standards, and avoid the risks of severe hypotension, hypertension, pheochromo-

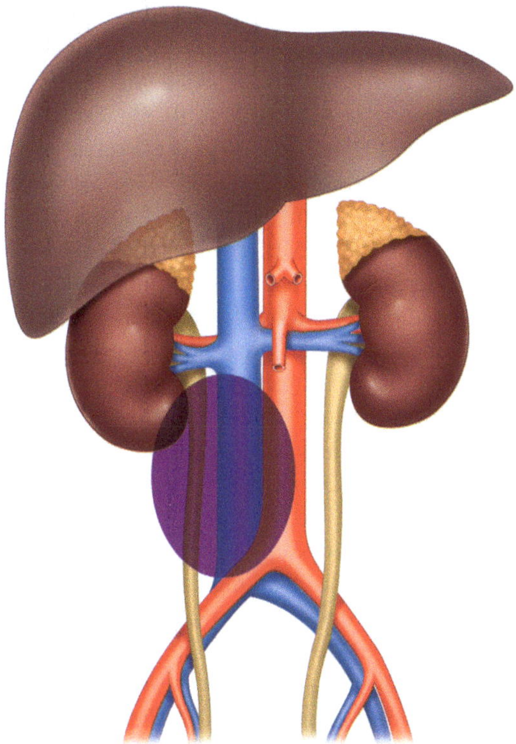

Fig. 7.14 Schematic diagram of the location of the mass

cytoma crisis, cerebral hemorrhage, shock, sudden death, etc.

7.5.6.3 Intensive Care Medicine

Patient has a high risk of surgery, and our department is willing to prepare a bed. Contact blood bank (6 U of red blood cells are currently available).

7.5.7 Surgical Approach (Fig. 7.14)

Laparoscopic exploration and resection of left retroperitoneal paraganglioma under general anesthesia

7.5.8 Postoperative Pathology

Lesions consistent with paragangliomas (paramesenteric arteries) (subméssentereal artery). Lymph nodes appear chronic inflammation (0/2).

Immunohistochemical results: AE1/AE3(−), CgA(+), Ki-67(index 2%), S-100(+), Syn(+)

7.6 Case 7.6

Patient: Male, 33 years old

7.6.1 Complaints

Episodic headache, palpitations, and heavy sweating for 5 years

7.6.2 History of Present Illness

The first hospitalization (November 11, 2018–December 21, 2018)

In 2013, the patient had sudden headache and palpitations with no obvious cause. He denied chest tightness, chest pain, abdominal pain, and diarrhea. He went to Dongguang County Hospital, Cangzhou City, Hebei Province. Symptoms were relieved after 2 h, and the patient reported no abnormality in subsequent imaging examinations. After that, enalapril maleate 10 mg QD and amlodipine 10 mg QD were taken orally. The BP was controlled at about 130/90 mmHg. In 2016, the patient had headache and palpitations again without obvious cause, accompanied by profuse sweating, nausea, pale complexion, and clammy limbs. He went to a local hospital to measure BP and found the BP of 210/140 mmHg. The symptoms were relieved after 1–2 h of infusion treatment (specific details are unknown). Then he continued to take the abovementioned antihypertensive drugs orally and control the blood pressure as above. On November 8, 2018, the patient drank a small amount of alcohol at noon, and in the early morning of the ninth, a severe abdominal pain occurred, accompanied by headache, nausea and vomiting, palpitations, profuse sweating, pale complexion, clammy and cold limbs, and the desire to defecate. He went to a hospital in Hebei Province to measure the BP. The highest blood pressure was 270/110 mmHg, and minimum blood pressure was 57/30 mmHg. No significant improvement was seen after dopamine and sedation (unknown). Then he was transferred to Cangzhou People's Hospital and Tianjin General Hospital. The aortic CTA showed an abdominal para-aortic mass, about the size of 8.8 cm × 7.5 cm × 7.1 cm, with clear borders and uneven density. Paraganglioma and secondary paraganglioma crisis were considered. It was recommended to seek medical treatment at a higher-level hospital. On November 10 at 2 am, he was admitted to the emergency room of our hospital, and the admission status was BP 44/22 mmHg, HR 156 bpm. ABG: pH 7.383, pCO2 19.9 mmHg↓, pO2 144.0 mmHg↑, HCO3–11.6 mmol/L↓, SBE-12.6 mmol/L↓, AG 9.9 mmol/L, Lac 3.6 mmol/L↑. Blood conventional: WBC 26.49 × 10^9/L↑, NEUT% 88.8%↑, HGB 211 g/L↑, HCT 58.1%↑, PLT 399 × 10^9/L↑. Biochemical: GLU 10.2 mmol/L, K 4.7 mmol/L, urea 14.53 mmol/L↑, Cr 309 μmol/L↑. Myocardial injury markers: CK 405 → 422 U/L↑, CKMB 6.7 → 6.3 μg/L↑, cTnI 3.625 → 3.53 μg/L↑. Myoglobin 981–1279 μg/L↑, NT-proBNP 22,423 pg/mL↑.

Due to low blood pressure, dopamine booster therapy was given. Because of the possibility of pheochromocytoma crisis, the NBP fluctuated at 44–237/22–163 mmHg. Rapid rehydration and yanidine pump therapy were given. The NBP started at 4 am. It tended to be stable and fluctuated between 70 and 120/40 and 90 mmHg. In the morning of November 10, the patient's abdominal pain, headache, palpitations, and other symptoms were relieved. He was transferred to the internal medicine ICU for a further diagnosis and treatment, continued to complete the relevant assessment, and confirmed the diagnosis. The results reported 24 h urine catecholamine to be 217.53 μg/24 h. Twenty-four hours urine NMN and MN were all elevated. Abdominal and pelvic enhanced CT, abdominal ultrasound, somatostatin receptor imaging, 131I-MIBG, and trunk PET/CT suggested a paraganglioma of abdominal aorta, secondary paraganglioma crisis, paroxysmal exacerbation of persistent hypertension, possible catecholamine cardiomyopathy, diabetes, acute kidney injury, and liver abnormal function. He was treated accordingly. After admission to the internal medicine ICU, BP was measured, and yanidine was given to lower blood pressure. From the morning of November 11, phenoxybenzamine 5 mg po Q12H was added. The phenoxybenzamine was increased to 10 mg Q12H on November 13, and the dose was increased to 10 mg on November 15 q8H. Monitor NBP: 130–160/80–100 mmHg, HR 80–120 bpm. HCT, Cr, BUN, CK, CKMB, cTnI, and NT-proBNP were decreased. Hypoglycemic Glibose 0.2 mg po tid and metformin 0.5 g po tid were taken. On November 16, he was transferred to endocrinology department for treatment and given phenoxybenzamine 10 mg q8H. On November 25, phenoxybenzamine was increased to 15 mg Q8H. Phenoxybenzamine was adjusted to 10–10–15–10 mg on December 3.

After that, dosage of phenoxybenzamine was gradually increased by 5 mg each time, adjusted to 15–10–15–10 mg (6–12–18–24) on December 5; 15–10–20–10 mg on December 7 (6–12–18–24); 15–15–20–10 mg (6–12–18–24) on December 10; and 15–15–20–15 mg on December 12 (6–12–18–24). On December 15, Betaloc was added to reduce the heart rate. On December 17, Betaloc was increased to 12.5 mg q12H. On November 16, subcutaneous injection of voglibose 0.2 mg tid + Lantus 8u before bedtime was given. On November 19, the hypoglycemic regimen was changed to voglibose 0.2 mg TID + Lantus 10u QN + Amaryl 2 mg QD. On December 4, Amaryl was reduced to 1 mg qd, Lantus 10u qn before bedtime, and Beixin 0.2 mg tid for the hypoglycemic therapy. On December 11, Amaryl was discontinued, and Beixin 0.2 mg tid + Lantus 10u qn for the hypoglycemic therapy were given. On December 17, the dose was reduced to 8 with the subcutaneous injection before bedtime, and oral Bexin 0.2 mg tid was continued. Smooth stool was noticed, and weight changed from 75 to 78.5 kg. Later, he was transferred to our department to evaluate the condition and explain the risks of the operation. The patient and his family expressed that they could not accept it and asked to be discharged first for drug preparation. Because of the stable conditions, he was discharged from the hospital.

Second hospitalization (January 18, 2019–January 31, 2019)

After discharge, the patient regularly took oral phenol benzylamine tablets 15–15–20–15 mg (6–12–18–24) and Betaloc 12.5 mg q12h. Monitored blood pressure was about 140/90 mmHg with a HR unknown. He denied of palpitations. Before going to bed, 8u subcutaneous injection was administered. Self-discontinuation of Bexin was reported. Monitoring fasting blood glucose was 5–7 mmol/L, and postprandial 2 h blood glucose was about 8–9 mmol/L. On January 13, 2019, the patient was more talkative, felt bloated, fatigued, denied palpitations, and sweating. Blood pressure was increased. At 20:48, the measured BPmax was 180/120 mmHg with a HR of 78 times/min. Phenol benzylamine 15 mg at 24-h point was orally taken in advance. The blood pressure was gradually decreased. It could be reduced to 143/102 mmHg with a HR of 95 times/min. On January 14–17, 2019, patient's monitored recumbent blood pressure at 103–177/80–109 mmHg, HR 73–128 bpm, and upright blood pressure at 99–104/74–76 mmHg with a HR of 74–76 times/min. On January 17, 2019, at the endocrinology clinic, the supine blood pressure measurement was 172/123 mmHg with a HR of 120 beats/min. The upright blood pressure was 133/103 mmHg with a HR of 142 times/min. Blood examinations: HCT 47.4%, Cr(E) 99 μmol/L, CK 62 U/L, BNP 6 ng/L, ALT 14 U/L, AST 13 U/L. Phenolic benzylamine was increased to 20 mg q6h and Betaloc to 25 mg q12h. He was admitted to hospital for a further diagnosis and treatment. After admission, monitored 24 h UCA was NE 67.31 μg/24 h; E 78.53 μg/24 h; DA 213.16 (μg/24 h). There were no significant abnormalities in myocardial enzymes. Echocardiogram: left ventricular hypertrophy, left atrium enlargement, aortic root widening, mild thickening of the aortic valve, decreased function of left ventricular relaxation. Monitored supine blood pressure was 120–145/70–100 mmHg with a HR of 70–100 times/min, and vertical blood pressure was 85–120/55–70 mmHg with a HR of 100–120 times/min. After the stable conditions, he was discharged.

Third hospitalization (March 1, 2019–Present)

Since the last discharge, the patient has been regularly and orally taking phenol benzylamine 20 mg qid (6–12–18-24). He self-reports that his blood pressure is stable, which can be controlled at about 135/75 mmHg with a HR of 70–80 bpm. There is no episodic headache, blackness, wet and cold limbs, chest pain, loss of consciousness, and other discomforts. He is now admitted to our department for a further treatment. In the past 3 months, the patient's mental, sleep, and appetite are acceptable. He urinates and defecates as usual. There is no obvious change in weight.

7.6.3 Past, Personal, Marital and Childbearing, Family History

The blood glucose was increased for 4 years. Currently, he takes an oral betaxin 0.2 mg per repas plus 8u insulin glargine qn. Fasting blood glucose is 7 mmol/L. Postprandial blood glucose is generally about 10–8-9 mmol/L. In 2016, he underwent the dissection of double lower extremity large saphenous vein. Nothing special for personal history and family history

7.6.4 Accessory Examination

Peritoneal enhanced CT + CTA (Fig. 7.15): A cystic solid mass on the left side of the abdominal aorta, which can be consistent with paraganglioma changes. Please combine with clinical presentations. Inferior mesenteric artery is pushed and pressed, and some part of it is closely related to the lesion. It is closely related to the mid-abdominal small intestine, with poor demarcation of the left lumbar major muscle. Hepatic artery comes from the abdominal aorta. There are bilateral pararenal arteries. Right kidney has double renal arteries. Abdominal aorta and its branches have atherosclerotic change. Small cysts of the right lobe of the liver exist. Possible cholestasis. Slightly thicker bladder wall. Enlargement of the prostate gland. Multiple small lymph nodes can be seen in retroperitoneum, supramensal, pelvic, and bilateral inguinal.

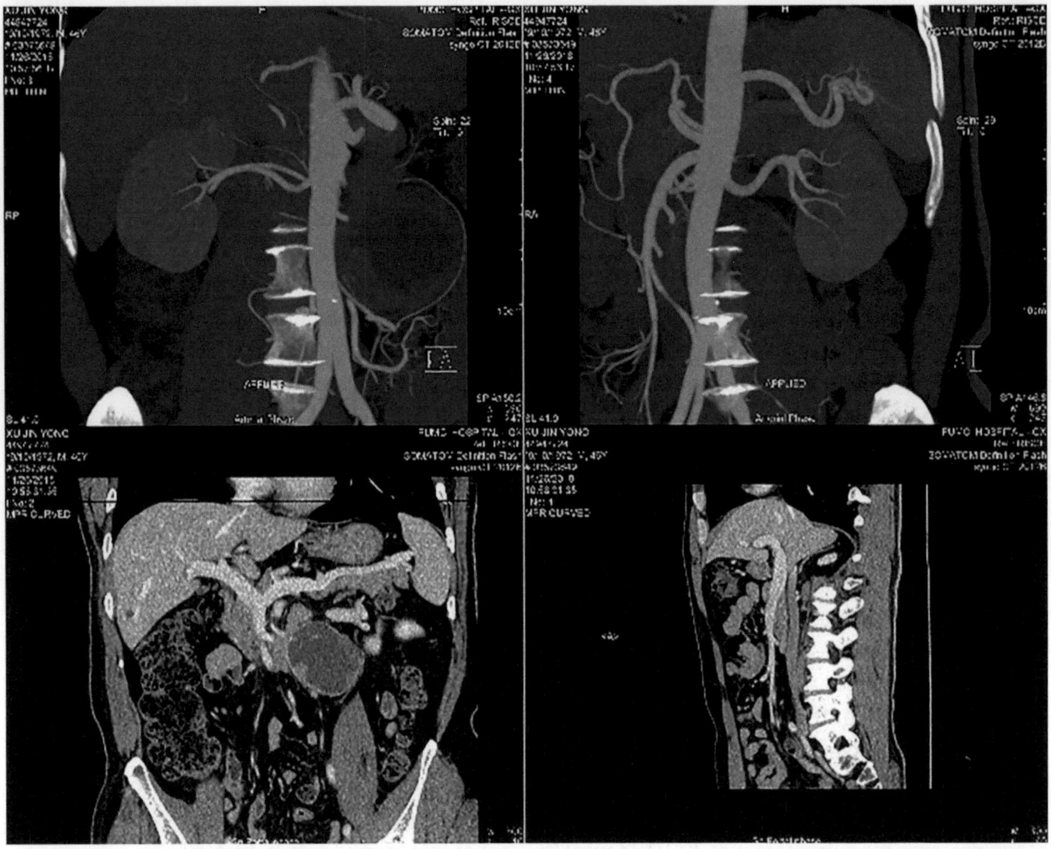

Fig. 7.15 Three-dimensional reconstruction of abdominal pelvic CT

Somatostatin receptor imaging: abnormal demonstration in the left mid-abdomen. Tomography fusion imaging is recommended.

131I-MIBG: area of radioactivity in the left mid-quadrant, a paraganglioma being considered, with possible central liquefaction

The inferior mesenteric artery is pushed, and some part of it is closely related to the lesion. It is closely related to the small intestine in the middle abdomen. The demarcation with the left lumbar major muscle is not clear.

7.6.5 Current Diagnoses

Left inferior mesenteric paraganglioma

Paroxysmal exacerbations of persistent hypertension

Catecholamine cardiomyopathy is not excluded

Diabetes

Nodules in both lung

Liver cysts

Enlargement of the prostate

Prostate cyst

Past exfoliation of the great saphenous veins of both lower extremities

7.6.6 MDT Discussion

7.6.6.1 Department of Anesthesiology

Patient with paragangliomas and paraganglioma crisis needs to be vigilant against catecholamine cardiomyopathy, complete the examinations before surgery, and make a step forward in assessing cardiac function. Anesthesia is prepared according to routine preparation for pheochromocytoma. Passage of arteries and veins is established. Vasoactive drugs are prepared, and intraoperative monitoring of changes in vital signs is strengthened. Perioperative cardiovascular and cerebrovascular accidents and risk of major bleeding are fully explained. Return to the ICU after surgery.

7.6.6.2 Endocrinology

Suggest high-sodium, diabetic diet, and instruct patient to avoid intake of sweets and liquid food and squeezing the abdomen and strenuous exercise. In terms of blood glucose, it is recommended to increase the amount to 10 U qn and to continue oral bexin with the same dose as before. The targets for blood glucose control are FBG 5–7 and PBG 6–10. Phenol benzylamine dose is not adjusted. Continue to monitor recumbent blood pressure and heart rate. If there is no episodic blood pressure increase and no obvious orthostatic hypotension, selective surgical treatment can be considered.

7.6.6.3 Basic Surgery

There is a palpable solid mass of about 4 cm × 5 cm in left upper quadrant with a poor mobility. CT shows that the mass is located in the lower edge of the pancreas. The upper part reaches the fine end of the colon. It is recommended to complete the intestinal preparation before surgery. Explain to the patient the risks that may involve colon and mesenteric vascular damage, postoperative pancreatic leakage, partial pancreatic resection, small intestine injury, spleen injury, and other risks.

7.6.6.4 Surgical Approach

Transperitonealoscopic resection of left retroperitoneal paraganglioma under general anesthesia (Fig. 7.16)

7.6.7 Postoperative Pathology

Lesions (left paraganglioma) are consistent with paragangliomas.

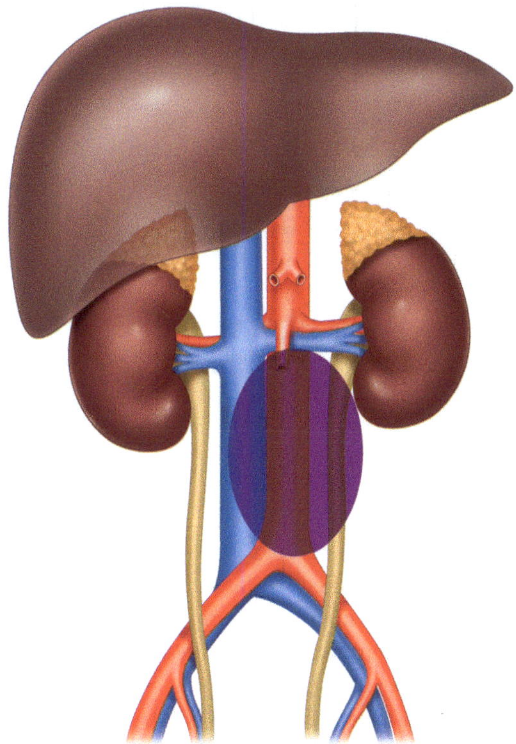

Fig. 7.16 Schematic diagram of the location of the mass

7.7 Case 7.7

Patient: Female, 43 years old

7.7.1 Complaints

Increased blood pressure for 1 year and right low back pain for 3 months

7.7.2 History of Present Illness

One year ago, the patient's physical examination showed an increase in blood pressure, up to 140/100 mmHg. There were no symptoms such as episodic sweating, palpitations, headache, and dizziness. Three months ago, the patient had, with no obvious trigger, a sudden right low back pain, with no radiation from other parts. It lasted for 3 h and was relieved after rest. The patient presented in the outer hospital. The abdominal

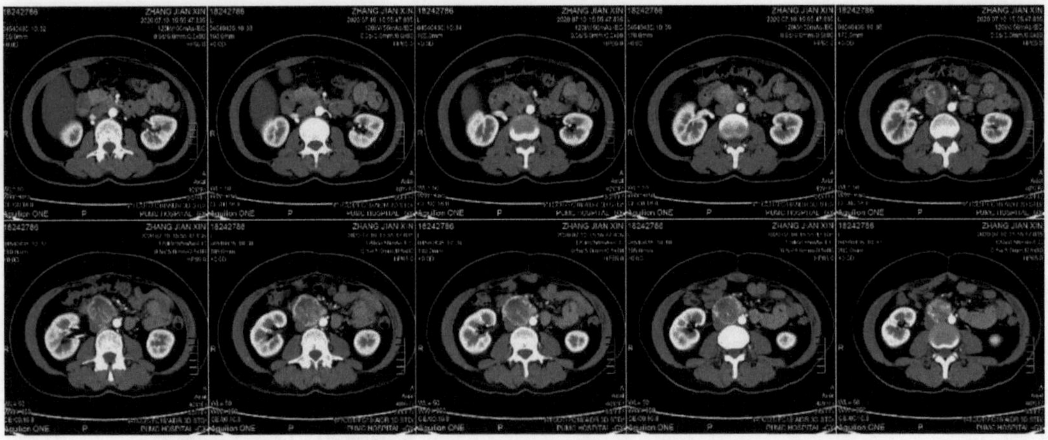

Fig. 7.17 Abdominal pelvic CT enhanced scan

CT scan was performed to show a retroperitoneal mass (specification unknown). The diagnosis of stromal tumor was considered. A further diagnosis and treatment were recommended. The patient visited the basic surgery department of our hospital (July 16, 2020). Abdominal enhancement CT + pancreatic thin scan +3D reconstruction (July 16, 2020) showed that the clump of soft tissue density was seen below the horizontal segment of the pancreatic head duodenum, the inferior vena cava, and the front of the abdominal aorta, with a size of about 4.8 cm × 4.1 cm × 4.3 cm. The diagnosis of a paraganglioma was considered. Further diagnosis and treatment was recommended. Two months ago, the patient presented at the endocrinology department. 3-methoxydehrepinephrine (NMN) was 19.85 nmol/L. Paraganglioma being diagnosed, the patient took phenolic benzylamine 5 mg every 8 h, increased to 10 mg every 12 h after 5 days, and increased to 10 mg every 8 h after 5 days. She is now taking phenol benzylamine 15 mg q8h treatment. Blood pressure is well controlled. For horizontal position, BP is 122/88 mmHg with a heart rate of 60 beats/min. For standing position, BP is 105/77 mmHg with a heart rate of 81 beats/min. One month ago, the liver function found (14 September 2020) ALT 64 U/L. It was reexamined and treated with glucuronolactone 100 mg tid. Currently, patient is admitted to the hospital for a further surgical treatment. Since the onset of disease, the patient's mental health, appetite, and sleep are normal. The patient has normal bowel and bowel movements and a weight gain of 6 kg.

7.7.3 Past, Personal, Marital and Childbearing, Family History

Bilateral salpingectomy was performed 8 years ago because of pelvic adhesions. From 2012 to 2013, she did IVF twice. The first time failed, and in 2013, she successfully became pregnant after IVF. She had gestational diabetes during pregnancy. She reported that OGTT 2 h was 12 mmol/L. Type 2 diabetes mellitus was diagnosed in March 2020. No medication was taken. Fasting blood glucose was 8.0 mmol/L. Nothing special for personal history and family history

7.7.4 Accessory Examination

Abdominal enhancement CT + pancreatic thin sweep + three-dimensional reconstruction (Figs. 7.17 and 7.18): There is a mass below the horizontal segment of the duodenum of the pancreas, the inferior vena cava, and the anterior abdominal aorta, locally accompanied by a cystic necrosis. Possible paraganglioma? Please combine clinical presentations. A small branch of the

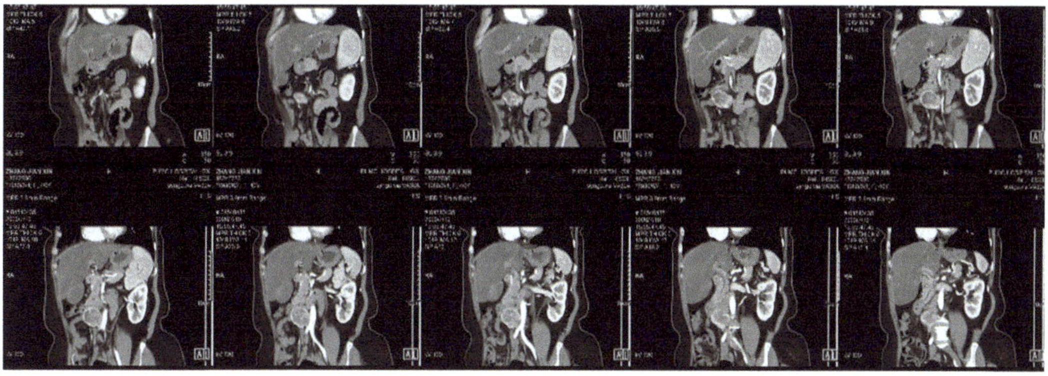

Fig. 7.18 3D reconstruction of abdominal pelvic CT

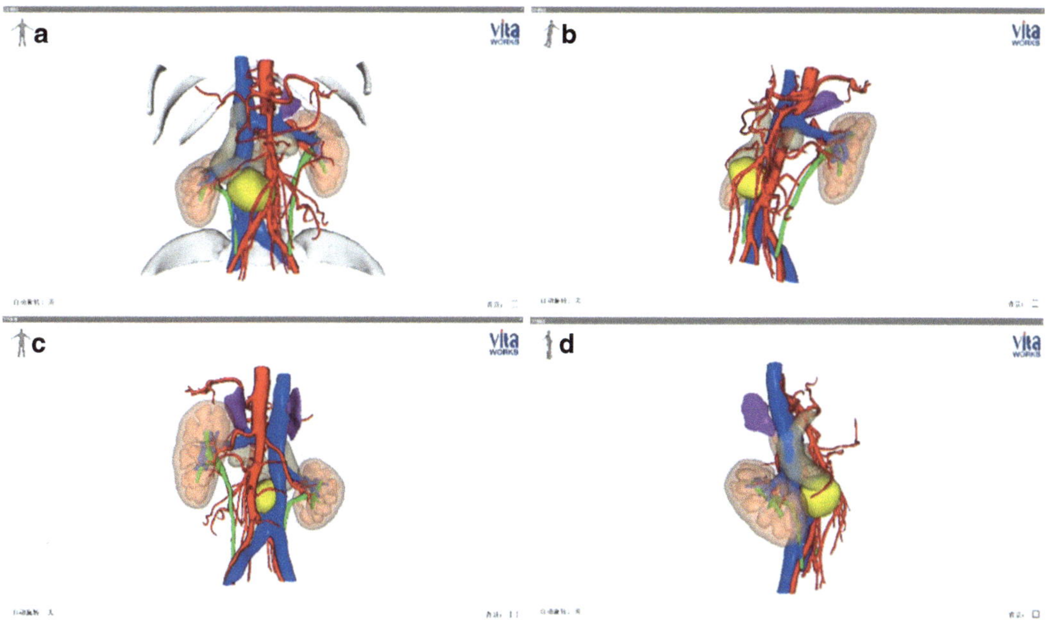

Fig. 7.19 (**a–d**) 3D visualization reconstruction

abdominal aorta provides the mass with blood supply. The lesion is close to the intestinal wall of the duodenal level. The local intestinal wall is compressed. **3D visualization reconstruction** (Fig. 7.19) showed that the inferior vena cava is slightly pushed toward the left by local compression. There are more tortuous and slightly thicker vascular shadows in the periphery of the spleen, which communicate with the spleen vein and the left renal vein. The lateral branch of the spleen-kidney vein is thickened and communicated. There is a severe fatty liver.

Somatostatin receptor SPECT/CT fusion imaging: right retroperitoneal hyperexpressive foci of somatostatin receptor. Neuroendocrine tumor is considered? Paraarthritis? Please consult to clinical presentations. The rest of somatostatin receptor imaging shows no abnormalities.

131I-MIBG: right-sided abnormalities seen in the middle and lower abdomen; paraganglioma is considered.

There is a mass below the horizontal segment of the duodenum of the pancreas, the inferior vena cava, and the anterior abdominal aorta, locally accompanied by a cystic necrosis; possible paraganglioma

A small branch of the abdominal aorta provides the mass with blood supply. The lesion is close to the intestinal wall of the duodenal level. The local intestinal wall is compressed. The inferior vena cava is slightly pushed toward the left by local compression. There are more tortuous and slightly thicker vascular shadows in the periphery of the spleen, which communicates with the spleen vein and the left renal vein. The lateral branch of the spleen-kidney vein is thickened and communicated.

7.7.5 Current Diagnoses

Right retroperitoneal paraganglioma
- Hypertension
- Type 2 Diabetes
- Micronodules of the right lung
- Fatty liver
- Osteoporosis

7.7.6 MDT Discussion

7.7.6.1 Endocrinology

(1) Monitor blood pressure and heart rate in the recumbent position at least two times a day, monitor the amount of intake and weight, repeat HCT once a week, and avoid infection, fatigue, severe postural changes, and compression of the abdomen. Avoid the use of morpholine, gastric rehabilitation, etc. (2) The patient's supine blood pressure has reached the standard, and the treatment of phenol benzylamine 15 mg q8h can be continued. Due to insignificant increase in body weight, the standing heart rate is significantly increased. The HCT level is increased in comparison with before. It is recommended to increase the daily drinking >2–3 L. (3) The patient's intravenous blood glucose is high. Please monitor the spectrum of blood glucose. If necessary, a diabetic diet is given. If water is fasted during the perioperative period, a certain amount of insulin in intravenous fluids is given. The blood glucose in the maintenance solution is 7–11 mmol/L. (4) Prior to surgery, consult with the Department of Anesthesiology and Critical Care Medicine to assist in perioperative assessment. (5) Postoperative follow-up by endocrinology outpatient. Selective recheck of glucagon. If necessary, complete genetic screening.

7.7.6.2 Department of Anesthesiology

Continue the current preparation, monitor blood glucose, strengthen blood glucose control, and stop taking phenol benzylamine 1 day before surgery and the morning of surgery. Explain the risks of perioperative cardiovascular and cerebrovascular events, malignant arrhythmias, heart failure, hemorrhagic shock, sudden death, etc. Return to the ICU after surgery.

7.7.6.3 Vascular Surgery

(1) The patient's mass is closely related to the vena cava, etc. The operation is finely performed, and the blood transfusion is fully prepared. (2) Explain the risk of vascular damage. If necessary, we are willing to assist during operation.

7.7.6.4 Basic Surgery

(1) The patient's mass is closely related to the vena cava, etc. The operation is finely performed, and the blood transfusion is fully prepared. (2) Explain the risk of vascular damage. If necessary, we are willing to assist during operation.

7.7.7 Surgical Approach

Transperitonealoscopic resection of right retroperitoneal paraganglioma (Fig. 7.20)

7.7.8 Postoperative Pathology

Lesions (retroperitoneal paraganglioma) are consistent with paragangliomas.

Immunohistochemical results: Melan-A(−), AE1/AE3(−), CgA(+), Syn(+), Ki-67(index8%), S-100(−), α-inhibin(weak+), SDHB(−).

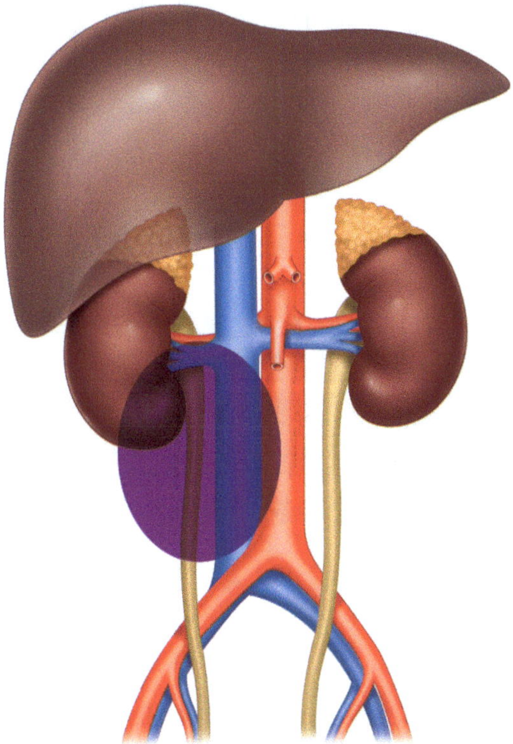

Fig. 7.20 Schematic diagram of the location of the mass

7.8 Case 7.8

Patient: Female, 47 years old

7.8.1 Complaints

Physical examination revealed a retroperitoneal tumor for 3 years.

7.8.2 History of Present Illness

In 2017, a retroperitoneal tumor was found in the B-ultrasound of the physical examination, and no tumor was found in the reexamination ultrasound. In 2018, patient experienced two times intermittent headache. Blood pressure was measured at 180/90 mmHg, with heart rate unknown. Symptoms could be relieved after a rest of 1–2 h. There were no heart palpitations, profuse sweating, and pale complexion. In 2019, a retroperitoneal tumor (not reported) was found during B-ultrasonography in a local hospital, and CT examination found a retroperitoneal tumor, about 4 cm in size, which could be heterogeneously enhanced. In June 2020, she came to the outpatient clinic of Peking Union Medical College Hospital, and the CT scan of the abdomen and pelvis showed a mass of slightly low-density nodule with a size of about 4.1 cm × 3.3 cm. The edge of the enhanced scan showed an obvious enhancement in the arterial phase, and no enhancement was seen in the center. It is located at about the L2–L3 level of vertebral of right anterior abdominal aorta, which may be a paraganglioma.

7.8.3 Past, Personal, Marital and Childbearing, Family History

Nothing special

7.8.4 Accessory Examination

CT scan of the abdominal pelvis (Fig. 7.21): A slightly less dense nodule on the right side of the abdominal aorta at approximately L2–L3 vertebral level, about 4.1 cm × 3.3 cm in size. Paraganglioma may be considered.

A slightly lower-density nodule was seen on the right anterior side of the abdominal aorta at about L2–L3 vertebral level, with a size of about 4.1 × 3.3 cm, and the arterial phase was significantly strengthened at the edge of the enhanced scan, and no strengthening was seen in the center. It suggests a right-sided anterior mass of the abdominal aorta at about L2–L3 vertebral level, and paragangliomas may be present.

7.8.5 Current Diagnoses

Right retroperitoneal paraganglioma

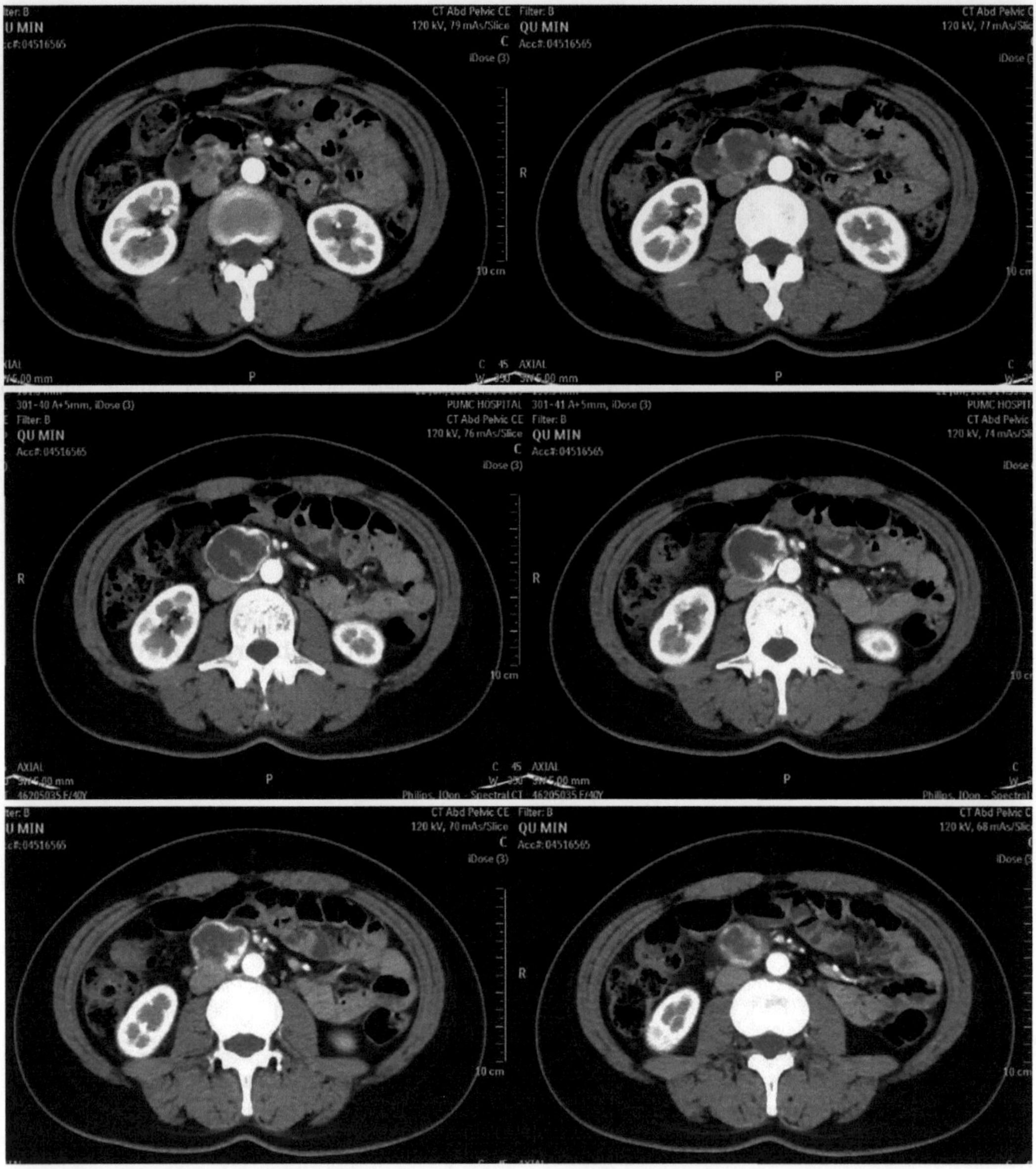

Fig. 7.21 Abdominal pelvic CT enhanced scan

7.8.6 MDT Discussion

7.8.6.1 Department of Anesthesiology

Case is regarded as an ASA Grade III, limited-duration surgery. Patient with paraganglioma is advised to complete preoperative cardiac evaluations. According to the routine preparation of anesthesia for paraganglioma, the following items should be performed to patient: the establishment of arteriovenous passage, administration of vasoactive drugs, strengthening the monitoring of changes in vital signs during surgery, maintaining the balance of myocardial oxygen supply and oxygen consumption, and ensuring the perfusion of important organs. Patient must be fully explained with the risk of perioperative cardiovascular and cerebrovascular accidents and major bleeding. Pay attention to the fluctuations of blood pressure, maintain water-electrolyte balance, and fully prepare blood supply. Postoperative return to the ICU.

7.8.6.2 Urology

Right retroperitoneal paraganglioma is highly likely. Surgery can be considered. Continue to complete preoperative preparations and maintain stable blood pressure.

7.8.7 Surgical Approach

Laparoscopic resection of right retroperitoneal tumor (Fig. 7.22)

7.8.8 Postoperative Pathology

Lesions (retroperitoneal tumors) are consistent with paraganglioma.

Immunohistochemical results: Melan-A(−), α-inhibin(−), AE1/AE3(−), CgA(+), Syn(−), Ki-67(index 1%), S-100(+), SDHB(+).

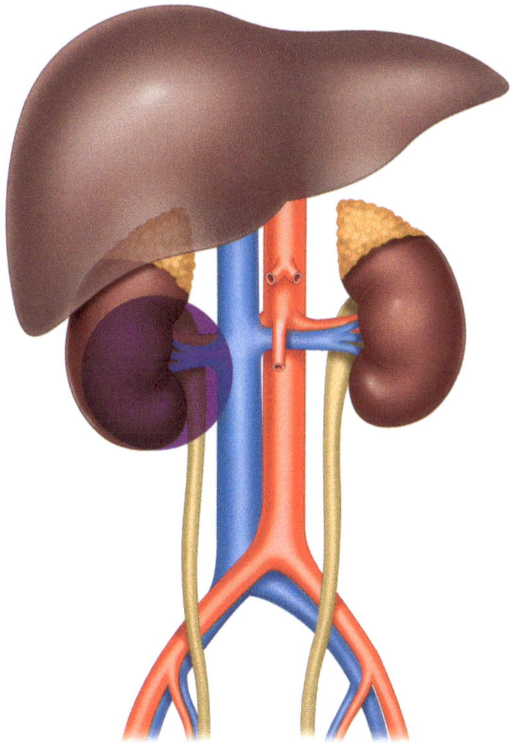

Fig. 7.22 Schematic diagram of the location of the mass

8 Multidisciplinary Treatment of Pelvic Paraganglioma and Metastatic Pheochromocytoma

Shi Rong, Lin Ma, Jin Wen, Hong Jun Li, Su Yan, Zhan Wang, Hai Wang, Xu Wang, and Guo Rong Li

8.1 Case 8.1

Patient: Female, 44 years old

8.1.1 Complaints

Paroxysmal dizziness, palpitations, and increased blood pressure for more than 6 years and a vaginal mass found 9 months ago

8.1.2 History of Present Illness

Paroxysmal dizziness and palpitations began to occur 6 years ago without obvious triggers, accompanied by increased blood pressure, with systolic blood pressure up to 240–250 mmHg and diastolic blood pressure 110–120 mmHg, sometimes accompanied by nausea, vomiting, and other symptoms. Each episode lasts about 10 min and is resolved spontaneously. The above symptoms occur once a day for the frequent episodes but usually once in 4–5 days. Most of the above symptoms occur in a resting state. There are occasional dizziness and discomfort during sex, but there are no other serious symptoms. At the end of 2019, the patient again had dizziness, palpitations, and blood in the vomit. The vagina was found to be occupied by a mass during the external hospital examination. The vaginal internal examination before the proposed gynecological surgery was carried out in the city hospital.

Symptoms of dizziness, palpitations, and increased blood pressure occurred when the tumor body was touched. The systolic blood pressure was up to 240–250 mmHg, accompanied by nausea and vomiting symptoms. Local endocrinology department checked 24 h urinary norepinephrine, with a slight elevation of 105.24 μg/day. In August 2020, our hospital's abdominal pelvis enhancement CT showed a shadow of soft tissue density of the left wall of the vagina. The maximum cross-section was 3.2 × 2.5 cm. The enhanced scan was significantly strengthened, and the boundary with the lower wall of the bladder and the anterior wall of the rectum was not clear. The vaginal mass of multi-blood supply was considered. At the same time, a small hamartoma of the right kidney, an uneven density of cervical enlargement, and a suspicious soft tissue density shadow in the left posterior rectum were found. In August 2020, for the completion of endocrine examination in our hospital, the blood NMN was 4.70 nmol/L, which was significantly elevated, and the 24-h urinary catecholamine NE showed 78.32 μg/24 h. In August

Shi Rong and Lin Ma contributed equally to this work.

S. Rong · L. Ma · J. Wen (✉) · H. J. Li · S. Yan
Z. Wang · H. Wang · X. Wang
Department of Urology, Peking Union Medical College Hospital, Beijing, China

G. R. Li
Department of Urology, University Hospital & University Jean Monnet, Saint-Etienne, France

J. Wen (ed.), *Surgical Management of Pheochromocytoma and Retroperitoneal Paraganglioma*,
https://doi.org/10.1007/978-981-99-8421-3_8

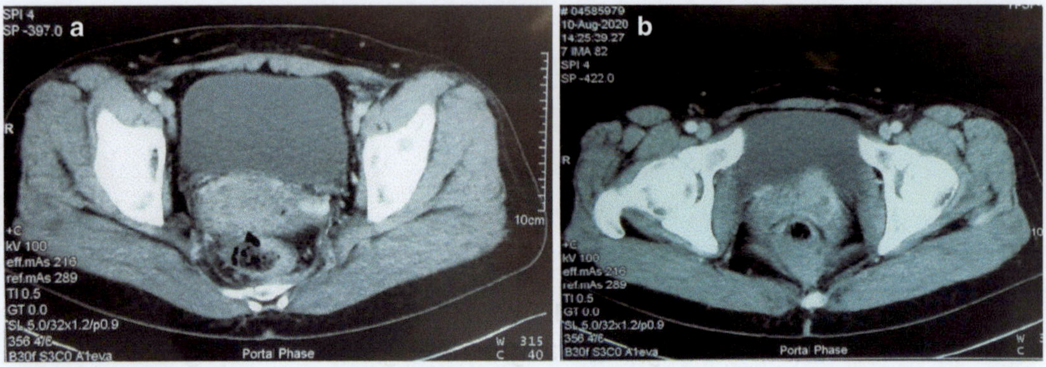

Fig. 8.1 (**a, b**) Abdominal pelvic CT enhanced scan

2020, during the nuclear medicine examination of our hospital, somatostatin receptor imaging and tomography imaging found negative. 131I-MIBG finds the equivalence of anomalies seen in the perineal region, suggesting that paragangliomas are more likely. Adrenal medullary tomography fusion imaging suggests abnormalities in the left wall of the vagina, which is more likely to be a paragangliomas in conjunction with the clinical history.

Since the end of August 2020, in our outpatient clinic, she began to take oral phenol benzylamine 5 mg q8h. Since starting oral medication, she has no paroxysmal palpitations, sweating, increase of blood pressure, and other symptoms. Currently, she continues to take the drug regularly. She gains about 5 kg. There is a mild nasal congestion.

8.1.3 Past, Personal, Marital and Childbearing, Family History

The patient's parents, an older brother, and two older sisters are in good health. She has a son and a daughter. Her son is a patient with Down syndrome.

8.1.4 Accessory Examination

Abdominal pelvic enhanced CT (Fig. 8.1a, b): soft tissue density shadow of the left wall of the vagina, maximum cross-section 3.2 cm × 2.5 cm

A shadow of soft tissue density of the left wall of the vagina. The maximum cross-section is 3.2 × 2.5 cm. The enhanced scan is significantly strengthened, and the boundary with the lower wall of the bladder and the anterior wall of the rectum is not clear, considering the vaginal multi-blood supply mass. The cervical enlargement is seen with uneven density. A suspicious shadow of soft tissue density in the left posterior rectum is suggested.

8.1.5 Current Diagnoses

Pass in anterior vaginal wall

Paraganglioma

The cause of cervical enlargement remains to be investigated.

Left posterior mass of the rectum

8.1.6 MDT Discussion

8.1.6.1 Incretion

Complete the screening for related endocrine syndromes.

8.1.6.2 Basic Surgery

Tumor is closely related to the rectum. Invasion cannot be excluded, and there is a risk of rectal damage.

8.1.6.3 Gynecology

A 4.0 × 2.5 cm mass on the left wall of the vagina. The lower pole is located about 3 cm (about the position of the bladder neck) to the external orifice of the urethra. It can be surgically removed, and there is a risk for urethral injury.

8.1.7 Surgical Approach

Resection of vaginal paraganglioma

Laparoscopic resection of presacral mass

8.1.8 Postoperative Pathology

Anterior vaginal wall tumor is consistent with paraganglioma.

Immunohistochemical results: Melan-A(−), AE1/AE3(−), CgA(+), Ki-67(index 3%), S-100(+), α-inhibin(−), Desmin(−), EMA(−), Syn(+), Vimentin(+), TTF-1(−), Braf(IHC)(−), SDHB(+)

(Mass of rectum) Cysts of the columnar epithelium and mucus columnar epithelium covered with false layers of ciliates and mucus columnar epithelium. The walls of the cysts can be seen with mucus glands and sebaceous adenoid structures. The lesion is considered to be a mature cystic teratomas.

8.2 Case 8.2

Patient: Female, 55 years old

8.2.1 Complaints

High blood pressure for 7 years and palpitations for 9 months

8.2.2 History of Present Illness

Increased blood pressure has been found 7 years ago. A right adrenal mass was found during physical examination (no report seen). In April 2019, coronary CTA found double adrenal masses, the left-side diameter of about 1 cm and the right-side diameter of about 2 cm. Blood pressure measurement is 140/90 mmHg.

From December 2019 to August 2020, she had intermittent sudden forehead and parietal occipital pains, VAS 5–6 points, with palpitations, no sweating, blood pressure measurement of 210/105 mmHg, and a heart rate > 100 bpm. After administration of Hyjaya + Betaloc + nifedipine + Urapidil, she still had attacks. During the course of the disease, the patient denies that the face has become red, presence of kidney stones, fracture history, intermittent hot flashes, and sweating. Since the onset of illness, diet and spirit are normal, but sleep is slightly worse. Previously, she liked salty in taste. Sodium intake has been controlled in recent years. Nocturia is three times. She lost a weight of 6.5 kg in the past 3 months.

8.2.3 Past, Personal, Marital and Childbearing, Family History

Pregnant hyperesthesia, allergic asthma, thyroid nodectomy, pituitary tumor, "total hysterectomy" for uterine fibroids in 2011, diabetes mellitus, history of allergy for cayenne pepper, high blood pressure with her mother, prolactinoma with one of her sons

8.2.4 Accessory Examination

CTU (Fig. 8.2): A nodular shadow of slightly less dense can be seen in the right adrenal junction, with a size of about 1.7 cm × 1.0 cm. The average CT value of the flat scan is about 16.2 Hu. The arterial phase of the enhanced scan is moderately strengthened, with an average CT value of about 47.2 Hu. The left adrenal gland is thickened. A small nodule shadow is seen in the lateral branch and the medial branch. The length and diameter of the lateral limb are about 7.1 mm, while those of the medial limb are about 9.0 mm. Mild strengthening is seen on the enhancement scan. Patchy iso-density filling defects can be seen on the right posterior wall of the bladder, about 4.0 × 3.3 × 3.9 cm, and patchy low-density shadows can be seen in the center of the lesion. A significant strengthening is seen on enhanced scanning, and no significant strengthening is seen in the central low-density area. Strengthening is seen near the lesion on the right wall of the bladder.

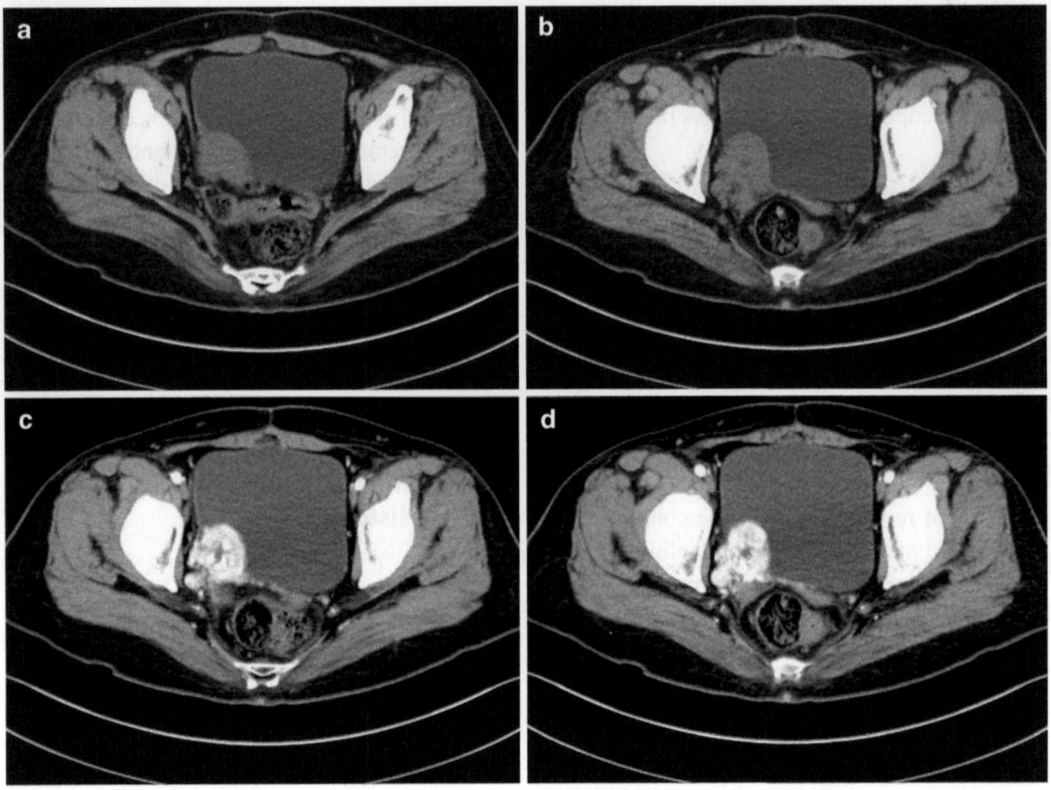

Fig. 8.2 Abdominal pelvic CT enhanced scan. (**a–d**) Patchy iso-density filling defects can be seen on the right posterior wall of the bladder, about 4.0 × 3.3 × 3.9 cm, and patchy low-density shadows can be seen in the center of the lesion. A significant strengthening is seen on enhanced scanning, and no significant strengthening is seen in the central low-density area. Strengthening is seen near the lesion on the right wall of the bladder

Somatostatin receptor imaging: right adrenal nodules, suspected mild somatostatin receptor expression

131I-MIBG: bilateral adrenal small nodules, pelvic masses, no definitive increase in radiopharmacy

PET-CT: slightly increased soft tissue density nodules in the right adrenal region. Malignant lesions cannot be excluded. SUVmax is 3.3. Small nodules of the left adrenal gland with no increase in metabolism are found with the benign possibility. There are masses of abnormally elevated soft tissue in the right wall of the pelvis, closely linked to the bladder, with SUVmax 21.5. The possibility of malignant lesions cannot be excluded. A slightly increased local metabolism is found on the left side of the saddle. SUV max is 5.0. It may be a microadenoma.

Endocrine examination: Blood NMN 13.61 nmol/L, MN 0.12 nmol/L

24 h urinary catecholamines: NE 639.67 μg/24 h, E 7.49 μg/24 h, DA 232.07 μg/24 h

MEN and tumor-related screening: anterior pituitary function (−) pituitary flat scan + dynamic enhancement

MRI: pituitary microadenoma may be possible.

Calcium and phosphorus metabolism, parathyroid ultrasound (−) **GAS**: 16 pg/mL; blood glucose, glucagon, chest and abdomen pelvic CT pancreas did not see significant abnormalities. Tumor markers AFP, CEA, CA199, CA125, CA153, CA72–4, CA242, SCC, AFP, NSE, Cyfr211, ProGRP (−)

Evaluation of complications: myocardial enzymes, 8hUAE, ACR, and 24 h total urinary protein quantification are in the normal range. In-room ECG: (−).

Carotid artery, vertebral artery ultrasound: thickening of the median membrane at the right carotid artery bifurcation and the formation of small plaques at the left carotid artery bifurcation. For renal artery, upper limb, and lower extremity artery ultrasound and inferior vena cava and hepatic vein ultrasound, no obvious abnormalities were seen. ECHO LVEF is 67% with reduced function of left ventricular relaxation.

8.2.5 Current Diagnoses

Bladder paraganglioma

Bilateral adrenal masses (adenoma)

Diabetes

Past resection of right lobe and isthmus of thyroid

Multiple small cysts with the remaining left lobe of the thyroid gland

Pituitary microadenomas may be possible.

8.2.6 MDT Discussion

8.2.6.1 Department of Critical Medicine

Fully account for the risks associated with the perioperative period and return to the ICU after surgery.

8.2.6.2 Urology

It is recommended to complete the CTU assessment of pelvic mass and bladder and ureteral position.

8.2.6.3 Gynecologic

The patient's pelvic cavity shows a SUVmax of 21.5, which alerts to the possibility of malignancy. If the operation is an open surgery, our department can participate at the same time to remove the mass first during the operation. Quickly frozen pathology examination is to be prepared.

8.2.6.4 Department of Anesthesiology

The patient is currently under stable blood pressure control and continues the current treatments. Prevention of colds in the near future. Antihypertensive drugs and phenolic benzylamine are taken in the morning of surgery. Continue follow-up. ICU Consultation Opinion: for surgery on Monday, please submit the relevant form, and reserve the ICU bed.

8.2.6.5 ICU

Fully account the risks associated with the perioperative period. Return to the ICU ward after surgery.

8.2.7 Surgical Approach

Resection of the paraganglioma of the bladder + laparoscopic resection of the right adrenal tumor

8.2.8 Postoperative Pathology

Bladder tumor in combination with immunohistochemistry; the lesion conforms to the paraganglioma.

Right adrenal tumors 1 and 2 are consistent with nodular hyperplasia of the adrenal cortex, accompanied by tumor 1 intracellular excess brown pigment deposition.

Immunohistochemical results: bladder tumors: AE1/AE3(−), CgA(+), Syn(+), Ki-67 (index 3%), S-100 (fine support Cell +), α-inhibin(+), SDHB(−). Right adrenal tumor 1: Melan-A (+), α-inhibin (partial +)

8.3 Case 8.3

Patient: Male, 20 years old

8.3.1 Complaints

Eight years after surgery for left adrenal pheochromocytoma, 4 years after the discovery of a right adrenal mass

8.3.2 History of Present Illness

In 2012, he was admitted to a local hospital for paroxysmal abdominal pain with a diagnosis of left adrenal pheochromocytoma. The resection of left adrenal pheochromocytoma was performed. Postoperative pathology was clearly a left adrenal pheochromocytoma. In 2016, the patient found a mass visible in the right adrenal gland; no treatment was provided. He visited our hospital in 2017 and performed chest-abdominal pelvic enhancement CT, which shows multiple round nodules of soft tissue density beside the lateral branch of the left adrenal gland and the medial branch of the right adrenal gland, at the L3 vertebral body level, on the right side of abdominal aorta. The edge was smooth, and the diameter was about 1.7 cm, 1.1 cm, and 0.9 cm, respectively. The arterial phase was significantly strengthened after enhancement. The maximum nodule density and strengthening were not uniform, and the strengthening of the portal pulse and the delayed phase was reduced. There was no abnormality in the aorta and its branches. Patient had no obvious symptoms at that time and was temporarily observed. Phenolbenzylamine drug preparation has lasted for more than 1 month, with a dose of 10 mg q12h. Symptoms of nasal congestion are found. There is no acral hot flashes. He gained a weight of 25 kg in the past 6 months. Supine blood pressure is 128/77 mmHg, and supine pulse is 75 times/min. Upright blood pressure is 102/75 mmHg, and upright pulse is 83 times/min.

8.3.3 Past, Personal, Marital and Childbearing, Family History

Nothing special

8.3.4 Accessory Examination

Abdominal pelvic CT enhancement scan + three-dimensional reconstruction (Fig. 8.3): Multiple round nodules of soft tissue density beside the lateral branch of the left adrenal gland and the medial branch of the right adrenal gland, at the L3 vertebral body level, on the right side of abdominal aorta. The edge was smooth, and the diameter was about 1.7 cm, 1.1 cm, and 0.9 cm, respectively. The arterial phase was significantly strengthened after enhancement. The maximum nodule density and strengthening were not uniform, and the strengthening of the portal pulse and the delayed phase was reduced.

131I-MIBG scintigraphy: abnormalities in the right adrenal region are seen, and pheochromocytoma is highly likely to be considered.

Endocrine examination: 24 h urinary catecholamines: NE 230.25 μg/24 h, E 2.84 μg/24 h, DA 145.32 μg/24 h; 3-Methoxy norepinephrine (NMN) 7.95 nmol/L; 3-Methoxyephrine (MN) 0.06 nmol/L

Multiple round nodules of soft tissue density beside the lateral branch of the left adrenal gland and the medial branch of the right adrenal gland, at the L3 vertebral body level, on the right side of abdominal aorta. The edge was smooth, and the diameter was about 1.7 cm, 1.1 cm, and 0.9 cm, respectively. The arterial phase was significantly strengthened after enhancement. The maximum nodule density and strengthening were not uniform, and the strengthening of the portal pulse and the delayed phase was reduced

8.3.5 Current Diagnoses

Polychromocytoma in the right adrenal region (metastatic pheochromocytoma)

Past surgery for left adrenal pheochromocytoma

8.3.6 MDT Discussion

8.3.6.1 Department of Anesthesiology

Relevant results of examinations have not been returned yet. If the results are significantly abnormal, please consult with the internal medicine department for diagnosis and treatment, and follow up with our department. The diagno-

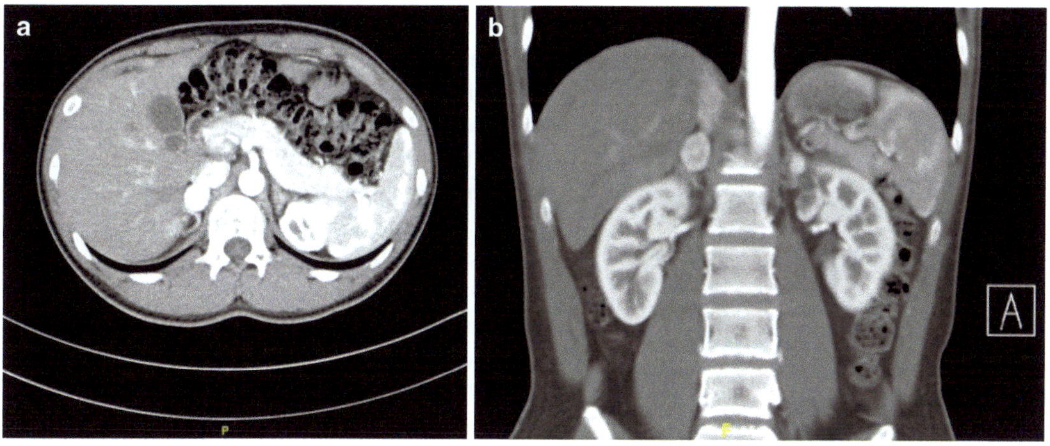

Fig. 8.3 (**a**, **b**) Abdominal pelvic CT enhanced scan +3D reconstruction

sis of pheochromocytoma is clear. The current blood pressure at recumbent position can be controlled. There is no orthostatic hypotension, finger warm, and hand not sweaty. There is a weight gain of 5 kg. The preoperative preparation is acceptable. There is a risk for perioperative chromophilus crisis. Please fully explain the risk to the patient and family. Our department prepares for an invasive artery monitoring, central venous catheter placement, and blood recovery device, if necessary. If there is a risk for major bleeding, please contact the blood bank to prepare blood supply. Return the patient to the ICU after surgery.

8.3.6.2 Endocrinology

(1) It is recommended to measure blood pressure and heart rate in the recumbent position three times a day, and it is recommended to complete the 24-h Holter ECG monitoring, monitor weight and intake and output, and recheck HCT once a week. Avoid fatigue, infection, severe postural changes, and compression of the abdomen. Avoid the use of morphine, gastric rehabilitation, etc. (2) When the patient experiences headache again, please retest the blood pressure in time, and clarify the correlation between the headache and PPGL. If necessary, complete the 24-h urine catecholamine test on the attack day and on the control day, and compare them. Patient's weight is 79 kg. He still has headaches and sweating. Orthostatic hypotension is obvious. It is recommended to increase phenol benzylamine to 10 mg q8h and to increase daily water intake to 3 L/day. Adequate criteria for preoperative preparation are no symptoms of episodic hypertension, no postural hypotension, decreased sweating, patency of stools, decreased HCT levels, and weight gain. Before surgery, the Department of Anesthesiology and the Department of Critical Care should be asked to assist in the assessment of perioperative risk. (4) Complete myocardial enzymes and echocardiography to screen for catecholamine cardiomyopathy. (5) Complete parathyroid hormone, calcitonin, alpha work 2 + 3, and thyroid ultrasound to screen MEN. Follow up with the endocrinology outpatient for the analysis of screening genes.

8.3.7 Surgical Approach

Laparoscopic resection of right adrenal pheochromocytoma (Fig. 8.4)

8.3.8 Postoperative Pathology

Right pheochromocytoma pheochromocytoma

Immunohistochemical results: Melan-A(−), α-inhibin(−), AE1/AE3(−), CgA(+), Syn(+), Ki-67(index 1%), S-100(+), SDHB(weak+).

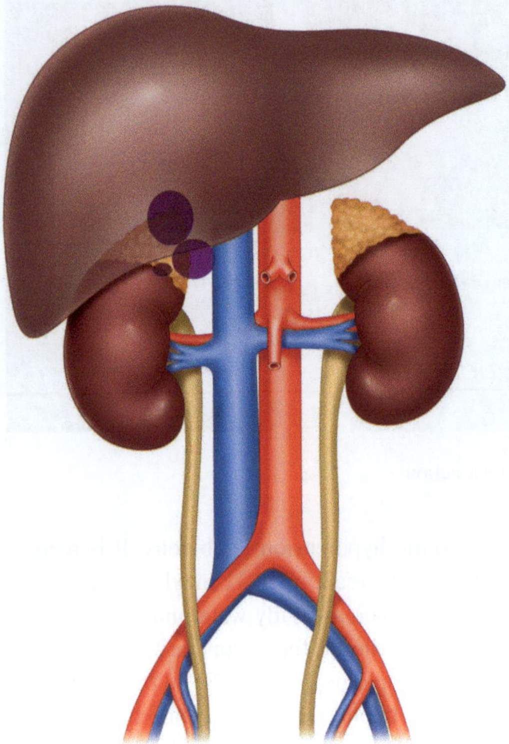

Fig. 8.4 Schematic diagram of the location of the mass

8.4 Case 8.4

Patient: Male, 32 years

8.4.1 Complaints

Sixteen years after resection of the left adrenal pheochromocytoma, and the tumor recurrence was found half a year's ago.

8.4.2 History of Present Illness

In 2006, the patient had a maximum hypertension of 180/140 mmHg. Due to an elevated blood pressure and headache, he took a CT examination at the local hospital, which suggests a left adrenal mass (3.3 cm × 3.0 cm × 2.4 cm). Left-sided pheochromocytoma was considered at the time. On August 5, 2006, laparoscopic resection of left adrenal pheochromocytoma was performed under general anesthesia, and the patient's blood pressure was stable after the operation. He did not take antihypertensive drugs again. In May 2020, the patient's blood pressure was found to rise again (up to 140/110 mmHg) during the physical examination, accompanied by symptoms such as general weakness and mental weakness. Patient presented to the hospital for reexamination of the abdominal and pelvic CT, which suggests a recurrence of the left pheochromocytoma. After the patient visited our hospital, the 24-h urinary catecholamine showed that norepinephrine and dopamine were significantly elevated. Somatostatin receptor imaging shows the possibility of recurrence of left adrenal pheochromocytoma and the possibility of right adrenal gland. Imaging of 131 I-MIBG suggests a possible right adrenal pheochromocytoma and no increased radionuclide uptake in the left adrenal mass. Adrenal enhancement CT and coronary sagittal reconstruction suggest that a left adrenal mass does not exclude tumor recurrence and that right adrenal junction nodule does not exclude pheochromocytoma.

Patient began preparation of oral phenolic benzylamine drugs at the end of September 2020. So far, weight gain has been 4 kg (54–58 kg). Nasal congestion is obvious, and the extremities are warm; 24 h urinary catecholamines: 24 hNE 1825.45 μg/24 h↑, 24hE 5.02 μg/24 h, 24hDA 935.45 μg/24 h↑. Plasma catecholamines and their metabolites: MN 0.11 nmol/L, NMN 12.15 nmol/L↑

8.4.3 Past, Personal, Marital and Childbearing, Family History

Nothing special

8.4.4 Accessory Examination

Adrenal enhancement CT + coronary sagittal reconstruction (Figs. 8.5a–d and 8.6a–d): Postoperative changes in left adrenal pheochromocytoma. There is a left adrenal mass shadow with cyst necrosis. Tumor recurrence cannot be

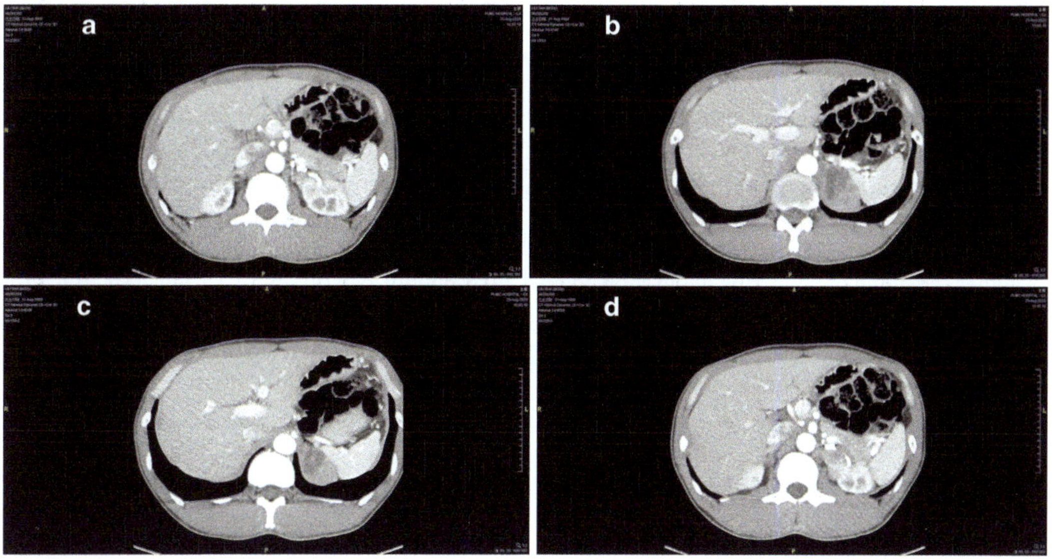

Fig. 8.5 Abdominal pelvic CT enhanced scan +3D reconstruction. (**a**–**d**) Changes after the surgery of pheochromocytoma in the left adrenal. There exists a left adrenal mass shadow with cyst necrosis. Tumor recurrence is not excluded

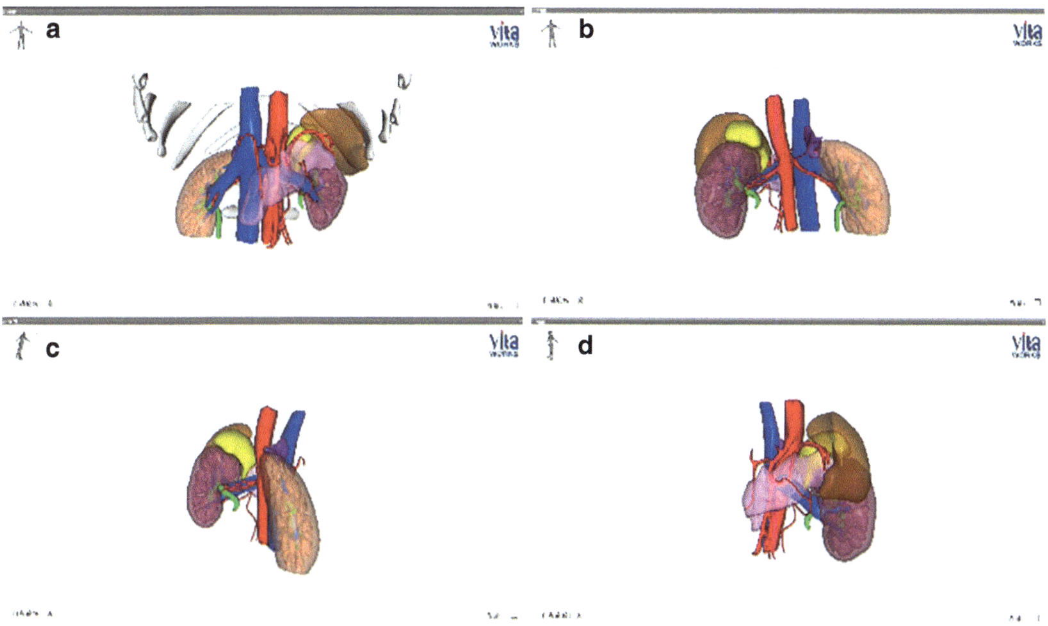

Fig. 8.6 (**a**–**d**) 3D visual reconstruction image

excluded. About the strengthening nodule in right adrenal junction, pheochromocytoma cannot be excluded. Intrahepatic scattered small cysts may be seen.

3D visualization of reconstructed images: a left adrenal mass shadow with cystic necrosis and a mass in right adrenal junction. Pheochromocytoma is not excluded.

Somatostatin receptor imaging (tomography): the left adrenal mass with cystic necrosis cannot exclude the possibility of postoperative recurrence of pheochromocytoma.

131I-MIBG (fault): abnormalities in the right adrenal are seen, and the possibility of pheochromocytoma is high. There is a mixed density mass in the left adrenal region, mainly cystic. No explicit increase in radiophernalia is seen, that is, no clear signs of pheochromocytoma are seen. It is recommended to combine clinical presentations to exclude the pheochromocytoma recurrence.

Other screening of endocrine gland showed no evidence of tumors.

A left adrenal mass shadow with cyst necrosis and a mass in the right adrenal junction

8.4.5 Current Diagnoses

Recurrence after the resection of left adrenal pheochromocytoma

8.4.6 MDT Discussion

8.4.6.1 Internal Medicine

The etiology of elevated ALT is unknown, and further completion of EBV/CMV DNA, hepatitis 1/IgG/IgM, AIH and PBC autoantibody profiles, and abdominal B ultrasound is recommended. In terms of treatment, continue the current treatment of Tianqing Luscious and Yi Shanfu. Closely monitor the changes of liver enzyme, and liver damage drugs should be taken with caution.

8.4.6.2 Department of Anesthesiology

Continue the current preparation of phenol benzylamine; advise patient to drink sufficient water; fully account for the risks of perioperative cardiovascular and cerebrovascular events, malignant arrhythmias, heart failure, hemorrhagic shock, etc.; and recommend returning to the ICU for the further treatment after surgery.

8.4.6.3 Endocrinology

(1) Increase the amount of intake; the daily amount should be greater than 3000 mL. Advise patient to take a high-sodium and high-protein diet. Monitor the blood pressure and heart rate in the recumbent position at least two times a day, in-and-out volume, weight, and stool. Repeat HCT once a week. Advise patient to avoid the increase of abdominal pressure such as forced defecation and gastric reassurance, morphine, and other drugs and (2) continue to take phenol benzylamine 15 mg q8h. Because the patient's orthostatic hypotension is obvious, it is recommended to further strengthen volume management. If necessary, normal saline or colloidal intravenous infusion may be given to improve volume. Currently, patient has no episodic symptoms. Blood pressure can be controlled, and surgical treatment can be considered after improving the volume. (3) Patient with high surgical risks and their families should be explained with the risks and recommended consultations by Department of Anesthesiology and ICU to assess the perioperative risks.

8.4.6.4 ICU

(1) The patient should be told to expect a large scope of surgery. There is a high risk of surgical complications such as bleeding. This should be fully explained to the patient. (2) Return patient to the ICU after surgery.

8.4.7 Surgical Approach

Laparoscopic resection of recurrent pheochromocytoma of the left adrenal gland (Fig. 8.7)

8.4.8 Postoperative Pathology

Adrenal pheochromocytoma (Left adrenal mass). Necrosis may be seen.

Immunohistochemical results: Melan-A(−), AE1/AE3(−), CgA(+), Ki-67(index5%), S-100(−), α-inhibin(−), Syn(+), SDHB(+)

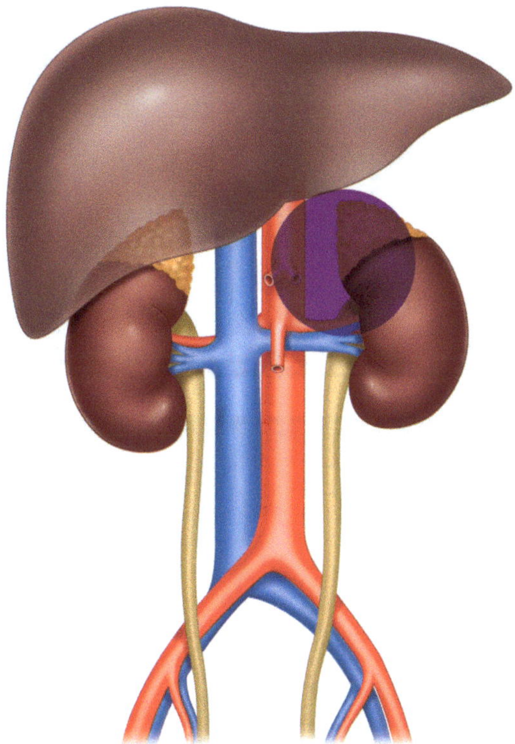

Fig. 8.7 Schematic diagram of the location of the mass

8.5 Case 8.5

Patient: Female, 26 years old

8.5.1 Complaints

More than 20 months after the resection of bilateral pheochromocytoma

8.5.2 History of Present Illness

From 2015, she feels a repeated headache, palpitation, and sweating. The frequency is one to two times per week. Symptoms last about 10 min. BPmax is 200/130 mmHg. The examination of NMN showed 14.77 → 41.89 nmol/L↑, MN 0.73 → 1.64 nmol/L↑, and embryonic RET mutation (+). In July 2015, laparoscopic resection of right adrenal mass was performed in the outer hospital, and the total resection of right adrenal gland was intraoperatively performed. In August 2019, imaging examination found that the right pheochromocytoma was recurred after surgery. In December 2020, she began to take phenol benzylamine 15 mg tid + Betaloc 12.5 mg bid.

8.5.3 Past, Personal, Marital and Childbearing, Family History

Fasting blood glucose: 6–7 mmol/L. Family history: her father has six brothers and sisters. Two aunts were diagnosed with bilateral pheochromocytoma. There is no recurrence found by 10 years' regular follow-up after surgery. She has one younger brother and is physically healthy.

8.5.4 Accessory Examination

2019 and 2020 abdominal pelvic enhanced CT scans (Fig. 8.8): postoperative recurrence of right-sided pheochromocytoma

CT scan of the abdominal basin in March 2021 (Fig. 8.9): Multiple abnormal signals in the lower and posterior section of the right lobe of the liver, between the hepatic and renal space, and around the right perirenal space. The tumor volume was increased significantly, and pheochromocytoma recurrence or metastasis was considered.

131I-MIBG abdominal tomography visualization: slightly less dense nodules with abnormally increased radiopheromic uptake between the liver and kidney, behind the right kidney, and on the side of the right inferior kidney. Some are partially fused, the largest about 3.3 cm × 2.1 cm, in line with pheochromocytoma metastases.

There are multiple abnormal signals in the lower posterior part of the right lobe of the liver, around the space between the liver and kidney, and on the right perirenal region. The tumor volume is significantly increased, and the recurrence or metastasis of pheochromocytoma is considered.

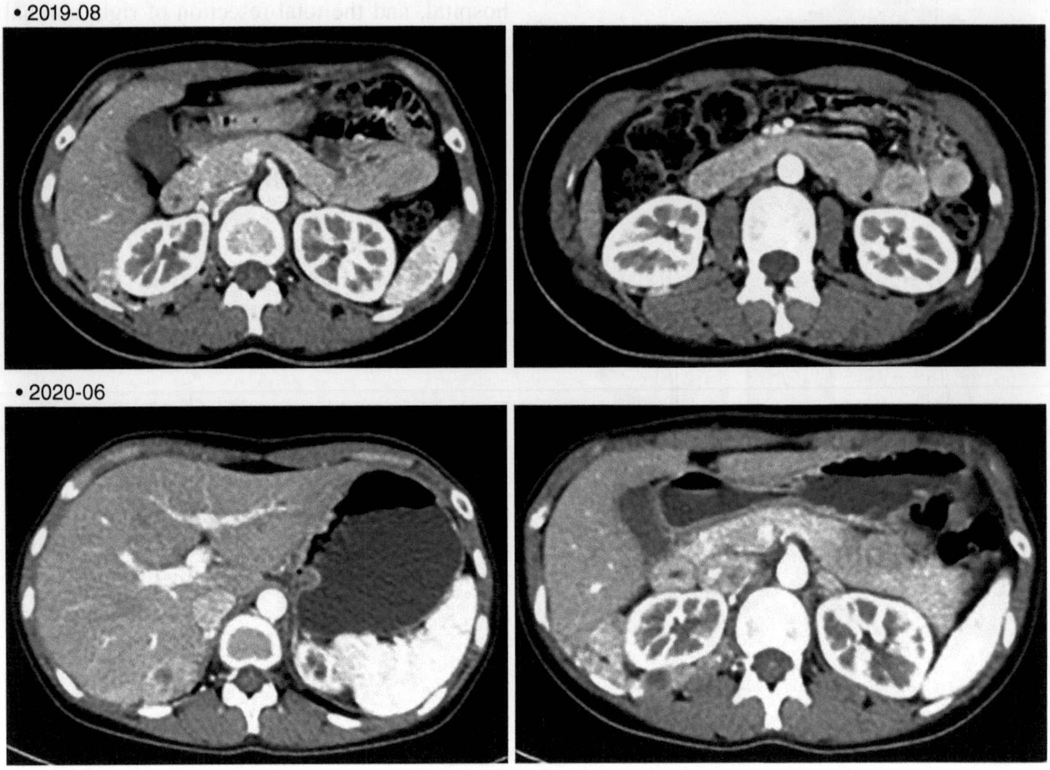

Fig. 8.8 Enhanced CT scan of the abdominal pelvis in 2019 and 2020

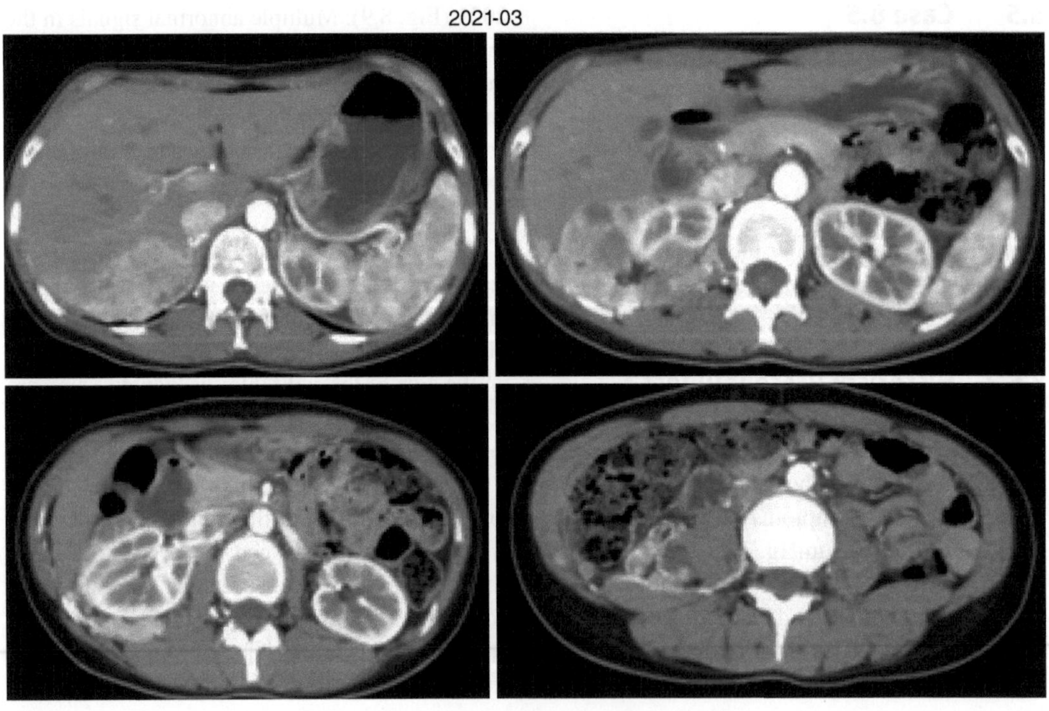

Fig. 8.9 Abdominal pelvic CT enhanced scan in March 2021

8.5.5 Current Diagnoses

Postoperative metastasis of right adrenal pheochromocytoma relapse

Past resection of the left adrenal pheochromocytoma

Solid thyroid nodules

Primary hyperparathyroidism is not excluded.

8.5.6 MDT Discussion

8.5.6.1 Endocrinology

Have the patient continue a high-sodium and high-protein diet, ensuring that the amount of intake is greater than 3000 mL; monitor the amount of inflow and weight, measure the blood pressure and heart rate recumbent position at least two to three times per day, and repeat HCT once a week. Avoid drastic postural changes, laborious bowel movements, agitation, exertion, and infection. Avoid medications such as gastric reassurance and morpholine.

Patient with normal blood pressure and mild orthostatic hypotension. Preoperative preparations are considered to be basically adequate. It is recommended that your department continue to strengthen the volume management. If necessary, intravenous injection of crystals or colloids can be taken. Adequate preoperative preparation criteria for pheochromocytoma include normal blood pressure, no paroxysmal increase in blood pressure, palpitations, hyperhidrosis, etc., no severe orthostatic hypotension, volume recovery, and improvement in hypermetabolic syndrome.

Explain the risk of surgery. Closely monitor the patient's vital signs and heart rhythm during the perioperative period, and be vigilant against hypertensive crisis and alternating high and low blood pressure. Preoperatively, demand consultations with the Department of Anesthesiology and the Department of Critical Care to assist in the assessment. Fully account for surgical risks.

Patient has thyroid nodules, followed by the results of the most recent calcitonin test. Close monitoring of changes in nodular size and close follow-up of the basic surgery clinic are recommended.

Patient is found with an elevated PTH and normal serum calcium. Primary hyperparathyroidism is not excluded. It is recommended to monitor closely the changes in serum calcium during the perioperative period and be wary of hypercalcemia. Postoperative follow-up by endocrinology outpatient is a must.

8.5.6.2 Basic Surgery

The nature of the thyroid nodule is to be determined. Malignance may be possible, and the patient is communicated with the disease, such as a malignant thyroid nodule. There are indications for surgery. Consultation by the basic surgical clinic is to be taken as soon as possible.

8.5.7 Surgical Approach

Laparoscopic resection of adrenal pheochromocytoma under general anesthesia

8.5.8 Postoperative Pathology

Right adrenal pheochromocytoma, intact envelope. Immunohistochemistry: weak positive for CgA, Syn+, Ki-67 1% +, S-100+, SDHB+, RET+

Left adrenal pheochromocytoma, tumor size 2.5 × 2.0 × 1.5 cm. The results of immunohistochemistry are the same.

8.6 Case 8.6

Patient: Female, 53 years old

8.6.1 Complaints

Episodic headache, palpitations, and sweating for 2 years and a retroperitoneal mass found 2 months ago

8.6.2 History of Present Illness

The patient had episodic dizziness, sweating, palpitations, and cold extremities 2 years ago.

BPmax was 180/100 mmHg. For nearly 2 years, she takes oral nifedipine 1# bid, Hygea 1# bid, Betaloc 25 mg bid, and other drug treatment. The control of blood pressure is not good. The above symptoms are not improve significantly. In April 2018, the patient visited the local hospital for abdominal CT, which showed multiple shadows in the left retroperitoneum. In April 2018, our hospital CT finds, between the medial side of the inferior pole of left kidney and the abdominal aorta, a circular cystic solid density shadow. The boundary was relatively clear. The maximum cross-sectional size was about 60 mm × 52 mm, The solid part of the enhanced scan was significantly strengthened. The boundary with the lower wall of the duodenal horizontal segment was not clear. The fat gap between the abdominal aorta existed, and multiple arteries for blood supply were originated from the abdominal aorta. Multiple cystic solid nodular shadows were seen at the lower edge of the lesion, distributed around the abdominal aorta, inferior vena cava, and adjacent to iliac vessels. They were partially strengthened after enhancement, with a short diameter of 2.5 cm for larger nodules. Paragangliomas are considered, and metastatic lymph nodes may be suggested. From May 4, oral benzylamine preparation was started. The current dose is of 20 mg tid. Supine blood pressure is monitored to be around 110–130/70–90 mmHg, and standing blood pressure is 70–90/60–80 mmHg. In the past month, she gained 2 kg of weight, and HCT decreased from 44% to 41%.

8.6.3 Past, Personal, Marital and Childbearing, Family History

Laparoscopic removal of uterine fibroid in 2005

8.6.4 Accessory Examination

Abdominal pelvic enhanced CT (Figs. 8.10 and 8.11): A circular shadow of cystic solid density between the medial of inferior pole of left kidney and the abdominal aorta, with a maximum cross-sectional size of about 6.0 × 5.0 cm. The boundary with the surrounding intestine is not clear. Below there are also several round cystic solid nodules, located next to the retroperitoneal abdominal aorta, bilateral iliac blood vessels, and in front of the sacrum. The larger ones are about 2.0 cm in size. Between the medial of left inferior extremum and abdominal aorta, there is a circular shadow of cystic solid density. The boundary is relatively clear. The maximum cross-sectional size is about 60 mm × 52 mm, and the enhanced scan shows that the solid part is significantly strengthened. The boundary with the lower wall of the horizontal section of the duodenum is not clear. There is a fat gap between the mass and the abdominal aorta. Multiple arteries for blood supply originated from the abdominal aorta. Multiple cystic solid nodules are seen at the lower edge of the lesion, distributed around the abdominal aorta and inferior vena cava and adjacent to iliac vessels. They are partially strengthened after enhancement, with a short diameter of 2.5 cm for larger nodules. Metastatic paraganglioma are considered.

PET-CT: circular shadow of cystic density between the medial of inferior pole of left kidney and the abdominal aorta. The maximum cross-sectional size is about 6.0 cm × 5.0 cm. The radiophernalia of the solid part is increased. SUVmax is 22.6, and the boundary with the surrounding intestine is not clear. Below are several round cystic solid nodules, located around the retroperitoneal ventral aorta, bilateral iliac vessels, and anterior sacroids. The larger ones are about 2.0 cm in size. The radioactive uptake of the solid part is increased. The SUV max is 3.3. The remaining nodules have mild radioactive uptake. Retroperitoneal malignancy is considered, and multiple retroperitoneal lymph node metastases are possible.

131I-MIBG: multiple episodes of abnormal radiotrophic uptake of varying sizes in the mid-abdomen

Somatostatin receptor imaging: multiple radiologically elevated shadows in the mid-abdomen

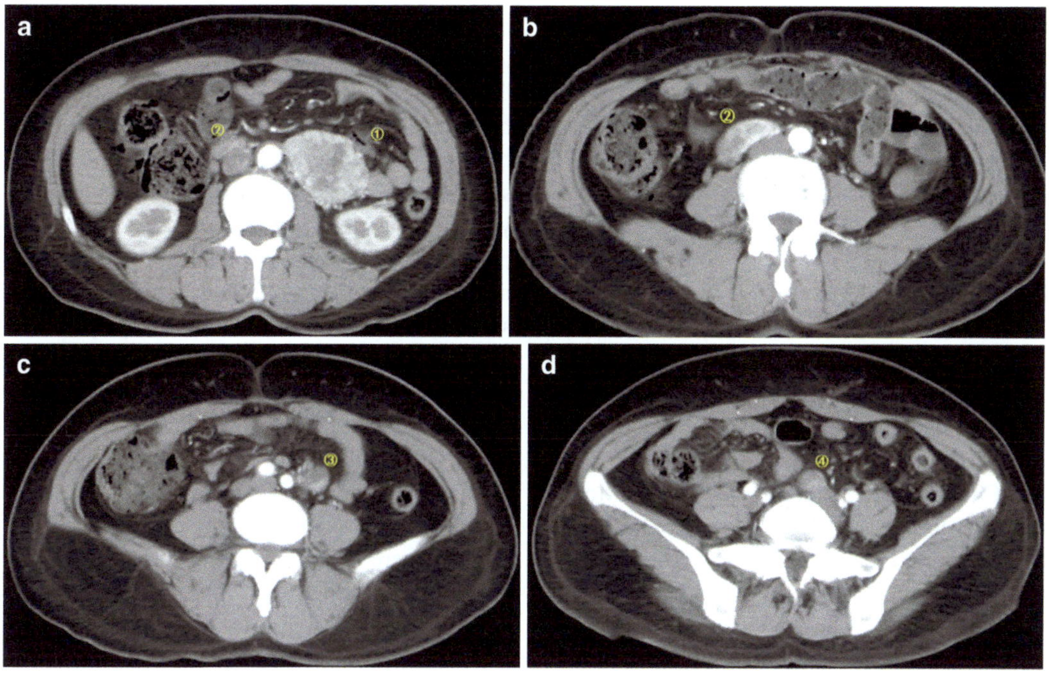

Fig. 8.10 Abdominal pelvic CT enhanced scan. (**a–d**) A circular shadow of cystic solid density between the medial of inferior pole of left kidney and the abdominal aorta, with a maximum cross-sectional size of about 6.0 × 5.0 cm. The boundary with the surrounding intestine is not clear. Below are also several round cystic solid nodules, located next to the retroperitoneal abdominal aorta, bilateral iliac blood vessels, and in front of the sacrum. The larger ones are about 2.0 cm in size. Between the medial of left inferior extremum and abdominal aorta, there is a circular shadow of cystic solid density. The boundary is relatively clear. The maximum cross-sectional size is about 60 mm × 52 mm, and the enhanced scan shows that the solid part is significantly strengthened. The boundary with the lower wall of the horizontal section of the duodenum is not clear. There is a fat gap between the mass and the abdominal aorta. Multiple arteries for blood supply originated from the abdominal aorta. Multiple cystic solid nodules are seen at the lower edge of the lesion, distributed around the abdominal aorta and inferior vena cava and adjacent to iliac vessels. They are partially strengthened after enhancement, with a short diameter of 2.5 cm for larger nodules. Metastatic paradondromes are considered

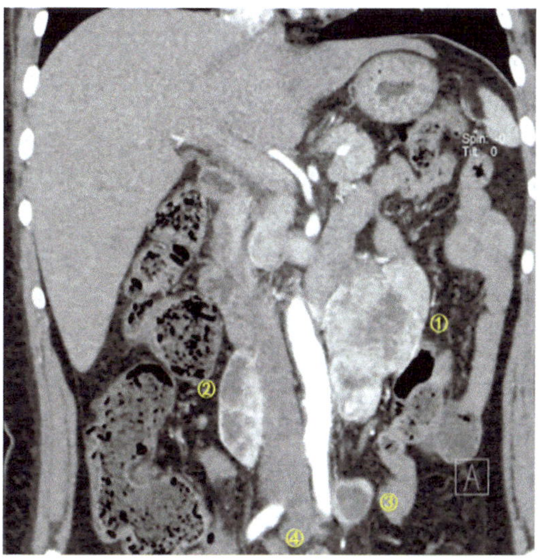

Fig. 8.11 Abdominal pelvic CT enhances coronary reconstruction

Endocrine examination: 24 h urine CA: NE 1023.75 μg/24 h, E 3.94 μg/24 h, DA 248.68 μg/24 h; methoxy norepinephrine >20.56 (normal range ≤ 0.9)

There is a circular shadow of cystic solid density between the medial of inferior pole of left kidney and the abdominal aorta. The maximum cross-sectional size is about 6.0 cm × 5.0 cm. The radiophernalia of the solid part is increased. SUVmax is 22.6, and the boundary with the surrounding intestine is not clear. Below are several round cystic solid nodules, located around the retroperitoneal ventral aorta, bilateral iliac vessels, and anterior sacroids. The larger ones are about 2.0 cm in size. Retroperitoneal malignancy is considered, and multiple retroperitoneal lymph node metastases are possible

8.6.5 Current Diagnosis

Multiple retroperitoneal paragangliomas
Hypertension (grade 3, very high risk)
Type 2 diabetes
Past uterine fibroid removal

8.6.6 MDT Discussion

8.6.6.1 Urology

Patient is a middle-aged woman, displaying a clinical manifestation of episodic hypertension. Accessory examination found 24 h urinary CA↑, and CT found left pararenal and retroperitoneal multiple masses. MIBG and somatostatin receptor imaging were (+). PET-CT showed that the uptakes of left pararenal mass and retroperitoneal multiple tumors were significantly increased. SUVmax was 22.6. Combining the patient's medical history, physical examination, and accessory examination, malignant paraganglioma is considered, and multiple retroperitoneal lymph node metastases were not excluded. Due to multiple occurrences of masses, large size, and close relationship with adjacent structures such as the left renal pedicle, duodenum, abdominal aorta, inferior vena cava, iliac artery, etc., the risk for surgical injury is high. In addition, the surgery is a tumor reduction surgery, so complete resection of tumors is not expected. The risk of recurrence in the short term after surgery is high, and it is necessary to cooperate with a MIBG isotope therapy. The diagnosis of multiple retroperitoneal paragangliomas in the patient is clear. Drug treatment has been fully prepared. She has no recent episodic symptoms. A recent surgery is planned. Because the patient had multiple occurrences of mass and previous laparoscopic surgery, the surgical approach is directly an open surgery. Before the operation, files to the medical office and blood bank will be sent. Fully prepare red blood cells, plasma, and platelets, and have the patient sign the informed consent form under the lawyer's notarization. Carefully dissect during the operation, and be vigilant against damage to the nearby large blood vessels and duodenum. Patient shall be returned to the ICU after surgery.

8.6.6.2 Department of Anesthesiology

Patient is regarded as ASA III level, limited-time surgery. Complete cardiac ultrasound and myocardial enzyme and blood gas tests. Please consult with the endocrinology department and ICU. Prepare routinely during the perioperative period according to pheochromocytoma's operation: establish arteriovenous passages, prepare vasoactive drugs, strengthen vital signs monitoring, maintain the balance of myocardial oxygen supply and demand, and maintain the perfusion of vital organs. Fully account for the risks of perioperative cardiovascular and cerebrovascular accidents, major hemorrhage, vascular embolism, reflux aspiration, delayed awakening, extubation difficulties, delirium, etc. Prepare adequate blood. Return to ICU after surgery.

8.6.6.3 Basic Surgery

The boundary between the mass and the duodenum and the small intestinal wall is not clear. Our department is willing to assist in operation.

8.6.6.4 Vascular Surgery

Fully explain the risk of vascular damage. If necessary, our department is willing to provide active support during operation.

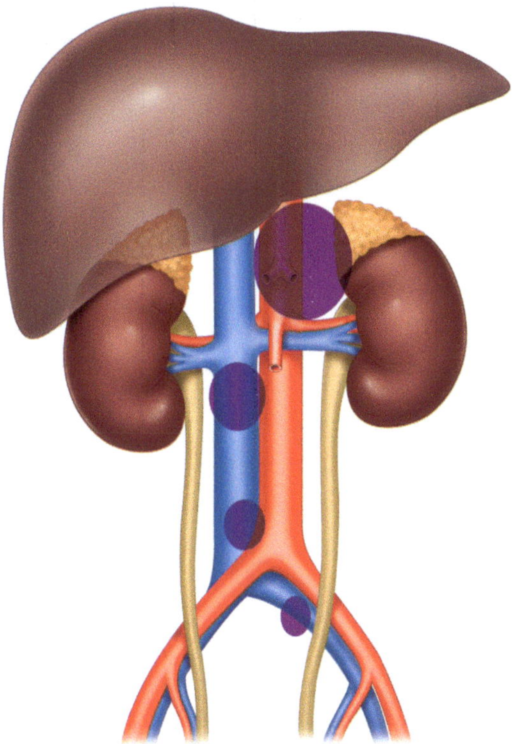

Fig. 8.12 Schematic diagram of the location of the mass

8.6.7 Surgical Approach

Laparotomy under general anesthesia and retroperitoneal resection of multiple paragangliomas (Fig. 8.12).

8.6.8 Postoperative Pathology

(Mass 1, 2, 3) Paraganglioma infiltration is seen in fibroadipose tissue. In combination with clinical practice, malignant biological behavior is not excluded. Immunohistochemical results: CgA (+), S-100 (partial +), Syn (+), Ki-67 (index <1%), Vimentin (+), α-inhibin (−), Calretinin (−), Melan-A (−), SDHB (+)

MIX
Papier aus verantwortungsvollen Quellen
Paper from responsible sources
FSC® C105338

If you have any concerns about our products,
you can contact us on
ProductSafety@springernature.com

In case Publisher is established outside the EU,
the EU authorized representative is:
Springer Nature Customer Service Center GmbH
Europaplatz 3, 69115 Heidelberg, Germany

Printed by Libri Plureos GmbH
in Hamburg, Germany